Neurology for Physiotherapists

Neurology for Physiotherapists

edited by

JOAN CASH
B.A., F.C.S.P., Dip.T.P.

FABER & FABER

London · Boston

First published in 1974
by Faber and Faber Limited
3 Queen Square London WC1
Reprinted 1975, 1976
Second edition 1977
Reprinted 1979
Printed in Great Britain by
Unwin Brothers Limited
The Gresham Press, Old Woking, Surrey
All rights reserved

British Library Cataloguing in Publication Data

Neurology for physiotherapists. – 2nd ed.
1 Nervous system – Diseases
I. Cash, Joan Elizabeth
616.8   RC346

ISBN 0–571–04928–1
ISBN 0–571–04948–6   Pbk

Acknowledgements

To all the contributors to *Neurology for Physiotherapists* both first and second editions, I would like to offer my most sincere thanks for the work they have put into their chapters and for their generous co-operation throughout its preparation. It has been a very real pleasure to work with them.

My thanks also go to the many people who have helped with advice and by reading sections of the manuscript: Mrs. H. W. Atkinson, Principal, School of Physiotherapy, Coventry and Warwickshire Hospital and her staff; Miss N. Bolam, Principal, School of Physiotherapy, Newcastle University Hospitals and Mr. I. Fell of the same hospital; Miss D. Caney, Principal, School of Physiotherapy, Queen Elizabeth Hospital, Birmingham and her staff; Mrs. Davies, Head Occupational Therapist, Hollymoor Hospital, Birmingham; Mrs. B. Goff, School of Physiotherapy, Oswestry; Miss H. Oakman, Superintendent Physiotherapist, the National Hospital for Nervous Diseases, London; Miss Shaw, Head Occupational Therapist, Selly Oak Hospital, Birmingham and her staff; Miss M. Stewart, Principal, School of Physiotherapy, King's College Hospital, London and her staff.

I would like to thank all those, too numerous to mention here, who through lectures and discussions have added great value to the book and made its completion possible. In addition I wish to thank Miss Hilary Baines for her patience and skill in typing and retyping the manuscript. My thanks also go to Mrs. Audrey Besterman, Medical Artist, for her illustrations, and to Dr. Oliver Sacks for Plate XVI/1.

I express my very great debt of gratitude to Miss P. Jean Cunningham, Miss Heather Potter, B.Sc. and Miss P. A. Downie, F.C.S.P., Editor of Nursing and Medical Books, Faber & Faber Ltd., for their unfailing patience and help in the production of this book.

J.E.C.

Mrs. Atkinson would like to express her thanks to all those who have helped her in her section of the book. She is particularly grateful to Miss M. Knott of Vallejo, California and Dr. and Mrs. K. Bobath of the Western Cerebral Palsy Centre, London, who are responsible for stimulating her interest in this field originally. Mr. James, the Medical Photographer of Coventry and Warwickshire Hospital, has been most helpful in preparing plates from her slides and she is most grateful to the parents of the children shown in the illustrations. The patient understanding of Miss J. Cash and the helpful criticism from Mrs. B. Goff have made these chapters possible. Lastly, Mrs. Atkinson would like to thank the patients she has treated and her students, since they are the best teachers of all.

Mrs. Compton would like to express grateful thanks to members of Southampton Social Services Department and Department of Community Health, and staff of Southampton General Hospital, Department of Rehabilitation, for their help and encouragement; and to her husband, John, for his patience in the role of student from which many helpful comments were made.

Mrs. J. Dodgson would like to thank Drs. D. R. Gander, D. C. Beatty and A. M. Edwards; Miss A. V. Greenaway, Superintendent Physiotherapist, and colleagues at Queen Elizabeth II Hospital, Welwyn Garden City for their criticisms and encouragements, and Mrs. A. Jones for her very efficient typing.

Mrs. B. Goff would like to thank Miss J. Cash for help and forbearance; the Management of the Robert Jones and Agnes Hunt Orthopaedic Hospital, Oswestry, for permission to publish photographs; her colleagues at the Orthopaedic Hospital, Oswestry including the following: Miss P. M. Jones for typing, Mr. and Mrs. David Jones of the Clinical Photography Department, Miss Susan Shaw, M.C.S.P., Senior Physiotherapist, Spinal Unit, and Mr. Ralph Kay, M.C.S.P., Dip.T.P., for proof-reading. Mrs. Goff would also like to thank the patients of the Midland Spinal Injuries Unit who co-operated with the photographers.

Acknowledgements

Mr. Hill would like to thank Mr. A. T. Scowcroft, M.C.S.P., Dip.T.P., Principal of the Nottingham School of Physiotherapy for information and advice concerning the formulation of a suitable syllabus in psychology for students of physiotherapy, and Mrs. D. Bunker for typing the script at short notice.

Miss Sheila Kelly wishes to express her gratitude to Mr. T. F. Dee, Chief Medical Photographer, Department of Medical Illustration, Birmingham Medical Centre, for Plates XV/1-6.

Miss Sophie Levitt would like to thank the Richard Cloudesley School, London, E.C.1., for Plates XII/1, XII/3 and XII/4, and Mrs. Glen Smerdan for typing the chapter.

Mrs. O. Nettles expresses her appreciation to the following: Mr. D. M. Forrest, F.R.C.S., for his medical help, advice and co-operation in the preparation of the chapter on spina bifida; the medical, physiotherapy and nursing staff of Queen Mary's Hospital, Carshalton for all their assistance and loan of charts and photographs; Dr. J. Lorber, M.D., F.R.C.P., for diagrams on which Figs. XI/1 and XI/2 are based; Dr. Chester Swinyard and Mr. Leonard W. Mayo, Executive Director, the Association for the Aid to Crippled Children, New York for diagrams on which Figs. XI/4 and XI/6 are based; Mr. H. B. Eckstein, F.R.C.S. and *The Lancet* for the diagram on which Fig. XI/5 is based; Mr. W. J. W. Sharrard, M.D., M.B., Ch.B., F.R.C.S. and the *Journal of Bone and Joint Surgery* for the diagram on which Fig. XI/8 is based; the Scottish Spina Bifida Association for reproduction of Plate XI/2.

Miss E. L. Renfrew wishes to express appreciation to Mr. K. E. Guest, F.R.C.S. (Edin.), Consultant Orthopaedic Surgeon, Mearnskirk Hospital, Glasgow and to Professor W. Bryan Jennett, F.R.C.S., Professor of Neurosurgery, Institute of Neurological Sciences, Glasgow for their advice in the preparation of the chapter on head injuries.

Miss B. J. Sutcliffe and Miss M. I. Salter wish to acknowledge the help and encouragement always available from Group-Captain Wynn Parry, M.B.E., M.A., D.M., F.R.C.P. and are grateful to the Director General Medical Services, Royal Air Force, for permission to publish their chapter on peripheral nerve injuries. The brachial plexus splint and the spider splint shown in Plates XIX/1 and XIX/7(b) were manufactured by Hugh Steeper Ltd., Roehampton.

7

Acknowledgements

Miss Todd and Miss Davies wish to express their appreciation to Dr. and Mrs. Bobath for pioneering the work on which their chapters are based. They would also like to thank Miss P. Aldridge for her patience in endless retyping.

Contents

Contents

Plates

Plates

Figures

Figures

Figures

Contributors

Helen W. Atkinson, M.C.S.P., DIP.T.P.
Principal, School of Physiotherapy, Coventry and Warwickshire Hospital

Jennifer Bryce, M.C.S.P.
Principal, Bobath Centre, London

Ann Compton, M.C.S.P.
Superintendent Community Physiotherapist, Rehabilitation Department, Southampton General Hospital

Patricia A. Davies, M.C.S.P., DIP.PHYS.ED.
Superintendent Physiotherapist, King's College Hospital, London

Joan M. Dodgson, M.C.S.P., O.N.C.
Psychiatric Unit, Queen Elizabeth II Hospital, Welwyn Garden City

Barbara Goff, O.N.C., M.C.S.P., DIP.T.P.
School of Physiotherapy, Robert Jones and Agnes Hunt Orthopaedic Hospital, Oswestry

Uta Greiner, DIP.P.T. (BERLIN)
Superintendent Physiotherapist, National Hospital for Nervous Diseases, London

David A. Hill, B.SC., M.C.S.P., DIP.T.P.
Reader in Health Sciences, Ulster College, The Northern Ireland Polytechnic

Sheila Kelly, M.C.S.P., DIP.T.P.
School of Physiotherapy, Queen Elizabeth Medical Centre, Birmingham

Contributors

Sophie Levitt, B.SC. (PHYSIOTHERAPY, RAND)
Supervisor of Therapy Studies, The Wolfson Centre, Institute of Child Health, University of London

Olwen Nettles, O.N.C., M.C.S.P.
formerly Appliance Officer, Association for Spina Bifida and Hydrocephalus, London

Susan Nosworthy, B.PHTY., M.A.P.A.
Assistant Superintendent Physiotherapist, National Hospital for Nervous Diseases, London

Elizabeth L. Renfrew, M.C.S.P.
Superintendent Physiotherapist, Mearnskirk Hospital, Glasgow

Maureen I. Salter, M.C.S.P.
Superintendent Physiotherapist, Joint Service Medical Rehabilitation Unit, RAF Chessington

Barbara J. Sutcliffe, M.C.S.P.
Group Superintendent Physiotherapist, Westminster Hospital, London

Jennifer M. Todd, M.C.S.P.
Superintendent Physiotherapist, Wolfson Medical Rehabilitation Unit, Atkinson Morley's Hospital, London

CHAPTER I

Applied Anatomy and Physiology

by HELEN W. ATKINSON, M.C.S.P., DIP.T.P.

The physiotherapist is frequently called upon to aid in the management of patients suffering from disorders of neurological origin. In order to give maximum assistance it is necessary for the therapist to understand certain basic physiological concepts and to have some knowledge of the general anatomy of the nervous system as a whole. Detailed anatomy and physiology is a preliminary subject in the training period and may be obtained from any of the standard textbooks. It is the intention in this section, therefore, to select only those concepts which are particularly applicable to therapy.

THE NERVOUS SYSTEM AS A TOOL

The nervous system is the tool used by the living creature in order to be able to react to its environment. The more complex the creature, the more complicated its nervous system and the more versatile are its reactions. The system is concerned with physical (motor, sensory and autonomic), intellectual and emotional activities and, in consequence, any disorder may involve any one or all three of these major functions.

Neurone

The nervous system is composed of an enormous number of neurones, connected together and following certain pathways, in order to make functional activity possible. The neurone is the basic unit of the nervous system and comprises the nerve cell and its processes. Each neurone has a cell body and two types of processes (see Fig. I/1), dendrites and axons.

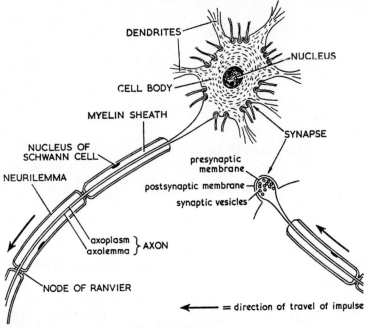

DENDRITES

NUCLEUS

CELL BODY

MYELIN SHEATH

NUCLEUS OF SCHWANN CELL

NEURILEMMA

SYNAPSE

presynaptic membrane

postsynaptic membrane

synaptic vesicles

axoplasm } **AXON**
axolemma }

NODE OF RANVIER

⟵ = direction of travel of impulse

Fig. I /1 Neurone

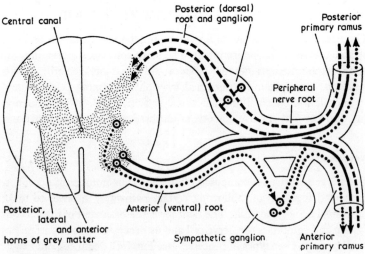

Lower motor neurone
Afferent (sensory) neurone
Sympathetic neurone

Central canal

Posterior (dorsal) root and ganglion

Posterior primary ramus

Peripheral nerve root

Posterior, lateral and anterior horns of grey matter

Anterior (ventral) root

Sympathetic ganglion

Anterior primary ramus

Fig. I/2 Neurones forming a mixed spinal nerve at thoracic level

Note in Fig. I/2 that each ramus carries motor, sensory and autonomic fibres, only one of each is used to represent many, and the sympathetic ganglion communicates with those above and below it in level and also sends fibres to the visceral contents. In Fig. I/3 note that the

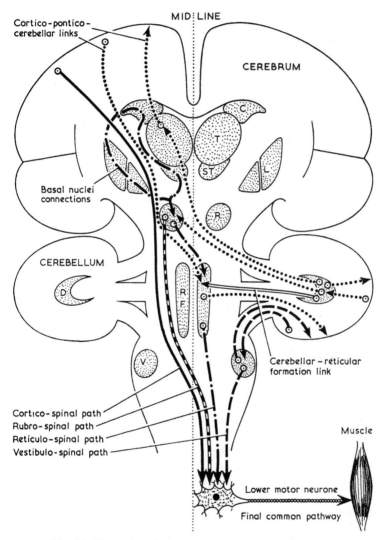

Fig. I/3 Examples of some motor neurone connections

23

corticospinal path represents the pyramidal system and other paths may be considered to be extrapyramidal.

The synapse

This is the term used to define the area where the process of one neurone links with another. The synapse is a point of contiguity but not of continuity. Synapses may occur between the terminal parts of an axon and the dendrites of another cell or with the cell body. The number of synaptic areas may be very vast in any one neurone. The synapse enables impulses from one neurone to be transmitted to another neurone by virtue of chemical changes taking place which bring about an alteration in membrane potential on the receiving neurone. Synapses have certain properties which are of importance. Some of the more important ones are:

1. *Synaptic delay.* When an impulse reaches a synapse there is a brief time-lag before a response occurs in the recipient neurone. Consequently conduction along a chain of neurones is slower than along one single neurone. Thus monosynaptic pathways conduct more rapidly than polysynaptic routes.

2. *One-way conduction.* Synapses permit conduction of impulses in one direction only, i.e. from the presynaptic to the postsynaptic neurone.

3. *Vulnerability.* Synapses are very sensitive to anoxia and to the effects of drugs. Polysynaptic pathways are very susceptible to anaesthesia.

4. *Summation.* The effect of impulses arriving at a synapse can be added to by other impulses. For instance the effect of impulses could be subliminal (insufficient to bring about adequate chemical change for depolarization of the postsynaptic neurone). If however another spate of impulses arrives before the effect of the previous one has subsided then the two effects may complement each other and the total change be sufficient to cause depolarization. Such a phenomenon is called summation. There are two types of summation, the type just described being dependent upon a time factor and being called temporal summation. The other type is called spatial summation. It is the result of the adding together of impulses from different neurones which converge upon the postsynaptic neurone and bring about depolarization of its membrane.

5. *Fatigue.* The synapse is thought to be the site of fatigue in nerve conductivity.

6. *Inhibition.* Certain neurones have an inhibitory effect upon the postsynaptic neurone, possibly because they use a different chemical mediator. Thus the effect of these neurones would be to discourage depolarization of the postsynaptic cell membrane and would be antagonistic to influences exerted by excitatory neurones. These effects can summate in the same way as the excitatory effects. Many interneurones have an inhibitory effect.

7. *Post-tetanic potentiation.* This occurs across synapses which have been subjected to prolonged and repeated activity. The threshold of stimulation of these junctions is thought to be lowered making transmission across it more easily brought about for a period of several hours. Facilitation of transmission is said to occur, and is an elementary form of learning and also forms an important part in the approach to physical treatment of patients showing disorders of the neurological variety.

Supporting tissue

Neurones are delicate, highly-specialized structures and require support and protection. This is afforded to them in the nervous system by specialized connective tissue called neuroglia. If neurones are damaged and destroyed their place is filled by proliferation of neuroglial material.

The axons are surrounded by a fatty sheath called myelin which has an important effect on the conduction of impulses. Because of this sheath bundles of axons give a whitish appearance and form the white matter of the central nervous system.

When the axon and its myelin sheath leave the central nervous system they become surrounded by a membrane called the neurilemma. This is of vital importance and it should be noted that the neurilemma is absent round the fibres of the brain and spinal cord whereas it is present as soon as they leave these areas.

Nerve fibres which are surrounded by neurilemma may regenerate if they are destroyed. Hence destruction of fibres in a peripheral nerve does not necessarily mean permanent loss of function whereas destruction of the fibres in the central nervous system will mean permanent loss of function of those fibres. It should also be noted that the nerve cell is resilient to injury and has considerable recuperative powers but, if it dies, it is incapable of being replaced. Thus destruction of cell bodies means permanent loss of function.

SOME PHYSIOLOGICAL CONCEPTS

Most patients suffering from neurological disorders show movement difficulties, and it is therefore important to consider the factors which are essential for the production of normal movement and activity.

Movement in its mature and skilled form is the result of complex teamwork between a multitude of muscles and joints so that balanced movement patterns are produced which can achieve an effect for the individual. Movement and postural attitudes are so closely related that it is impossible to distinguish one from the other.

The muscles concerned in the production of movement receive their ultimate stimulation from the motoneurone pools or masses of cells housed in the anterior horns of the spinal cord or, in the case of the cranial nerves, in the motor nuclei of the brain stem. Axons from the motoneurone pools pass to the muscles and constitute the lower motor neurones or final common pathways.

Many neurones converge upon and synapse with the lower motor neurone, some coming from the extrapyramidal and pyramidal pathways, some being spinal interneurones and some coming direct from the peripheral afferent system. Whether or not impulses pass along the final common pathways depends upon two very important factors:

1. the integrity of the pathway;
2. the influence being exerted upon the cells of the motoneurone pool.

If the lower motoneurone pathway is not intact there is no route for the impulses to take. Fortunately each muscle is supplied by many neurones and only a severe lesion in the pathway would involve every lower motoneurone passing to any one muscle. However, this can occur and the result is a muscle which cannot be made to contract via activity in its own motor nerve supply and therefore one which is unable to participate in any team work towards functional activity.

Since many neurones are converging upon the cells in the motoneurone pools, including interneurones, it is possible that two types of influence may be exerted. These are *excitatory* – encouraging depolarization – and *inhibitory* – discouraging depolarization. The ratio between these two influences is the deciding factor as to whether the motoneurone pools are activated or not. The muscles they supply will, therefore, contract or remain inactive according to the balance of excitatory *versus* inhibitory influences being exerted upon their motoneurone pools.

When contraction occurs its intensity is dependent upon the number of muscle fibres brought into action. The number of fibres activated depends upon the number of cells in the motoneurone pool which have conveyed impulses. Thus the greater the excitatory influence on the motoneurone pool and the lower their threshold of stimulation, the greater the number of active motoneurones and the greater the resultant degree of muscle contraction.

The factors exerting an influence on the motoneurone pools

These are many and varied. Pathways which are of importance are those of the pyramidal and extrapyramidal parts of the central nervous system which convey impulses resulting in volitional, postural and equilibrium reactions. Also of importance are the lower reflex pathways which give rise to withdrawal and stretch responses which are the result of more direct influences from the afferent side of the peripheral system. The interrelationship between one and the other is very important and can be illustrated by a simple account of the stretch reflex mechanism.

Skeletal muscles may be divided into two types of fibres. The large, ordinary fibres are known as extrafusal fibres and the smaller fibres which lie parallel to the extrafusal fibres and are encapsulated are known as intrafusal fibres. The intrafusal fibres are part of the stretch reflex mechanism of muscle and the one illustrated in Fig. I/4 has a non-contractile part and a contractile part.

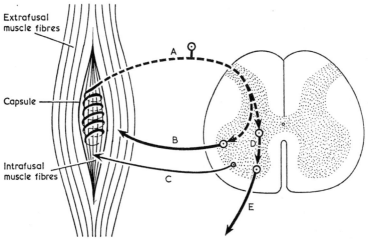

Fig. I/4 The simple stretch reflex mechanism

The non-contractile part of the intrafusal fibres is concerned with stretch reception and is linked to the central nervous system by an afferent neurone (called a Ia fibre) which makes direct synapse with a large anterior horn cell in the motoneurone pool of the same muscle to which the intrafusal fibres belong. Stretch to the muscle and therefore to the non-contractile part of the intrafusal fibre has an excitatory effect on the stretch receptor, and impulses travel along the Ia fibre to the motoneurone pool where the large anterior horn cell is stimulated and conveys impulses to the extrafusal fibres causing them to contract. The large anterior horn cell is said to send an Alpha efferent to the extrafusal muscle fibre. In this way the stretch on the intrafusal fibres is reduced. The afferent fibres also influence other associated motoneurones and by means of interneurones they may exert an inhibitory influence on the motoneurone pools of antagonistic muscles.

The contractile parts of the intrafusal fibres have their own nerve supply from the motoneurone pools by means of small anterior horn cells. The axons of these cells are called fusimotor fibres (Gamma efferents) to distinguish them from the fibres of the large anterior horn cells. Impulses passing along these fusimotor fibres to the intrafusal muscle fibres will cause them to contract and make them exert tension upon their own non-contractile areas. Thus they are able to make the intrafusal non-contractile area more sensitive to stretch by their activity or less sensitive to stretch by their inactivity.

In other words a bias can be put upon the sensitivity of the stretch reflex mechanism depending upon the degree of activity in the intrafusal contractile tissue and the fusimotor fibres. This bias depends upon the influences being exerted upon the small anterior horn cells which are particularly linked to the extrapyramidal pathways from the central nervous system, which in turn incorporates the balance and postural mechanism. Through this system the stretch reflex mechanism in muscle can be made sensitive or less so according to the postural needs of the moment. Thus there is interaction between excitation and inhibition and between lower reflex activity and higher control.

The stretch reflex mechanism is in fact more complicated than this. There are at least two types of intrafusal fibres (nuclear bag and nuclear chain). There are also two types of stretch receptors, Ia and II, and there are at least two types of fusimotor fibres. This rather complicated mechanism makes the muscle sensitive to both velocity and degree of stretch, enables it to adjust its resting length and to be sensitive to stretch to a varying degree whatever its resting length happens to be. Fig. I/5 illustrates the simple stretch reflex mechanism and the effect of contraction of the intrafusal fibres.

Thus it may be seen that the influence of the fibres from the extra-pyramidal system can adjust muscle activity to a fine degree and since certain righting, postural and equilibrium reactions are integrated

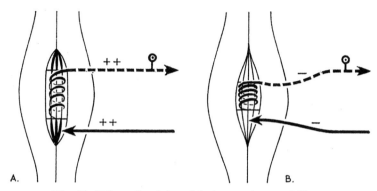

Fig. I/5 Effect of activity of fusimotor (gamma) fibres

into the extrapyramidal system it is not difficult to see that these reactions exert their influence upon the motoneurone pools via these fibres.

These postural mechanisms and reactions make possible a variety of automatic responses to various situations. The normal human being can, however, encourage or inhibit these activities at will and can carry out activities which are not entirely automatic but are dependent upon some automatic adjustments. When these background automatic adjustments are not available normal willed movement becomes inco-ordinate, posturally unsound and wellnigh impossible.

Some useful points to note when considering the production of volitional movement

SENSORY INPUT

All volitional movement is triggered off as a response to some type of *afferent information*. Without input there can be no adequate motor output.

The types of afferent stimulation which give rise to movement are many and varied. The following few examples may be of some help in the appreciation of a need for sensory stimulus. We move if we feel discomfort, excessive pressure or insecurity; we move in response to basic needs such as hunger and thirst; we move if we see something we desire to investigate further; we move because of the stimulus generated by memory, thought or idea.

We must have stimulation to move and we must have suitable pathways available to receive, transmit and interpret the stimulation. Without the available pathways movement would not occur to any purpose.

The importance of input is not fully appreciated until we consider its effect on where and how we move. Unless we have a knowledge of our position in space (conscious or subconscious) it is impossible for us to change our position.

If we do receive a stimulus to move we must know where we are in order to change our position, how we should feel during the movement and how the completed movement should feel. There has to be a constant 'feed-back' of information if our movements are to be successful.

AROUSAL OF IDEA OF MOVEMENT

The ingoing sensations must be able to arouse the idea of movement. This is probably done via the arousal part of the reticular formation which alerts the higher centres of the brain to the onslaught of ingoing information. It may also link with the non-anatomically defined centrocephalic area thought to be related to the initiation of the idea of movement. This area is connected with both the pyramidal and extrapyramidal cortical regions.

STIMULATION OF PYRAMIDAL AND EXTRAPYRAMIDAL PATHWAYS

The pyramidal pathways need to be put into action but not before the extrapyramidal system has been informed of the intended movement. These two systems work closely together to give us the desired movement patterns with correct synergy and postural reactions.

Many theories have been put forward to explain the production of voluntary movement. The following factors are needed:

1. initiation of the idea to move;

2. stimulation of the main motoneurone pools involved in the pattern of activity;

3. modification or controlled inhibition of the antagonists;
4. activation of synergistic and fixator muscles;
5. the necessary postural adjustments and alterations in postural patterns to make the movement possible;
6. continuous 'feed-back' regarding progress.

The function of the pyramidal pathways. These are thought to be responsible for initiating the movement which has been conceived as an idea by the centrocephalic area. If these pathways worked alone without the aid of the extrapyramidal system the movement produced would tend to be a mass movement without synergy. Thus unwanted components might occur.

The function of the extrapyramidal pathways. The extrapyramidal cortical cells are thought to be also stimulated by activity in the centrocephalic area and as they are rapidly conducting they prepare the way for impulses passing down the pyramidal pathways. They send impulses to the extrapyramidal masses of grey matter (basal ganglia, red nucleus, substantia nigra etc.) so that necessary patterns of excitation and inhibition of motoneurone pools are already initiated preparing them for action or preventing unwanted activity when the impulses via the pyramidal pathways reach them. In this way the appropriate excitation and inhibition of synergic activity may be brought about.

The extrapyramidal cortical cells also inform the cerebellum of intended activity via the cortico-pontico-cerebellar pathways. This enables the cerebellum to exert appropriate influences upon the red nucleus and brain stem nuclei helping the synergic selection activities and postural adjustments needed. A 'feed-back' exists between cerebellum and cortex via the thalamus.

To summarize this particular theory, it can be said that the pyramidal pathways will demand the main movements and extrapyramidal pathways will influence the motoneurone pools in such a way as to make the required movement possible without involving unwanted activity.

This gives rather a clear-cut difference between pyramidal and extrapyramidal systems which may be excessively dogmatic. The student must appreciate that movement is the result of an extremely complex combination of excitation and inhibition giving a desired effect.

SOME OBSERVATIONS ON REFLEXES

Reflexes and reactions play an important part in the activity of the nervous system. In fact the reflex arc may be called the basic functional unit of the nervous system. It consists, essentially, of a receptor organ and its neurone which makes synaptic connection with an efferent neurone which, in turn, connects with an effector organ. Such an arc would be monosynaptic and, in man, is only found in the phasic stretch reflexes of muscle, i.e. the so-called 'deep reflexes' elicited when a muscle is stretched by tapping its tendon such as the knee, ankle and elbow jerk.

Most reflex arcs are polysynaptic and because of this they are a little slower in conduction rate than those of the monosynaptic variety. Although the afferent supply enters the central nervous system at a given segmental level, according to the position of the receptor organ, the motor response may occur at many levels because of linkage by interneurones conveying impulses to many motoneurone pools at lower and higher levels. An example of such a reflex would be the protective withdrawal reflex which is a response to undesirable stimulation. The plantar reflex response to scratching the skin over the sole of the foot and the abdominal contractions following skin stimulation over the muscles would also be examples. These are commonly called superficial reflexes, due to the fact that the receptor organs lie at a superficial level.

There is only one reflex arc which involves one neurone only and it occurs outside the central nervous system. This is the axon reflex which is a protective mechanism against skin irritation.

Reflexes have been classified in many ways and it is not the intention to reclassify them in this particular work. Certain mechanisms will be named and some described in order to give the student a greater understanding of the problems faced by the neurological patient.

Normally the reflex mechanisms are kept under control and inhibited or semi-inhibited by higher reactions and volitional control. However it must be remembered that the lower reflex mechanisms are like the bricks from which the foundations are made – not obviously useful by themselves, but, as built-in members of a whole, they are of vital importance. In certain neurological disorders the inhibitory and controlling mechanisms may be at fault and some of the reflex mechanisms may manifest themselves in an unrestrained way, dominating the activities of the individual.

The segmental reflexes

These are so called because they tend to have arcs in which afferents and efferents lie in the same segmental level in the central nervous system. The phasic stretch reflexes fall into this category.

The intersegmental reflexes

Here the arcs may travel by interneurones to different levels in the spinal cord and brain stem. The protective withdrawal reflexes are examples. The area and intensity of stimulus determines how far above and below segmental level it spreads. This is an important fact as it can have an important bearing on the management of patients in whom this type of reflex is relatively uninhibited.

The suprasegmental reflexes

These are mainly concerned with postural activities. Some are concerned with the maintenance of the upright position against gravity whilst others are concerned with the obtaining of the upright position and body alignment.

ANTIGRAVITY MECHANISMS
A. The myotatic extensor reflexes
These depend upon an intact peripheral system, intact spinal cord and intact brain stem up to and including the pons. The vestibular nuclei are particularly important to the reflex arcs concerned, in that they have an excitatory influence upon the small anterior horn cells which supply fusimotor fibres to the intrafusal muscle fibres which, by their contraction, put a positive bias on the stretch reflexes of the extensor groups concerned.

Thus the responses are really those of stretch reflex of the tonic or static variety. Such reflexes include the extensor thrust (positive supporting reflex) which is the response of a limb to a compression stimulus preferably applied along their long axis – e.g. compression applied to the palmar surface of the hand and to the sole of the foot. Such stimuli encourage an extensor response or 'thrusting away' from the stimulus.

Under this heading would also come the crossed extensor response.

This occurs when one limb is flexed giving an extensor response in the opposite limb to enable it to support the additional weight thrust upon it.

B. *The tonic postural reflexes*
These are many and include the following mechanisms which require the same amount of brain stem and spinal cord to function as those mentioned in section A.

i. *The tonic labyrinthine reflex.* The receptor organs in this case are the labyrinthine canals of the inner ear. The afferent pathway influences the vestibular nuclei and causes these neurones to send excitatory impulses to the fusimotor fibres of the extensor muscles so contracting their intrafusal fibres and making them more sensitive to stretch stimuli. This reflex, therefore, increases extensor activity. The position of the head has a profound effect on this reflex since the labyrinths are lodged in the skull. The receptor organs are most intensely stimulated when the face is directed upwards and forwards at about 45° to the horizontal regardless of the position of the rest of the body (see Fig. I/6.i).

ii. *The tonic neck reflexes.* These relate to the position of the cervical spine wherein the receptor organs are considered to lie. The afferents influence the vestibular nuclei as before but the pattern of increase in tone differs as follows:

a. The symmetrical tonic neck reflex. This occurs if the cervical

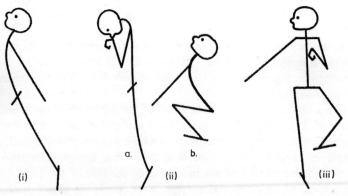

Fig. I/6 (i, ii, iii) Patterns of increased activity imposed by some tonic reflex mechanisms

spine is flexed or extended. If it is flexed extensor tone increases in the lower limbs and decreases in the upper limbs which flex. If it is extended extensor tone increases in the upper limbs and decreases in the lower limbs which, therefore, now flex (see Fig. I/6.ii a and b).

b. The asymmetrical tonic neck reflex. This is related to rotation of the cervical spine. If the head is turned to the right there is an increase in extensor tone in the limbs of the right side (jaw limbs) and a decrease in extensor tone and therefore a degree of flexion in the limbs of the left side (skull limbs). If the head is turned to the other side the situation is reversed (see Fig. I/6.iii).

REFLEXES CONCERNED WITH OBTAINING AN UPRIGHT POSITION
AND BODY ALIGNMENT

These are termed righting reflexes and require the peripheral system, the spinal cord and the brain stem up to and including the red nucleus, to be intact. The vestibular nuclei and reticular formation are very important grey areas. A combination of righting reflexes constitutes a righting reaction and enables an animal to obtain an upright position from any position of recumbency and very closely influences the rotational elements in movement. These are noticeably absent in certain neurological disorders.

The righting reflexes have been listed as follows:

a. the labyrinthine righting reflex;
b. the neck righting reflex;
c. body on head righting;
d. body on body righting;
e. optical righting (not complete at brain stem level).

The receptor organs required are the labyrinths, the muscles and joints, the skin and the retinae.

The labyrinthine righting reflex. This is the reflex which brings the head into the accepted upright position with eyes facing forward and eyes and ears level. Thus many pathways are involved.

The neck righting reflex. Rotation of the head or movement of the cervical spine stretches the neck muscles and triggers off a reflex mechanism to bring the body into alignment with the head so that shoulders and hips face forwards in complete harmony with the face. Obviously the response of the head to labyrinthine righting may, in turn, trigger off this mechanism.

The body on head righting reflex. Pressure on the side of the body will cause the head to right itself even if the previous two mechanisms are destroyed. It is a response to tactile stimulation and is dependent upon skin sensation.

The body on body righting reflexes. This is the response of the body to pressure stimulation. It will right itself whether the head can do so or not.

The optical righting reflexes. These require the presence of the visual cortex and are therefore more complex. Man particularly makes use of these reflexes but can manage without if need be. If there is a deficiency in the other reflexes, because of break in the arcs, man will substitute by using the optical righting mechanism almost entirely provided this is intact. This reflex fails him when it is dark or his eyes are closed.

It should be noted that these righting mechanisms work in conjunction with each other. The receptors and arcs concerned with the one response work to endorse or countermand another. The pathways linking the receptors for neck, optical and labyrinthine responses are carried in the medial longitudinal bundle of nerve fibres which link appropriate cranial nerve nuclei.

The righting reactions also work in conjunction with the tonic reflexes and segmental mechanisms. This interaction and integration of reflex mechanisms to gain functional adjustment is largely the function of the cerebellum working in conjunction with the cortical originating extrapyramidal system.

EQUILIBRIUM AND TILTING REACTIONS

These also need consideration. They are very complex mechanisms. The normal human reactions to disturbance of balance depend upon many factors amongst which are the following:

    a. the state of maturity of the central nervous system;

    b. the mobility of the joints of the limbs and vertebral column;

    c. the relative muscle power in different parts of the body.

These reactions have been grouped in many ways and the following is only one approach.

    1. *Those which widen the base and lower the centre of gravity.* These include the use of the arms in protective extension (sometimes called the parachute reaction). Both arms or one may be used passing in a forwards, sideways or backwards direction. These occur in response

to a shift of the centre of gravity in the appropriate direction. They are rather primitive reactions since they prevent the use of the hands for skilled activity because of preoccupation with equilibrium.

2. *Those which move the base to keep it under a moving centre of gravity.* These include the stepping reactions in which stepping may occur forwards, backwards, sideways and across midline. Also in this category come the hopping reactions which particularly occur when only one limb is free to receive weight. The placing reactions related to skin contact with obstacles (e.g. if the dorsum of the foot strikes an object, the foot is lifted to prevent tripping) may also be included here for want of a better place.

3. *Those which endeavour to keep the centre of gravity over the base.* These include the movements of upper and lower limbs and trunk in order to adjust the relative overall position of the centre of gravity. Also included are the torsional movements of the vertebral column which are closely related to the righting reactions.

The last two groups can be considered to be more mature than the first group. Any reactions which leave the upper limbs free from obligation to equilibrium and therefore available for skilled function are relatively mature in nature.

In the normal course of events these reactions occur in conjunction with each other all the time and the vestibular apparatus, cerebellum and extrapyramidal system are all involved in their control. Each individual gives a reaction to any given disturbance of balance in his own individual manner, which is dependent upon the three factors mentioned above.

There are many other reflex mechanisms and reactions which have not been mentioned. Some of these will be dealt with in other sections of this book and those particularly relevant to the developing child will be considered in Chapter II.

Developmental Background to Physiotherapy

by HELEN W. ATKINSON, M.C.S.P., DIP.T.P.

In Chapter I much has been said about the complexities of the nervous system and the way in which the ability to perform movement is brought about. However, we are not born with the ability to perform skilled movements. These have to develop gradually over a relatively protracted period of time.

At birth the central nervous system is not completely myelinated and it is therefore incapable of functioning in a mature manner until this process is complete. It may be said that maturation of the nervous system is dependent upon myelination. Connections between the mid-brain and cerebral cortex are not complete and, for this reason, the newly born child is inclined to behave in a manner which indicates that its reactions are being controlled by the subcortical regions. Movements tend to be relatively random and purposeless and specific reflex responses may be clearly demonstrated.

As the nervous system starts to develop shortly after conception it should be remembered that early reflex activities and movement responses develop long before birth. The child is, in fact, adapting his reactions to his environment right from the start. The influence of gravity upon the unborn child is not strong because of the fluid medium which supports and protects it in the uterus. This, added to the effect of the tonic labyrinthine reflex (which is quite strong at this stage), may explain why the child has so much difficulty in countering the effect of gravity during the early months of postnatal life.

As the nervous system matures some reflex pathways become more dominant for a period of time before becoming modified and integrated into more mature movement patterns. There are many early reflex mechanisms which are well developed in the full term infant and are very important to it for survival.

The Rooting Reflex. This is a mechanism whereby the child can find a source of nourishment. It is a response to the touch stimulus applied to the outer aspect of the cheeks, lips and nose. The motor response is to 'root around' until the lips contact the nipple of the mother's breast. The reflex then gives way to the sucking reflex.

The Sucking Reflex. This is a response to stimulation of the lips and in particular to their inner aspect. It gives rise to a sucking activity which in turn will trigger off the swallowing mechanism.

Swallowing is a response to stimulation of the soft palate by the fluid which has been sucked into the mouth. The motor response is the contraction of the muscles which guide the fluid into the oesophagus and temporarily close the glottis.

The Grasp Reflex. This is a mechanism whereby touch stimulus in the palm of the hand encourages flexion of the fingers giving the infant a grasp which clings to whatever touched the hand. In this way the child may cling to the mother's clothing by the same mechanism as a baby monkey clings to his mother's fur.

The Traction Reflex. This is often associated with the grasp reflex and is a mechanism whereby traction applied to the limbs encourages a flexion response. It is often demonstrable by placing the fingers of the demonstrator's hands into the palm of the hands of the infant. The child will respond with a grasp reflex. If traction is now exerted by lifting the child with its grasping hands the degree of grasp will increase and flexor tone in the upper limbs will increase to counter the traction. Many children can be made to support their own body weight for a minute or so by means of this grasp and traction mechanism.

The Startle Reflex occurs in response to a loud noise or a jerk of body position. It is basically an extensor response. The upper limbs are carried upwards and outwards whilst the lower limbs extend and the head jerks into extension.

Reflex Stepping or the Walking Reflex. This occurs if the infant is supported in standing and his body weight is gently pushed forwards. The child will respond by stepping forwards in an exaggerated walking pattern. This reflex is present prior to birth and may well influence the position of the child in utero.

Placing Reactions. If the dorsum of the foot or hand is touched or placed so that it touches an obstruction the limb will be flexed and placed onto or over the obstruction.

Many of these primitive mechanisms are apparently lost during the first few months of life. Some become apparent again in a modified and integrated form whilst others may reappear under conditions of duress.

The postural reflexes, righting and equilibrium reactions are by no means completely developed at birth and many of the infant's activities are related to the development and integration of these, so that they are eventually able to give the correct malleable postural background to all our mature activities. The child has to develop the mechanisms and gain control over them before they can fulfil a useful function. Thus much of the maturation process is related to the ability to inhibit or modify the unwanted, whilst allowing desirable activities to occur.

CEPHALOCAUDAL DEVELOPMENT

It should be remembered that the maturation process occurs in a cephalocaudal direction. This means that the ability to control the posture and movements of the head, upper trunk and upper limbs occurs before control of the lower trunk and lower limbs. It is also true to say that control extends proximally at first and proceeds distally.

The fact that the child develops in a cephalocaudal direction means that control of the head, neck and upper limbs will always be in advance of the lower limbs and that the upper part of the body may be entering one phase of development whilst the more caudal area is still trying to develop a more primitive stage.

Early development is directed at reducing the dominance of the flexor muscle groups and gaining the ability to extend. At first only the cervical spine extends, but, as the child matures, the upper limbs, upper trunk and lower limbs all go into extension. When this occurs in prone lying the child is said to show a Landau reaction. This response is gained by pressure on the anterior aspect of the thorax, as might occur if the child is placed in prone lying or supported by placing a hand under the lower thoracic region. Such a response is unlikely to occur before 4 to 5 months of age and will not be available in full strength until about the tenth month after which time it subsides and becomes integrated into the general body patterns. The exact time and age at which any activity develops is not so important as the order in which it develops. The following paragraphs give an abbreviated outline of some of the landmarks in development.

FIRST SIX WEEKS

During this time the child is influenced quite strongly by the asymmetrical tonic neck reflex and by the neck righting reflex. Both of these have been described in Chapter I. In addition to these the child is, of course, influenced by primitive grasp and traction, rooting, sucking, startle and stepping reactions. The child may be said to be in a stage of asymmetry. He is unable to keep his head in midline and thus the head is turned to one side or the other. There tends to be a preferred side in many children. The limbs often adopt the asymmetrical tonic neck reflex posturing and this appears to show more often in the lower limbs than in the upper, possibly because the control of the lower limbs is less mature (see Plate II/2a). Movements occur in rather an asymmetrical and random manner using stereotyped mass flexion or extension patterns.

The neck righting reflex which is present means that the child will turn from supine to side lying if his head is turned towards the side. The trunk follows as a whole and there is no spiralling at this stage.

In Prone Lying the hips and knees still retain a degree of flexion but the child will attempt to prevent himself from suffocating by turning his head away from the supporting surface (see Plate II/1a). In addition the labyrinthine righting reflex is beginning to develop and this means that the child will try to bring his head towards an upright position. Success is a long way off at this stage but the attempt is there. Ventral suspension does not give a Landau response (see Plate II/4a).

In Supine Lying the child may be pulled by the hands towards sitting. There will, however, be a complete head lag indicating no control over the head position at this stage (see Plates II/2b and II/3a).

41

SIX WEEKS TO THREE MONTHS

During this period the strong influence being exerted by the asymmetrical tonic neck reflex gradually weakens whilst the symmetrical tonic neck reflex gains in strength. The neck righting mechanism is still quite strong and the labyrinthine righting mechanism is steadily gaining in strenth. Because of these facts gradual changes in the child's abilities begin to occur.

Placed in Prone Lying the child will gradually begin to be able to lift his head further from the supporting surface and also to bring it towards midline. By three months the head and shoulders may be lifted and the elbows used to support the shoulders. The lower limbs may still show traces of the influence of the asymmetrical tonic neck reflex pattern, but this will not occur so frequently. Head lifting is brought about by the labyrinthine righting reflex and the extension produced may also influence the movements of the hands and feet (see Plate II/1b).

Placed in Supported Sitting the head will drop forwards frequently but towards the third month the child will be lifting the head and holding it steadily (see Plate II/3b). If, however, the trunk is inclined backwards from sitting towards supine lying, there will be a considerable head lag.

Because the child is gaining more head control in midline he is able to use his eyes for watching objects held for him to see. He is also able to place his hands in midline and can observe them, thus building up body image.

The gradually rising influence of the symmetrical tonic neck reflex encourages symmetry and the child is often said to be entering a stage of symmetry for this reason (see Plate II/2c). Because of this the ability to respond to primitive stepping or walking gradually subsides. If weight is put onto the feet the lower limbs go into bilateral extension and cannot work reciprocally.

FOUR TO SIX MONTHS

During this period the asymmetrical tonic neck reflex is still weakening in its influence whilst the symmetrical tonic neck reflex is gaining in strength. The labyrinthine righting reflex is strong but neck righting is gradually coming under some degree of control. The Landau reaction is beginning to be demonstrable.

When Placed in Prone Lying the child is able to rest on his forearms with his head lifted high (see Plate II/1c). He will occasionally lift the forearms clear and extend the head, shoulders and arms, supporting his weight completely on the lower thorax. This is an attempt at a Landau reaction. During this process the hips and knees also extend.

When in Supine the head is held in midline and often lifts forward. The hands meet in midline and attempts are made to grasp objects when the hands are free.

Placed in Sitting, the head is held well and only the lumbar spine shows flexion (see Plate II/3c). There is now no head lag if the child's trunk is inclined backwards or if the child is pulled towards sitting (see Plate II/2d).

At this stage the child gradually develops the ability to grasp objects deliberately. This is only possible because the grasp reflex has now been integrated so that release of grasp can occur in order to open the hand prior to closing on the desired object.

SIX TO EIGHT MONTHS

During this period many interesting things are happening. The neck righting reflexes which have become weakened in dominance work in conjunction with the stronger labyrinthine righting mechanisms and also with the symmetrical tonic neck reflex to make rolling from prone to supine possible, and later from supine to prone (see Plate II/5). At the same time the important body rotating activities also develop giving a special action to rolling over.

The child is now doing many different things (see Plate II/2e). He will help if he is pulled from supine to sitting, so that his head and shoulders come forward. If he is placed in sitting he is able to balance by placing his hands in front of him with extended elbows.

If he is placed in prone he will bear weight on extended elbows and will weight-bear on one arm whilst reaching forward with the other. Thus he is developing equilibrium reactions (see Plate II/3d). The Landau reaction occurs frequently (see Plate II/4b). He may attempt to creep using flexed elbows and allowing his legs to follow as passengers (see Plate II/1d). Nearer to the end of this time the legs may attempt to participate using rather primitive patterns. His elbows will be now extended, and the upper limbs will be working reciprocally. He may then be said to be crawling when his knees are able to support some weight and his legs are able to progress in a reciprocal manner.

EIGHT TO TEN MONTHS

The righting and equilibrium reactions are developing rapidly at this stage. They become available to the child in a variety of ways and equilibrium reactions may be seen in prone lying, supine lying and in sitting. At first the child could only lean forward in sitting but by this time he is able to support himself with a sideways extension of the upper limb.

This improvement in balance enables the child to move from prone lying to sitting and *vice versa*. Body rotation becomes very important. As the child is able to roll over and sit up quite early in this period he is also able to sit up and rotate freely without hand support before the tenth month. This enables him to play in sitting and to investigate toys and objects around him. He will pick them up, investigate them by mouth and hand before casting them aside. Mouthing is important as an afferent stimulus as the tongue is a highly sensitive structure and plays an important part in the learning process. Casting away of objects helps in gaining spatial perception and is therefore another form of learning.

The weight is borne on upper and lower limbs (see Plate II/1e), crawling is gaining as a method of progression and many children change to the pattern of walking on hands and feet (bear walking). The child is also likely to attempt to stand using his hands to help him pull himself up and may begin to lift one foot off the ground so long as he has hold of his support. He is now developing equilibrium reactions in standing.

Some children do not crawl but develop a method of progression which can only be described as shuffling along on the bottom! Provided no other abnormality is present this is acceptable and is then designated as benign shuffling.

TEN TO TWELVE MONTHS

The child is still likely to walk on hands and feet and when standing he may cruise around furniture. By this stage the child's upper limbs have gone from a period of behaving in a rather reciprocal manner to a period of freedom. The lower limbs are still learning reciprocal activities and for this reason balance in standing is not yet secure and walking may be delayed until reciprocal stepping activities are available again.

As the righting and equilibrium reactions become fully integrated the child's ability to walk unaided develops. At first a wide base is used and the hands may be held upwards or the scapulae retracted with elbows flexed. As balance becomes more secure and movement patterns more available the child ceases to use a wide base and adopts body rotation as a means of maintaining walking equilibrium.

At first the child will rise into standing by rolling to prone and then progressing upwards. Later he will half turn before rising and eventually he will rise symmetrically as in adulthood. The symmetrical method may not develop until he is about three years of age.

Steps and stairs present a problem. At about one year of age the child will virtually crawl up, whilst at two years he may ascend one step at a time, one foot coming up to join the other. He may well be four years of age before he is able to go up and down steps in a truly reciprocal manner. The ability to descend always lags behind the ability to ascend.

Maturation of movement continues for a protracted period of time. The most rapid progress occurs within the first three years but complexity of movement continues to improve throughout adolescence into early adulthood. It has been found that although stimulus and environmental influences may stimulate the perfection of activities they in no way affect the rate of myelination. In other words the child will not roll over unaided until the nervous system has sufficiently matured to enable the pathways to be used no matter how much external environmental pressure is exerted. Equally well demonstrated is the fact that if the child is held fixed and prevented from demonstrating movements to which its nervous system has matured they will be produced immediately the body is free to respond.

The above summary by no means covers all the aspects of motor development. It should be noted that mature movements are complex permutations of the basic flexion and extension synergies. Until the child can mix flexion and extension components of movement, only mass patterns can be produced. The ability to stabilize the trunk and proximal part of the limbs whilst allowing distal parts to move is important where skilled activity is concerned and cerebellar activity is very important to this. Equally well, the ability to retain a fixed distal extremity while the proximal segments and trunk move over it is also essential. Much of the child's developmental progress is related to the ability to produce these two varieties of movement, not only as distinct entities, but going on at the same time.

Let us take two examples to illustrate the points mentioned in this paragraph:

1. *The mixture of flexion and extension components.* A simple example may be seen when the sitting position is considered. This requires *extension* of the vertebral column, but *flexion* of the hips and knees. If it is impossible to extend the column unless a total extension pattern is used then the child is unable to maintain a sitting position.

A more complex example may be seen if the lower limbs are considered in the walking synergies. Mass movement patterns of a more reflex variety follow certain stereotyped synergies. When the hip and knee flex the lower limb also abducts and may laterally rotate and the foot dorsiflexes. However, to walk forward we require to flex the hip and knee whilst adducting the limb. This is followed by extending the knee whilst dorsiflexing the foot. Here, alone, are some interesting synergies. The leg then prepares to take weight, when it extends at the knee and hip and abducts to prevent a Trendelenburg sign (drop of the pelvis on the non-weight-bearing side) (Fig. II/1) while the foot is dorsiflexed – another mixture of synergies. In Fig. II/1a the abductors of the weight-bearing limb are working to prevent the pelvis from dropping on the non-weight-bearing side. In Fig. II/1b the abductors are not working and so the pelvis has dropped into adduction on that side, causing a compensatory lurch of the trunk. This is called a Trendelenburg sign.

The push-off requires more extension of the hip, flexion of the knee and plantar flexion of the foot. This is a very complex series of synergies. This ability is not immediately available. The child who has recently

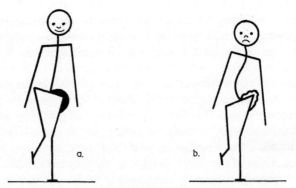

Fig II/1 (a, b) Role of abductors in weight-bearing

started walking flexes and abducts his hip. Only later does he keep it adducted as the leg comes forward.

2. *Proximal fixation and distal freedom and vice versa.* A simple example may be seen when we consider the child in prone lying. When he is able to take weight on one elbow whilst playing with a toy with the other hand he is demonstrating distal fixation of the supporting limb with the trunk free to move over it, whilst the free limb is moving distally against the proximal support of the steady trunk.

A more complex example of the same thing occurs with the much more mature pattern of writing. Here the supporting arm is offering distal stability to the trunk which is free to move over it. The hand which is putting pen to paper is working freely with a more proximal area of stability in the forearm. However, the forearm must also be partly free to move for each word and so movement at the shoulder has to occur. The shoulder is functioning as a stable and mobile structure at one and the same time against the stable background of the trunk which, in turn, is free to move over the other, or supporting limb. This is a very complex synergy. Little wonder that we cannot write at birth!

Many learning processes depend upon the ability to move. We require movement to be able to explore our environment and unless this is possible our mental processes cannot develop normally. Head control is essential to movement but is also essential for the ability to make maximum use of the sense of sight. If we cannot control our head position it is difficult to gain control over our eye activities. The eyes also need to have a stable base from which to work. Eye movements are similar to limbs. They can remain stable while the head moves, or they can move whilst the head stays still, or the two activities may go on at once. None of this is possible if head control is absent.

Assessment of spatial relationships depends upon movement. The relationship between hands and eyes depends upon the ability to move and explore, and the perception of depth, space, height, size and shape have all to be learned by experiences dependent upon movements of different areas of the body.

Balance activities basically start by the balance of the head upon the shoulders in prone lying. Progression is then made by balancing the shoulders over the elbows which offer a forward support in prone lying. In sitting it should be noted that the body is at first inclined forward so that head balance on the shoulders is still an extension activity and the arms are in a supporting forward position, but with extended elbows.

Later the ability to balance with the arms supporting sideways develops and much later the arms may support by being placed behind as when sitting in a backwards leaning position. This requires flexor activity in the head and neck to maintain the balance of the head on the shoulders.

Before the child is able to give a backwards support to the sitting position he is developing rotatory ability in the trunk which is the precursor to more skilful balance activities. Maturity of balance is seen when the upper limbs can carry out skilled activities, whilst the legs and trunk are dealing with maintenance of equilibrium without the aid of the upper limbs.

The development of motor skills is not complete until the hands can be used in prehensile activities and much work has been done by various authors on the development of prehension. As a summary it may be pointed out that the hand activities are inclined to develop from ulnar to radial side. The grasp and release activities of the early stages in development appear to commence with activity of the little finger and radiate out towards the thumb. Gradually the radial aspect of the hand becomes more dominant and eventually the pincer grasp between thumb and index finger develops whilst the ulnar side of the hand takes up a more stabilizing function. Much more mature is the 'dynamic tripod' posture described by Wynn Parry in 1966 and explained by Rosenbloom and Horton in 1971. Here the thumb, index and middle fingers are used as a threesome to give fine co-ordinated movements of the hand. The classic example of the use of this tripod is in writing, although it may be seen in many other functional activities.

The development of body image and awareness occurs in conjunction with the ability to move. At first, because of lack of myelination of the cortical pathways, the child is only able to know whether he is comfortable or not without necessarily knowing why. There is no discrimination of where the discomfort lies or what is causing it. Socially at

48

this stage the child is only able to communicate by crying and consequently discomfort of any kind will be voiced by crying. Comfort or pleasurable sensation is indicated by a silent and contented-looking child.

Gradually the child starts to learn about himself. Body awareness develops cephalocaudally as one might expect and head control, hands in midline and the ability to bring the hands to the mouth give the child the ability to see and feel his hands and to become aware of them as part of himself. He may also be able to discriminate between the people who are handling him. Mother recognition comes fairly early and the child is usually able to register pleasure by this stage in the form of smiling at his mother.

The ability to discriminate between what is part of oneself and what is part of one's surroundings is an important part of perceptual development. Much is dependent upon the opportunity given to explore. When a child is being carried by an adult he often tries to explore the adult's face with his hands and can cause considerable discomfort doing so! This is his method of learning to perceive whether or not the face is his or someone else's. He cannot, at this stage, be expected to appreciate discomfort in others since he is not yet aware of it fully in himself. At the same time he will gain some social perception since there will inevitably be a reaction to his activities of some kind or another and early communication will occur.

As time passes the child becomes aware of other parts of his body and can often be seen lying with his feet lifted up towards his mouth where there can be contact between feet, mouth and hands. Incidentally, when he lies supine with his feet in contact with his hands he is also exercising his equilibrium reactions and can frequently be seen to roll from supine to side and back, still holding his feet. Control of trunk position is being developed while he is learning about body image.

By this time the child is more aware of his surroundings and able to communicate not only by smiling and crying but also by making gurgling noises, coughing, cooing, etc. He is also able to show likes and dislikes regarding food. The sense of taste and smell are early basic mechanisms and develop early in life. The child also learns to appreciate the tone used and the word 'No'.

The process of improving body image and social contacts continues for many months and the child is usually about fifteen months old before he is able to indicate discomfort regarding wet pants accurately to his mother. Since development occurs cephalocaudally this is hardly surprising. After this has occurred he is likely to learn gradually to control his bladder activities, but may be three years of age before he is more or less reliable.

The physical, intellectual and social development of the child are so clearly linked with each other that it would take several volumes to give a complete and detailed account. Interested readers are advised to consult some of the references at the end of Chapter VI for further details.

The physiotherapist makes most use of the physical aspects of development but needs some understanding of the intellectual and social aspects to appreciate fully the whole problem.

As a brief summary it may be said that the process of integrating certain reflex mechanisms involved in movement occurs over a period of time and eventually makes controlled purposeful movement possible. The control develops in a cephalocaudal direction. It is closely linked with perception of body image, intellectual and social behaviour and, although it is not dependent upon environmental factors, these may influence the rate at which perfection develops. Motor development starts with control of the head position in prone with the upper limbs most able to take weight in a forward or elbow support position. Later development includes rolling and supported sitting with the weight supported forwards on the hands at first, and later at the sides and even later behind. Body rotation begins to be perfected as rolling occurs and limb rotation follows trunk rotation as a rule.

Movements at first follow primitive patterns of synergy but later the ability to combine flexion/extension patterns to give more complexity of movement develops. Ultimate maturity of movement is reached when the hands are totally free from an obligation to balance mechanisms, so that they can be freely developed as skilful tools and used in conjunction with visual and other sensory feed-back mechanisms.

It should be noted that the child's development mechanisms are so arranged that he is preparing for balance in a position before he is able fully to adopt the position and certainly before he is able to use it as a base for activities of his hands. Most usually the mother plays with the child so that he experiences advanced activities before he is able to perform them. In other words, he is being prepared for the activity in addition to making his own 'in-built' preparations.

Let us take an example. A child may be seven to eight months old before he is able to get himself into a sitting position. To sit in a balanced manner he needs to flex at the hips and extend at the trunk. He needs head control and the ability to support himself forwards on his hands. These are minimum requirements. He is prepared for this naturally by the early development of head control, the elbow and hand support prone positions, and by lying on his back playing with his feet. His mother also helps him by propping him into a sitting position so that he experiences it prior to achieving it. Help in this manner makes him experiment and he tries to balance when he is put into sitting and in fact learns to do so.

In the meantime his rolling and rotatory activities are developing. The child gradually develops the ability to get into sitting *after* he has learned to balance in that position.

The clinical value of a knowledge of developmental sequence

When working with handicapped children and, in particular, with the very young, it is easy to see that this information is exceedingly valuable.

When treating babies with movement defects it is important to start as early as possible and to bear in mind the normal sequence of development so that one can, as far as possible, channel the child's reactions along suitable lines and encourage step by step progress without leaving gaps which may lead to abnormality. The earlier the abnormal child is given help the more successful is the treatment likely to be. It is much more difficult to correct abnormal habits than it is to prevent them from occurring. The child's nervous system is very malleable and able to adapt very readily. Consequently it can be most easily influenced before it is fully matured. It is a great mistake to wait until the child can consciously co-operate. By this time irretrievable abnormalities will have developed. The skilled physiotherapist is able to exploit her knowledge of the nervous system to stimulate suitable responses in the child long before it is aware of co-operating.

However, many physiotherapists deal only with adults or, at least, the greater bulk of their patient load is adult. Where then does this knowledge have value? The answer is simply that injury or disease to the central nervous system frequently brings about demyelination of certain areas and may damage or destroy the nervous pathways which have been used to control certain activities. The patient frequently shows a regression of motor skills to a more primitive level. Certain of the reflex mechanisms, which have hitherto been integrated into mature movement patterns, may be partly released from cortical control and may exert an excessive influence over the patient, dominating these movement patterns into abnormality or even preventing them from occurring at all. The patient will frequently show absence or disturbance of normal equilibrium reactions, poverty of movement synergy, perception difficulties and diminution of sensory discrimination. If the physiotherapist is going to help the patient to make full use of such nervous connections as are left, she is more likely to be successful if she has a knowledge of the way in which more skilled activities develop in the first place so that she can, to some extent, simulate the conditions to facilitate redevelopment.

A SIMPLE EXAMPLE TO ILLUSTRATE THIS POINT
A patient with neurological symptoms can often maintain a sitting position but, on attempting to stand, he pulls himself up by placing his hands on a rigid forward support or by pulling on a helper who is standing in front of him. Frequently the head is flexed forwards or, conversely, it may be thrown back so that the nose is pointing upwards. In the first instance the patient is using the symmetrical tonic neck reflex pattern to aid him into standing and in the second his legs are making use of the tonic labyrinthine effect. Neither of these is acceptable as the patterns are those of total reflex synergy and balance in standing will never be achieved using these patterns. Such a patient has his movement excessively influenced by the tonic reflex mechanisms and requires training to modify them and to start early balance activities. He requires help in receiving weight onto his arms in a forward position. Such activities as elbow support prone lying are suitable, progressing to hand support forward side sitting, leading to prone kneeling and hand support forward standing (standing but resting hands on a stool or low support in front of him). He needs to feel the sensation of weight being received forwards instead of pulling back. There are many other facets to this patient's problems which need attention but the above example makes the point.

Many head injury cases regress to an enormous degree and intellectual and social abilities regress also. Motor training along developmental lines is accompanied, in many cases, by a brightening of intellectual activities and the beginning of social communication. The patient may never achieve behaviour patterns which are mature but he is more likely to make balanced progress if a developmental approach is used.

CHAPTER III

Disturbances of Normal Physiology

by HELEN W. ATKINSON, M.C.S.P., DIP.T.P.

On reading the previous two chapters it will have become obvious that injury or disease of the nervous system may cause a wide variety of problems according to the area and extent of the lesion. This chapter will attempt to outline some of the more common problems which the physiotherapist may meet when dealing with this type of patient.

DISTURBANCE OF AFFERENT INFORMATION

Loss of, or imperfection in, afferent supply may give rise to several problems. It may be the result of definite interruption of afferent pathways, giving areas of anaesthesia or paraesthesia. If the interruption lies within a peripheral nerve then the area affected will be that specifically supplied by that particular nerve. If, however, it is more centrally placed the lesion may have more diffuse effects because many fibres from different areas tend to travel together in the spinal cord.

Sensory disturbance may be due to disease processes pressing on afferent pathways giving distorted input. It may be due to faulty linkage between thalamus and cortex, which would prevent discriminative assessment of sensory information.

Disturbance in the link between spinal cord and cerebellum would give rise to inadequate information to help the cerebellum in its postural activities.

One must also remember that visual, auditory and vestibular afferents may be affected in addition to those conveying joint sensation. These latter factors give rise to the most potent symptoms of disorientation and loss of body image.

54

The results of afferent disturbance vary from very slight effects to total loss of body image, disorientation and rejection of the affected area. Skin anaesthesia makes the patient vulnerable to injury since pain is absent and there is no withdrawal from harmful stimuli.

Patients with a reduction in afferent information may have difficulty with spatial perception. The relative positions, size, heights and depths of objects may be difficult for them to perceive. This, of course, is closely linked to visual impressions. Ability of hand/eye control depend to some extent upon binocular vision.

Appreciation of shapes, textures and weight is also important and depends upon eyes, hands and manipulative skills in addition to skin and kinaesthetic sensation. Loss of this variety of sensory perception magnifies the loss of body image and the patient may forget the affected area or even reject it.

Disturbance of sensory perception may, in some cases, be aggravated by lack of experience. If the patient is prevented from experiencing certain afferent stimuli because of the disability then some measure of deprivation must occur. For example, the human being normally carries the hand towards the face for a multiplicity of reasons. If the movements of the upper limb are so impoverished that this cannot occur then the link between hand and face becomes weaker and some degree of body image is lost due to lack of repetitive experience.

Conversely other disturbing things may happen. If a patient experiences an abnormal sensation often enough, he may well eventually accept this as normal and may resent any attempt to adjust or correct this. Let us take an example to illustrate: the patient's disability may make him inclined to lean his weight, when sitting, consistently on to one side. If this is allowed to continue he will accept the one-sided pressure as being natural and normal and interpret the position as being one of safety and one in which he feels secure. If attempts are then made to encourage him to take weight evenly on each side he will feel that he is leaning dangerously towards the side which has not been accustomed to receiving weight. He will not feel safe until he has regained his own 'normal' position. Thus he may reject attempts to correct his posture to a more normal one and much patience and understanding will be required to gain his co-operation.

Paraesthesia is a term used to signify disturbed and diminished sensory information. It refers to tingling and numbness of the affected area and may be the result of lesions of any part of the afferent system.

However, it is most obvious in peripheral problems. Paraesthesia should not be confused with para-anaesthesia, which is a term used to denote *loss* of sensation in both lower limbs.

Dissociated anaesthesia refers to the loss of appreciation of pain and temperature whilst tactile information is still available. This is most often due to interruption of the lateral spinothalamic tracts within the cord and is seen in cases of syringomyelia.

Hypalgia refers to a reduction in sensitivity to pain. This occurs in certain disorders of the afferent system. Where all afferent information is reduced or lost there will obviously be hypalgia but it is most noticeable in association with dissociated anaesthesia. These two phenomena lead to damage as a result of major and minor trauma since they reduce the stimulation of protective mechanisms.

When afferent information reaches the brain it is received and interpreted. The brain processes the information so that appropriate reactions may occur. Any defect at this level makes the production of appropriate reactions difficult or impossible. The patient cannot recall, learn or relearn basic patterns of movement and may be very difficult to treat for this reason. It is important for the physiotherapist to appreciate this, since many patients are thought to be unco-operative or 'not trying', when in fact the problem is in the processing of afferent material.

ABNORMALITIES OF MOVEMENT

These may take several forms according to the area of damage.

MUSCLE FLACCIDITY OR PARALYSIS

This is the result of disturbance in the lower motor neurone. The muscle or group of muscles affected may be totally paralysed if all their available neurones are put out of action. If, however, only some anterior horn neurones are involved the muscles will show partial paralysis and will appear to be very weak. Any muscles affected in this way would be unable to function as members of a team and consequently movement synergies requiring their participation would be abnormal and substitute patterns would be produced. If only a small muscle group is affected in this way the abnormalities are minimal, but if many groups are involved, substitution can be grotesque or even inadequate, in which case the subject is rendered relatively helpless.

Totally flaccid muscles have no lower motor neurone supply because of damage or injury to all the cells in their motoneurone pools or to all the fibres passing peripherally. Such muscles cannot be brought into action voluntarily, or as an automatic reaction or in a reflex action. They feel soft and flabby to the touch, are non-resilient, offer no protection to the structures adjacent to them and are unable to support the joints over which they pull. Because of lack of use, and therefore of blood supply, they atrophy quite rapidly losing the greater part of their muscle bulk.

HYPOTONIA

This term is used here to denote the reduction in preparedness for action found in the muscles when there are defects in certain areas of the extrapyramidal part of the central nervous system. In this case the excitatory influence exerted by the extrapyramidal system upon the motoneurone pools is diminished and, as a result, the muscles show a reduction in sensitivity to stretch. This may, at first sight, be confused with muscle paralysis because the muscles may appear to be totally or almost totally flail. It is however, very different. The muscles have a normal lower motor neurone supply but the factors exerting an influence upon the motoneurone pools are seriously disturbed. There is a reduction of excitatory influence upon the small anterior horn cells which give rise to the fusimotor fibres. Because of this the fusimotor fibres are inactive and therefore activity of the intrafusal muscle fibres is diminished. Thus the muscles are less sensitive to stretch – particularly if it is applied slowly. Quick exaggerated stretch will bring about a response via the spinal stretch reflex but the bias on the receptors is low. If the muscle is stretched by distortion of its tendon, as in the knee jerk, the response will occur but will not be quickly checked by a reciprocal response in the hamstrings because their stretch reflex mechanism will also be sluggish. The lower leg will swing backwards and forwards like a pendulum before it finally comes to rest again.

Hypotonia never affects muscle groups in isolation because it is not a peripheral problem. It is usually found as a general feature or, in some cases, it may be unilateral. The most common reason for hypotonia is disturbance in function of the cerebellum. It may be the result of damage or disease in the cerebellum itself or in the links between the cerebellum and the brain stem extrapyramidal mechanisms.

The cerebellum is thought to exert its influence upon the postural reflex mechanisms by its link with the extrapyramidal system. If it fails to encourage excitation in these tonic mechanisms the fusimotor system will fail to function adequately and the stretch reflex bias will be low. This gives a background of postural instability and makes proximal fixation for distal movements unavailable. Movements therefore tend to be slow in forthcoming and when they do commence they are of an unstable, ill-controlled nature, inclined to overshoot the mark and show intention tremor. This term is used because the tremor occurs when a movement is being carried out and is not present when at rest.

Balance reactions are also disturbed and when they occur they are inclined to overcompensate. The patient may, in fact, fall because of his exaggerated balance reactions. These are occurring against a background of unstable postural tone due to diminished fusimotor activity.

ATAXIA

A patient who has hypotonia inevitably shows a form of ataxia. The symptoms described under the heading 'hypotonia' are also those of ataxia. Ataxia means that movements are inco-ordinate and ill timed, giving a deficiency of smoothness of movement. Ataxia related to hypotonia occurs partly because of the defective postural tone as a background and partly because of the phenomenon of *dyssynergia*.

Dyssynergia is the term used to describe the loss of fluency in a movement. The balance of activity is upset because of faulty synergy. The teamwork between muscles is lost, giving a jerky appearance to the movements, which may well be split up into a series of jerky, separated entities. Both stopping and starting of movements are difficult and overshooting occurs.

These symptoms may also be noted when hearing a patient speak. Speech is a very mature ability, requiring intricate control of co-ordination of the appropriate muscles. Dyssynergia and accompanying problems lead to speech being broken up in the same way as was described for movement. Speech affected in this way is said to be 'scanning'.

Ataxia may also be linked with the sensory problems mentioned earlier in this chapter. It may be due to deficiency of afferent information to the cerebellum and to the cortex, making the individual unaware of his position in space. In this case the cerebellum cannot bring about the necessary postural adjustments, nor is the central nervous system receiving a feed-back regarding the success of the movements. A person with this problem will show very similar symptoms to the previous form of ataxia, but he may be able to mask his problem by using his eyes and ears to excess as substitutes for his loss of skin and joint position sensation. If he is temporarily deprived of the use of his eyes – as in the dark – or of his ears – as in a noisy environment – he may be much more ataxic than when he is able to make full use of them. This is often called *Rhombergism*.

The ataxias are often accompanied by *nystagmus*, which is a form of dyssynergia in the eyes.

Occasionally ataxia may be accompanied by vestibular disturbance which gives rise to vertigo. This is a condition in which the patient's appreciation of head position is disorientated. The subject feels giddy and nauseated. These symptoms can add greatly to the problems of the ataxic patient.

Dysmetria is a term often applied to the ataxic patient. It refers to the difficulty in assessing and achieving the correct distance or range of movement. It is seen in the overshooting symptoms mentioned earlier.

HYPERTONIA

This denotes the opposite state of affairs to hypotonia. In this case the excitatory extrapyramidal influences upon the motoneurone pools are present to excess and the stretch reflex excitatory bias is high. The muscles are therefore more sensitive to stretch and are said to be hypertonic.

Let us refer back to the stretch reflex mechanism. Muscle spindles contain stretch receptors which can influence the large anterior horn cells in the motoneurone pools by means of the Ia afferent fibres. Stimulation of these stretch receptors creates impulses which pass via the Ia fibres to the motoneurone pools where they stimulate the large anterior horn cells to convey impulses to the extrafusal muscle which contracts in response to these impulses.

In addition to the extrafusal muscle fibres there are intrafusal fibres which form a contractile element to the stretch receptor. Their function is to keep the stretch receptor in a receptive state whatever the length of the extrafusal muscle fibres. To do this they require to be held in a state of contraction sufficient to keep the stretch receptor area sensitive to stretch. They receive a nerve supply via the small anterior horn cells of the motoneurone pool. These nerves are called fusimotor fibres and are influenced by the extrapyramidal system.

If the inhibitory influence is dominant the stretch receptors are less sensitive because the intrafusal fibres are less active. This is what happens in hypotonia.

If the excitatory influence is dominant then the stretch receptors are much more sensitive because they are being held taut by the contracting intrafusal fibres. This is the situation in hypertonia.

Under normal circumstances an appropriate balance of excitation and inhibition is maintained to keep the stretch receptors suitably sensitive according to the circumstances of the moment.

There are some additional factors which should now be mentioned. In addition to the Ia fibres from the stretch receptors, there are secondary receptors in the spindle which give rise to fibres belonging to a group known as group II. These are also sensitive to stretch and if stimulated they have been found to inhibit slow-acting motor units and facilitate fast-acting motor units.

Another factor which has so far not been introduced is the Ib group fibres, which arises from the tendons or aponeuroses of muscle. These fibres arise from sensory receptors in the musculo-tendinous junction (Golgi organs) and are receptive to stretch. They are known to have an inhibitory effect upon motoneurone pools of their own muscle supply – an autogenic effect. These effects of inhibition are brought about via interneurones.

In order to appreciate fully the phenomenon of hypertonicity it is necessary to consider the stretch reflex in this way: the stretch reflex is said to have both phasic and tonic components. The phasic stretch reflex occurs when the muscle spindles are stimulated briefly and give rise to a synchronous motor response. The tonic reflex mechanism is the effect which is gained by a slow stretch of the muscle so that an asynchronous firing of motor units causes a sustained contraction of varying degree according to the sensitivity of the muscle to stretch.

There are two types of hypertonia, *spasticity* and *rigidity*.

SPASTICITY

As was stated before, the fusimotor system is rendered excessively active by the influence of the excitatory extrapyramidal system. The sensitivity of the stretch receptors is excessively high to both slow and quick stretch stimuli. In its milder form the sensitivity to quick stretch is most noticeable, when a 'clasp-knife' phenomenon may be demonstrated. In this situation the muscles respond to quick stretch in a phasic manner when there is synchronous firing of the primary receptors, which in turn gives a synchronous contraction of extrafusal muscle in response. The primary receptors fire synchronously because their threshold has been made low due to the excessive activity of the fusimotor system. The term 'clasp-knife' phenomenon is occasionally used because the opposition of the muscle to stretch seems to build up to a climax and then to subside suddenly. The sudden reduction in opposition may be attributed to the inhibitory influence exerted by the group Ib Golgi tendon organs, when tension is applied to the musculo-tendinous junction. Many explanations have been offered for this phenomenon and studies are by no means complete.

The response to slow stretch is that of steady opposition to the stretch stimulus which, in some cases, may build up to a tremendous level whereas in other milder cases it may be very slight indeed. On the whole passive movements to joints, where the muscles are showing spasticity, are more likely to be successful if conducted slowly so as to avoid eliciting a phasic response.

This form of hypertonicity is associated with the release of reflex activity from cortical control. If the lesion has occurred at a high level in the central nervous system then the tonic postural reflexes may be released in addition to the spinal reflexes. The released reflexes will exert a relatively uninhibited effect upon the motoneurone pools and cause patterns of increase in tone relevant to the reflexes released. For example, the released asymmetrical tonic neck reflex will cause spasticity to show in the extensor groups of the limbs on the side towards which the face is turned and in the flexors of the opposite side. The tonic labyrinthine reflex will incline the patient to show spasticity in the extensor groups if his head is in the appropriate position. The symmetrical tonic neck reflex will cause appropriate spastic patterning according to the position of the cervical spine – i.e. if the cervical spine is flexed the upper limbs will flex and the lower limbs extend etc.

It is rare to find one reflex mechanism released in isolation and a confusion of patterns is more likely to occur. However, knowledge of these factors enables the physiotherapist to interpret what is happening at any one time more accurately.

Spastic patterning varies from moment to moment depending upon many factors. One factor is the general position of the patient. Another is the nature of the stimulus being applied to the patient and yet another is how much effort the patient is making to obtain a voluntary movement. Strong volition often simply facilitates the excitation of the spastic patterning. This is possibly because the threshold of the appropriate motoneurone pools is already low, due to reflex release, so that the slightest volitional effort triggers them into action.

If the damage to the central nervous system is lower in level so that only the spinal reflexes are released then the spastic patterning may well be more related to flexion withdrawal. According to the stimulus applied there may be flexion or extension patterning but flexion is more likely to be predominant. Withdrawal is a response to noxious stimuli, but in this type of case it can be the response to almost any stimulus: touching of bedclothes on the affected areas, vibration, noise, sudden movement. It is well to bear this in mind since such patients must be dealt with very carefully if flexion withdrawal is not to become a permanent position for the patient.

Spasticity is never isolated to one muscle group. It is always part of a total flexion or total extension synergy. Let us take a lower limb example. If the lower limb is in extensor spasticity it will tend to adopt hip extension, adduction and medial rotation, knee extension and foot plantar flexion. Thus if one detected spasticity in the adductor groups one should expect it in all the other groups in the pattern.

It should be noted that the limb is not put into a good weight-bearing position by this patterning. The heel is unable to touch the supporting surface and the adducted limb is unable to support the pelvis adequately. Thus the patient showing this patterning is not able to experience the appropriate stimuli which will give the slow-acting postural muscles the appropriate guidance to support the limb.

For sound supporting posture we require the normal afferent stimulus of compression upon the heel of the foot. In this way the appropriate malleable postural mechanisms giving balanced co-contraction of both flexors and extensors can be encouraged. If this occurs we do not show the hyper-extended knee of the mildly spastic or the complete inability to get the heel onto the ground of the severely spastic case.

The spastic patient of this type may be deprived of experiencing the very afferent stimulation which could make his postural tone more normal. This occurs in many ways to the patient with this abnormal patterning and is an important factor in his treatment. The physiotherapist must help the patient to experience afferent stimulation which he is, by his condition, denied.

Reflex release mechanisms are more often than not incomplete. It is because this is so that many patients have interesting variations in patterning and also have some voluntary control. Obviously, the more control the patient has, the less severe is the residual problem. However, some patients require time to make use of such control as may be available and meanwhile bad habits, if unchecked, could mar the patient's eventual result.

RIGIDITY

In this type of hypertonicity the fusimotor system is also excessively active giving an increase in sensitivity to the stretch receptors in muscle. The disturbance is thought to lie at a different level from that causing spasticity since there is a considerable difference in the type of change in response to stretch.

It will be remembered that the subcortical nuclei comprising the basal ganglia are thought to help in the production of postural fixation by exerting their influence upon the stretch reflex mechanism via the reticular formation. They help to maintain adequate postural fixation whilst allowing the necessary malleability for voluntary movement. If, however, they become too effective as factors in postural fixation the stretch reflex mechanism may lose its malleability due to excessive fusimotor action. Damage in the area of link between the cortex and basal ganglia may well lead to excessive postural fixation to the detriment of volitional activity. The rigidity which ensues is different from spasticity in that it does not adopt the patterns of any particular reflex mechanism because the reflexes of tonic posture are not released. The pathways in the brain stem may still be intact and consequently some control of the stretch reflex mechanism may be available. The 'clasp-knife' effect seen in spasticity is not available in rigidity because phasic stretch does not appear to be suddenly inhibited. This may be because the control centres in the brain stem exert a suppressor action upon the inhibitory mechanisms.

In rigidity the muscles respond to slow stretch by steady resistance which does not particularly build up or relax off. There is a tremor which is said to give a 'cog-wheel' effect, or the limbs may feel like lead when moved, giving rise to the term 'lead pipe' rigidity. Explanations of this phenomenon are not complete and it must be remembered that, at present, there are many questions which remain unanswered.

Patients showing rigidity usually have lesions in the subcortical areas and show a typical posture which becomes progressively more flexed. They do not rotate in any of their movements and lack of axial rotation seriously interferes with their balance reactions.

The 'rigidity' patient shows movement problems in which automatic adjustment and activities do not occur freely and therefore voluntary movement is slow and impoverished because it is unaccompanied by automatic balance reactions and because it occurs so slowly against the ever-resisting stretch mechanisms.

In spasticity movement impoverishment also occurs. Balance reactions cannot be produced against the spastic patterns and mature permutations of flexion versus extension patterns are not available, only the stereotyped reflex patterns being produced in voluntary movement.

ATHETOSIS

When this occurs the patient shows disorder of movement because of fluctuation in the level of postural fixation. The patient adopts a succession of abnormal postures which may be quite grotesque. The condition is made more severe by excitement and emotional stress. It is thought to be due to lesions within the basal ganglia and in particular in the putamen. In this instance the basal ganglia are failing in their ability to encourage adequate postural fixation and fluctuations therefore occur.

Involuntary movements occasionally occur but the symptoms are always made worse by voluntary activity.

CHOREIFORM ACTIVITY

This is a series of involuntary movements, which occur in the face and limbs. They are quicker than those of athetosis and are also made worse by voluntary movement. Many patients show a combination of choreiform and athetoid activities. The basal ganglia are considered to be at fault in choreiform problems.

BALLISMUS

This is a term used to describe wild flinging movements which may occur to such an extent that they throw the patient off balance. The condition usually occurs as a result of a lesion in the subthalamic region and only affects one side. In this case it is called hemiballismus.

DYSTONIA

This is a term used to describe an increase in muscle tone that is antagonistic to the intended movement. The symptoms tend to prevent movement and may pull the individual into grotesque postures. It may affect one part of the body or the body as a whole. Spasmodic torticollis is thought to be a type of local dystonia. The lesion is thought to lie in the putamen.

TENDENCY TO DEVELOP DEFORMITIES

Whenever there is a tendency to adopt habitual postures of one part of the body or many parts there is a danger of adaptive shortening of some soft tissues and lengthening of others. In this way joints may become stiff and give deformities which are very difficult to correct. The least vulnerable patients are the athetoids and choreiform types since these patients are rarely still, but the spastic, rigid and flaccid types of patient may develop severe deformities if left untreated.

VULNERABILITY TO INJURY

Sensory loss leads to obvious dangers. Pain produced by damage is a protection against continuation of the damage. If pain is not felt then damage can occur with no protective reaction. Many cases of skin lesion and ulceration are due to this problem.

Many of these patients have sphincter problems and are incontinent. This renders the skin soggy and even more vulnerable. Pressure sores are a common complication.

If pain is felt and the patient is unable to move away from its cause damage will also occur.

Muscle flaccidity, dyssynergia, and spasticity may all lead to ill-controlled joint positioning so that joints are put to undue strain and ligaments permanently stretched. The hyperextended knees of extensor spasticity are an example of this. The joint distortion may in some cases be great enough to cause subluxation.

Malposturing may also lead to undue pressure on nerves and blood vessels. This may give rise to secondary neuropathy, defects of venous return and oedema.

CIRCULATORY PROBLEMS

These exist in various forms in most neurological disorders.

When muscle paralysis is present the muscle pump action is defective and venous return is reduced. This may not have a noticeable effect if only small groups are affected, but if large areas of muscle are paralysed the effect may be great enough to case oedema and may have the effect of reducing the rate of growth in the child. A peripheral problem of this type also gives rise to autonomic defects involving the control of blood vessels and sweat glands. Skin changes corresponding to this occur. Atrophy of the skin may develop causing it to become dry, scaly, thin and more vulnerable.

Disorders of the spinal cord will interfere with the autonomic control of the blood vessels and may have a general effect on the patient's ability to give correct blood pressure adjustments. The higher the level of cord injury the more severe the effect. This is seen most dramatically in paraplegic and tetraplegic cases.

Hypotonia will also give rise to defects of muscle pump activity although the effect may not at first be noticeable because it is more general and there is no 'normal' for comparison.

RESPIRATORY PROBLEMS

The patient may show paralysis in the respiratory muscles and will then obviously have respiratory difficulties. Those who have paralysis or severe hypotonia in the throat musculature will also have difficulty, since the inspiratory movements tend to suck the walls of the pharynx inward unless muscle tone braces against this effect. Thus the patient may choke for this reason or because the throat muscles are incoordinate in swallowing so that inhalation of food occurs.

Respiratory movements may be so impaired as to make speech difficult and coughing impossible. Communication is therefore a problem and lung secretions gather.

The patient showing rigidity may have impaired respiratory function due to the difficulty in obtaining thoracic mobility.

SPEECH DISORDERS

These may be the direct result of respiratory problems, due to paralysis of speech muscles, or due to more complex problems of dyssynergia, spasticity and speech perceptual problems. A patient is said to be *dysphasic* when he has inco-ordination of speech and is unable to arrange his words in correct order. He is said to be *aphasic* when he is unable to express himself in writing, speech or by signs and is unable to comprehend written or spoken language. There are many different forms of aphasia and each one is very distressing to the patient.

DISTURBANCE OF EXERCISE TOLERANCE

This is inevitable. Only the most minor neurological changes would leave this undisturbed. The dysfunction of normal movement necessitates uneconomical substitute movements which undermine exercise tolerance. If this is not apparent because the patient is relatively immobile due to his disorder, his exercise tolerance will be reduced because of lack of exercise. The chair-bound patient who is wheeled about by relatives, quickly loses such exercise tolerance as he had because his circulatory and respiratory mechanisms are not put to any stress. Added to this he may be inclined to overeat and will put on unnecessary fat which will further reduce his condition of tolerance.

Any patient whose respiratory capacity is reduced must have diminished exercise tolerance.

Since there are many reasons for this problem they should be noted by the physiotherapist who may be able to minimize them in some cases.

PAIN

This is a factor in neurological cases but is not so prevalent as might at first seem likely. Pain can only be felt if there are pathways to convey the sensation.

Pain is most likely to occur in irritative lesions when the threshold of pain reception is low. Thus pain is a feature of neuritis. Other reasons are those connected with raised intracranial pressure giving rise to headache and throbbing sensations.

Some patients with lesions in the thalamic region show intractable thalamic pain which is difficult to understand until it is appreciated as a centrally placed lesion and is not due to damage in the peripheral area from which the pain is interpreted as coming.

Discomfort and pain from habitual bad posturing also occur and patients who have sudden waves of increase in muscle tone will complain of pain.

REFERRED PAIN

This is a term used to denote pain interpreted as arising from an area which is not, in fact, the site of the trouble. For example pressure on the roots of origin of cervical 5 and 6 spinal nerves can give pain which is referred to their dermatomes, myotomes and sclerotomes. The patient will complain of pain over the deltoid area, lateral aspect of forearm and over the radial side of the hand. He may complain of deep pain over the scapula, lateral aspect of humerus, radius and over the bones of the thumb. The site of this problem is, in this case, in the cervical region but the patient suspects disease or injury where he feels the pain. This type of referred pain is often called root pain.

Referred pain does not always relate to surface structures but may also relate to viscera. For example, in cardiac disease pain may be referred to the left shoulder.

It is well known that pain in the otherwise normal individual will give rise to protective muscle spasm and abnormalities of movement and posture. It must, therefore, be appreciated that pain will do the same to the neurological case provided the nervous pathways are available to react. Thus the abnormality induced by pain will be superimposed upon those already existing.

CAUSALGIA

This is a term used to describe a severe sensation of burning pain which accompanies some peripheral problems. The patient shows hyperaesthesia or increased sensitivity, trophic changes and over-activity of the autonomic supply of the area.

The pain is aggravated by exposure and heat or cold and also by emotional crises. Because of the hyperaesthesia the patient protects the affected area to an extreme degree and does not move it at all. Even cutting the finger nails, if the hand is affected, may prove too painful and gloves, shoes and stockings and other items of clothing may be intolerable.

The skin shows atrophy and scales, and vascular changes occur ranging from vasoconstriction to vasodilation. The skin appearance will relate to the condition of the vessels. If vasoconstriction is present the skin is mottled and cyanotic and usually moist due to activity of the sweat glands. If the vessels are dilated the skin will be pink, warm, dry and later may become very glossy.

Muscle atrophy and joint stiffness are frequent in these cases and osteoporosis may be evident.

The exact cause of this condition is not fully understood. It is known to occur when the peripheral injury is incomplete and may be due to deflection of nerve impulses from efferent nerves to afferents so that more impulses are reaching the posterior nerve roots. This could happen in a nerve crush situation where the traumatized area may form a kind of pseudo-synapse between various nerve fibres. It is generally thought that the autonomic disturbances are secondary to the hyperaesthesia.

Loss of consciousness

We are said to be unconscious when we are unaware of sensations such as seeing, hearing, feeling, tasting, smelling, etc. The reticular arousal system in the midbrain and subthalamic region awakens the cerebral cortex to the reception of sensations. If this formation is damaged or if the cortex is diffusely damaged we may lose consciousness.

Sudden changes in movement may cause temporary loss of consciousness by causing torsional strain on the midbrain. Space-occupying lesions like tumours and haemorrhages may press upon the midbrain either directly or indirectly.

The reticular arousal system is very sensitive to deficiencies of oxygen and also of glucose and these may therefore bring about unconsciousness.

It is most important to realise that there are various levels of unconsciousness and that many patients who are apparently totally unconscious are, to some extent, aware of their external environment. They do not appear to be aware of it because they cannot react, but they may have a level of consciousness which makes them semi-receptive.

Careless management of such a patient could be detrimental to his recovery. He may hear discouraging information about himself or be treated in a way which he may resent. He should always be talked to when he is being handled and in an adult manner so that he may as far as possible understand what is happening around him. The physiotherapist should never talk about the patient in front of him.

Epilepsy

This is a recurring disturbance of cerebral activity in which there is a sudden flood of discharge of impulses from neurones which have, for some reason, become uninhibited. If the area affected is near the reticular arousal area consciousness may be lost. Exact events depend upon the area affected.

Seizures may be major or minor in nature and may complicate many neurological problems, particularly those related to head injuries and tumours.

Urine retention and incontinence

These distressing problems may complicate some of the more severely affected patients.

Sphincters may remain closed leading to retention of urine, which eventually leaks out due to overfilling of the bladder. Such a condition often gives the appropriate stimulus for flexion withdrawal and may increase flexor spasticity.

The recumbent position added to urine retention may lead to back pressure into the kidneys with further complications. It is always wise to allow such patients to adopt a vertical position periodically to relieve this effect.

Incontinence of urine may lead to skin breakdown since, inevitably, the skin will become soggy and more vulnerable.

Some patients may develop 'automatic' bladder-emptying mechanisms but others may have to have some permanent help in the management of the problem.

There may also be problems related to defaecation although these can often be managed by careful control of the intake of food and fluids in addition to developing a routine of timing of likely bowel activity.

Loss of normal functional independence

This is likely in most neurological problems except in the most minor. In slowly progressive disorders loss of function appears late since, subconsciously, the patient substitutes for each disability as it appears. In sudden disorders functional loss is dramatic, since the patient has suffered sudden physiological trauma which requires time for adjustment in addition to the psychological trauma associated with sudden disability.

Many patients show rejection of the area most severely affected or at least disassociation from it and they manage as best they can with what is left. Sometimes this is a necessity but there are occasions when such a drastic adjustment is detrimental to the ultimate result and should therefore be discouraged.

Simple functions may be lost because of lack of balance reaction or postural fixation.

The patient may not be able to move around in bed, transfer himself from bed to chair, dress, wash or feed himself.

If functional independence is permanently lost a great burden is placed upon the relatives and on the community as a whole. The patient may live an excessively confined life and have, therefore, limited horizons. This must be avoided and dealing with this aspect plays a large part in the patient's treatment programme.

CHAPTER IV

Assessing the Patient

by HELEN W. ATKINSON, M.C.S.P., DIP.T.P.

This is a most important aspect of the management of the neurological patient since the ultimate goal and treatment programme to obtain it depend upon the findings.

It is worth spending two or three treatment sessions in obtaining an assessment, particularly if the patient has widespread problems. Indeed most workers find that they are learning new facts about their patients all the time and adjust their approach accordingly.

It is necessary to have a period of initial assessment with all patients and to have intermediary assessments at intervals of a suitable length throughout the whole period of time during which the patient is receiving help.

A final assessment should be made at the time he ceases to receive any further help so that should he later be thought to have deteriorated since discharge, there is some record of his condition at that particular time.

Emphasis will be placed, in this chapter, on the assessments most suitably made by the physiotherapist. At the end of the chapter some of the more common medical and surgical investigations are indicated.

Prior to assessing the patient the physiotherapist should have studied the medical history and any pertinent aspects of the medical examination which will already have occurred.

The physiotherapist's assessment should include some or all of the following points depending upon the nature and extent of the condition of the patient.

A general impression of the patient's condition

It should be noted whether the patient is ambulant, chair-bound or confined to bed and whether he requires any assistance if he is ambulant or chair-bound. His general appearance should be observed for build, muscle atrophy, skin coloration, signs of obvious ill-health or malnutrition and the overall condition of his hair, skin and nails. If he has any pressure sores or is likely to develop them his skin should be carefully examined and areas of breakdown noted.

At this stage it is also important to note the general impression of the patient's mental attitude to his problem and also whether he appears to be a social individual or more introverted in nature.

Interrogation of the patient

This is an important part of the examination as the experienced person can learn a great deal from the patient at this time. He should be questioned about his own particular difficulties which are the result of his illness. It is very important to find out from the patient what he finds to be the most serious drawback since his views may be quite different from that of those who are examining him.

If the patient has noticed some difficulty in fulfilling a function it is most important to examine this carefully and to try to find some way of alleviating the problem in the treatment programme. In this way the patient's co-operation is much more readily gained for this and many other aspects of his management.

The patient's hopes and fears must be noted and some idea of what he *wants* to be able to do must be obtained.

The physiotherapist should find out details of the patient's occupation and get some idea of what it involves in the way of physical and mental activity. In some cases it may be possible to enable the patient to resume his normal work but in many instances this is not possible. It is important to avoid holding out false hopes to a patient.

There will be some information concerning the patient's family and responsibilities in the medical notes but, if this has been omitted, it may be wise to find out as much as possible and to note the patient's attitude to those members of his family he mentions. Family relationships can have an important bearing on the desire to recover some functional ability.

The patient should be asked about pain and discomfort and he should also be asked about its quality and when and where it is felt.

The patient must be given time to tell his problems since, if he is rushed, he may omit some very important fact.

Whilst carrying out this interrogation the physiotherapist can note many other aspects of the problem without the patient being conscious of her doing so. She can notice any problems of speech or hearing and whether the patient is able to interpret her words easily and reply quickly, or slowly and with difficulty. She can note his respiratory control, expression changes on his face, whether he can control the saliva in his mouth and whether he is able to swallow easily.

The physiotherapist should also notice whether the patient can make automatic position adjustments whilst conversing.

It is not always possible to hold a two-way conversation with some patients since speech or hearing may be difficult. It may be necessary to arrange a signal system and question the patient on a yes/no basis. In some cases the written word may be of help.

If the patient is unconscious or too young to participate relatives may be needed to help to answer some of the queries.

Assessment of hearing

This is not really the province of the physiotherapist but it is important for her to know whether the patient can hear ordinary speech or whether this is difficult. She also needs to know whether he can hear himself moving against the bedclothes or chair or his feet on the floor, since the ability to do so makes a difference to his ability to move in a co-ordinate manner and with assurance.

Assessment of eyes and vision

Although this is the province of the highly qualified specialist, it is helpful for the physiotherapist to know whether the field of vision is limited or full, whether the pupils are able to react to light and whether there are inco-ordinate movements of the eyes such as nystagmus.

It is also important to know whether the patient has normal vision or requires the help of glasses to enable him to see near or distant objects. If the eyes are to be used to help in the production of movement it is important to know how much they can be expected to help. The medical notes may give most of the information that is required and should be studied carefully.

Visual fields can be roughly tested by holding two different coloured pencils some distance apart and asking the patient how many he can see. If he only claims to see one then the one he can see can be identified by colour (provided he is not blind to colour). This gives some indication of the visual field. The pencils can be moved about to find the extent of defect of field and the search can be narrowed down to the field of one eye by masking the other.

There is also the possibility of double vision and this can be assessed by holding up one object and asking how many the patient can see. If the patient has difficulty of convergence of the eyes he is likely to show double vision which can be distressing and make him insecure. Covering one eye will prevent double vision from being too troublesome and can be used to help patients who have no hope of correcting the problem in any other way.

Assessment of other sensory information

SKIN SENSATION

It should be noted whether the patient can distinguish between different types of sensation such as blunt and sharp, hard and soft, hot and cold etc.

It is possible to map out areas of defect on line diagrams of either the whole patient or the part requiring attention.

Two-point discrimination can be assessed for some patients but it must be remembered that this is variable in accordance with the area being examined. In the normal person two-point discrimination is better on the palmar aspect of the hand than it is on the dorsum. Thus one must expect discrepancies even in the normal individual. By two-point discrimination is meant the ability to distinguish two distinct areas being stimulated at any one time and noting how close the stimuli can be to each other before they are interpreted as one.

VIBRATION

This can be applied by a vibrator or by a tuning fork and is detected as a sensation by receptors in skin and bone. Because vibration has been found to have an important influence on muscle activity this is an interesting test to try. After the vibration stimulus has been given muscles working over the vibrated area may be seen to contract although they have not been stretched or stimulated in any other way. It is thought that the vibration is transmitted to the muscle spindles via the bone and gives a rapidly repetitive mild stretch stimulus. This may, incidentally, be one reason for the need for compression force of weight-bearing (giving a vibration) if one wishes to encourage co-contraction of muscles over a joint.

JOINT POSITION

This should be checked carefully and it may be done in various ways:

1. The patient may have the movements of a joint named for him – e.g. 'this is called bending the elbow and this is stretching' etc. Then he may be put through a passive range of movement whilst his eyes are closed and asked to state whether bending or stretching etc. is occurring. When moving the joint passively the physiotherapist must not indicate change of direction by moving her hands as the patient could otherwise detect discrepancies in direction because of this and give a false impression of his ability.

2. If the patient is sufficiently co-ordinate he could be asked to keep his eyes closed and to move a free limb into the same relative position as a limb being moved by the physiotherapist.

3. His limbs and trunk could be positioned by the physiotherapist and the patient could be asked to draw a pin man diagram of his position or to put a 'bendy toy' into a similar position. A 'bendy toy' is a toy doll made of sorbo rubber round a malleable wire frame which can be bent to any shape. These last methods do more than test joint sensation – they test body image interpretation and are suitable for only certain disabilities.

STEREOGNOSIS

This is the ability to recognize objects by feel and manipulation. It requires the ability to feel with the hands and to assess size and shape by the position of the joints. It also involves the ability to move the hands over and around the object.

It can be checked by putting objects into a patient's hand or hands whilst he is blindfolded and asking him to state what it is. Everyday articles should be chosen such as money, buttons, pens etc.

Another method would be to put a number of simple articles into an opaque bag and ask the patient to bring out only the pen or coin or button etc.

Closely allied to stereognosis is the ability to recognize texture of material and weight of identical-looking objects. Thus the patient may be asked to identify different materials such as wool, silk, paper, wood etc. The patient may do so by moving his hands over the material or having the material placed into or moved over his hands or other part of the body. Identical-looking objects but with different weights may be arranged in order of heaviness. This requires touch, pressure and joint sensation as well as some interpretation of the muscle activity needed to support the weight.

Areas of lost sensation should be recorded and also any areas of paraesthesia should be noted. Numbness and tingling give false sensation and dull sensory perception and so need to be taken notice of as they are indicative of disturbance occurring in sensory pathways (see Fig. IV/1 on p. 78).

Joint mobility and soft tissue length

The available range of movement in the joints should be noted. In some cases the range should be accurately measured but in most cases of neurological disorder this is not really necessary.

Passive and active range should be assessed since many patients cannot move the joints because of muscle weakness, hypotonia or hypertonia. When assessing the passive movements available the physiotherapist should remember to check the biological length of two-joint muscles as well as individual joint ranges.

If the patient is known to be spastic it should be remembered that certain positions of the head and neck could make movement of joints less available. For instance, supine lying could make hip and knee flexion very difficult for either the patient or the operator.

The physiotherapist should try to ascertain the reason for limitation of movement, note any fixed deformity and also any habitual posturing.

Variations in muscle activity

Here the physiotherapist is looking for flaccidity, hypotonicity, hypertonicity and the fluctuations associated with athetosis and ballismus etc.

Some information will already have been gained if the other assessments mentioned above have been carried out. However, discrepancies in muscle activity can also be assessed in the following ways:

PASSIVE MOVEMENTS

Relaxed passive movements give the following information:

a. That the muscles are flail and are allowing movement to occur

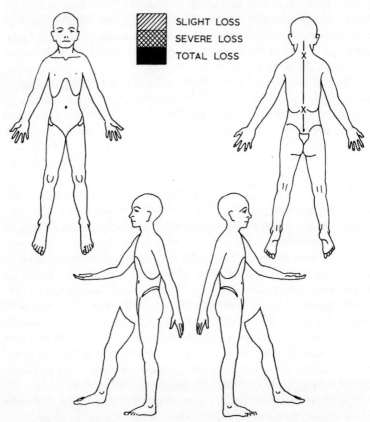

SLIGHT LOSS
SEVERE LOSS
TOTAL LOSS

Fig. IV/1 Sample chart for recording afferent information

with no opposition and may even be allowing an excessive range of movement to occur. If many muscles are involved the limb may feel heavy as there is no support from normal muscle activity.

b. That the muscles are showing excessive opposition to stretch. If they are showing spasticity they may show the clasp-knife phenomenon and will certainly oppose movements away from the spastic patterns.

If they are showing rigidity all movements will feel stiff and the cog-wheel phenomenon may be detected.

Passive movements should be performed both slowly and quickly to detect any difference in the response of muscles to slow and quick stretch.

If hypotonia is present the passive movements may feel similar to the effect given by flaccid muscle. However, quick passive movements to joints controlled by hypotonic muscles may initiate a stretch response which is not available in flaccid muscle.

PALPATION

Handling of muscles in varying states of tone can give helpful information. The flaccid muscle usually feels non-resilient, soft and atrophied. The hypotonic muscle feels soft but not really non-resilient. It does not usually show much atrophy. The spastic muscle feels tight and hard particularly if it is put slightly on the stretch. Its tendon may be felt to stand out from underlying structures. Muscles showing rigidity feel solid and the limbs are rather leaden to move about.

REFLEX TESTING

This is a common method of assessing muscle tone and the condition of the various neurological pathways.

Superficial reflexes may be tested by scratching the skin over an area and watching for muscle contraction. If the skin of the abdomen is stroked the abdominal muscles contract. If no response occurs there is either an interruption of the lower reflex pathway or a state of central shock in which the motoneurone pools are not receptive to stimuli. The response may be exaggerated if flexor spasticity is present, sluggish if there is hypotonia, and difficult to see if there is rigidity because the muscles will not be adequately relaxed to start with.

Scratching the sole of the foot has a similar effect. There is a withdrawal from the stimulus involving dorsiflexion of the foot. In the normal situation the great toe of the mature individual will plantar flex whilst the rest of the foot dorsiflexes. However, if hypertonicity of a spastic nature is present there will be dorsiflexion of the whole foot accompanied by flexion of knee and hip. This is often called a 'Babinski sign'. In hypotonicity the response will be sluggish and in the case of flaccid dorsiflexors there will be no response of these muscles but there may be flexion of knee and hip if these muscles are working and the limb is free to move. Again, as for the abdominal reflexes, if there is a state of spinal shock the reflex will be absent.

Tendon reflexes may be tested by tapping the tendon of a muscle. This does not stretch the tendon but by putting a momentary kink into its shape and by vibrating it the muscle fibres attached to the tendon are suddenly stretched. The normal response to this is for the muscle fibres to contract together giving a jerk of tone in the muscle. Hence we talk of the knee, ankle and elbow jerks. In these cases the patellar tendon, tendo achilles and triceps tendons are struck once with a tendon hammer and the appropriate response is awaited. The lower limb, foot and forearm must be free to move if the full effect is to be observed. This method can be applied to any muscle tendon but these are the ones most commonly tested.

If there is no response there may be interruption of the motor pathway between the spinal cord and the muscle indicating a flaccid paralysis of the muscle. It is possible also that sensory interruption has occurred which may or may not mean flaccid paralysis depending upon whether the motor pathway is also involved.

No response will occur if there is a state of spinal shock which may occur temporarily in injuries to the brain or spinal cord.

If the response is exaggerated it means that an excessive contraction of muscle occurs, then some hypertonicity of a spastic nature should be suspected.

A pendular or oscillating response indicates hypotonicity and lack of postural fixation to steady the limb after the initial jerk. The limb swings back and forth several times before settling down.

If hypertonicity of a spastic nature is suspected the physiotherapist should look for dominant reflex patterning and could well make use of her knowledge of the tonic postural reflexes to assess the severity of the condition. By placing the patient in the various postures which will most readily elicit a static reflex response, she can assess the dominance of the reflexes by the spastic patterning which occurs or by the increase in tone she feels in the muscles. For example, if the patient is placed in supine lying and the tonic labyrinthine reflex is therefore allowed free rein, the patient showing spasticity will show an increase in extensor tone and flexion will be difficult. If the head is then flexed forwards there may be more extensor tone in the lower limbs but an increase in flexor tone in the upper limbs indicating a symmetrical tonic neck reflex patterning.

Head turning may give extension of the limbs on the side to which the face is turned and flexion of the others indicating the influence of the asymmetrical tonic neck reflex. It should be noted that full patterning into spastic patterns may not necessarily occur. There may be a simple, slight increase in tone into the patterns, or movement out of the patterning may just be made slightly more difficult in the milder cases.

Fluctuations of tone as seen in the athetoid, chorea and ballismus case can usually be readily seen as involuntary movements.

Assessing for quality of movement

These assessments are most relevant to patients showing hypertonicity, ataxia and hypotonia, athetosis, chorea and ballismus etc.

Assessment is made of the patient's ability to give various permutations of movement, to balance adequately with suitable equilibrium reactions and to carry out smoothly co-ordinate movements with suitable postural background (see Appendix 1, p. 483).

MOVEMENT PERMUTATIONS

By this is meant the ability to mix flexion and extension movement components so as to get a balance of activity. It will be remembered that the spastic pattern of extension of a lower limb is extension, adduction and medial rotation of the hip, extension of the knee and plantar flexion of the foot. The reversal of this is flexion, abduction and lateral rotation of the hip, flexion of the knee and dorsiflexion of the foot. Mature movements involve a mixture of these two limb synergies so that every time the hip extends it does not also have to adduct but can remain abducted etc.

A quick method of assessing the patient's overall ability is to encourage movements through some fundamental and derived positions which are all, in fact, mixtures of flexion and extension synergies.

The quality of the movements and positions is the point to be observed. The positions most related to neurodevelopmental sequence are probably most useful. Let us take as an example the use of the lying position.

a. Prone lying. Is the patient able to take up elbow support prone lying? If not can he be put into the position and is he able to hold it when he is placed there?

b. Is he able to remain in prone lying with his legs abducted and laterally rotated?

c. Can he roll from prone lying to supine, leading with different parts of his body, e.g. head and neck, arms, or lower limbs – and does his body spiral as he turns or is it a solid mass going over as a whole?

d. Is he able to lie in supine with his legs abducted and laterally rotated and also his arms in a similar position?

e. Is he able to roll from supine to prone, leading with different parts of his body?

f. Does he have balance reactions in side lying if gently pushed backwards and forwards?

These points can be charted.

It must be remembered that disturbance in movement permutation need not necessarily be the result of neurological problem but may be related to an orthopaedic or traumatic problem or even simply to pain.

ASSESSING BALANCE

Good balance requires a well-integrated nervous system with adequate afferent information, mobile joints and sound muscles. Faults in any of these factors will influence the patient's ability to balance.

The ability to balance needs to be assessed in various postures and during movements from one posture to another. The earliest balance activity involves balancing the head over the upper trunk in prone lying and supported sitting, whereas a very advanced balance activity could be walking, carrying a tray full of glasses whilst avoiding and talking to people who are passing by! Obviously circus artistes perform many more advanced balance activities but few of us aspire to their heights.

Thus it would take a complete volume to assess every posture and movement for balance. However, having selected a position for assessment suitable for the patient the following procedure may be adopted:

a. How much help does he need to maintain the position?

b. Test his conscious balance responses by applying pressure and telling him to 'hold' or saying 'don't let me move you'. Give pressure in various directions and note his stability.

c. Try the same approach with his eyes closed. If he has been relying on eyesight he will be less stable or may fall when his eyes are closed.

d. Let him have his eyes open and test his automatic reactions to balance disturbance. Ask him to let you move him and tilt him backwards, forwards, sideways and rotate him – all gently – so as to disturb the position of his centre of gravity. Notice whether he moves his head, trunk, upper limbs or lower limbs or all of them to maintain his equilibrium. Try disturbing his balance this way by moving him at the shoulders, or using his arms as handles or by using his legs. The reaction you will get will depend upon what is available to the patient and what part of him you have left free to react.

e. Try the same reactions with his eyes closed. Be careful to prevent injury should his ability be poor in this situation. Record the reactions you obtain and relate them to those which should be obtainable. For example you do not expect stepping or hopping reactions if you have tested the patient in sitting.

f. Now test his reactions when carrying out a movement of some part of the body. For example in sitting, movements of the arms require balance adjustment. Try this with the eyes open and then closed.

g. Objective activity test. This requires the use of the position for a function such as dressing or any simple activity which takes the patient's mind off balancing and puts it on to the fulfilment of purposeful activity.

The various reactions obtained will depend upon the condition being examined. If there are many flaccid muscles exaggerated reactions will be seen in the normal parts of the body as compensation. If there is hypotonicity balance will be precarious, reactions slow to occur but exaggerated when they do occur and of rather a primitive nature (putting hand down onto a support and using a wide base).

If there is spasticity, disturbance in balance will give exaggerated reactions to any normal part and spastic patterning of the rest of the body.

If there is rigidity, balance reactions will probably be almost entirely absent except for forward stepping and protective extension. The reactions will occur very slowly.

It must be remembered that balance reactions may be altered by joint stiffness and account must be taken of this in any patients who are likely to have limitation of movement.

ASSESSING CO-ORDINATION AND PRECISION

Well co-ordinated purposeful movement requires i. a variety of movement permutations, ii. good balance reactions and iii. the ability to stabilize one part of the body whilst moving another part so that

83

movement occurs smoothly. In assessing i. and ii. a large part of iii. has already been examined. However, smoothness of movement needs to be checked, the ability to move the trunk on the limbs and the limbs on the trunk needs checking, and the ability to stop and start movement is very important.

This can be done by examining the patient's ability to move from prone lying to supine and from supine to prone in a slow smooth manner stopping and starting on the way. If suitable, he may be required to take up side sitting from prone lying and then proceed to all fours, kneeling, half kneeling and standing with stops and starts throughout. Whilst doing this, precision and smoothness are being checked and any tremor, overshooting or lack of precision is noted. These are gross co-ordinate activities and provided the patient is capable of coping with the various positions and movements they make a good starting point.

It should be remembered that slow movements are very often more difficult for the inco-ordinate patient and so both fast and slow movements should be assessed.

More detailed checks can be made regarding the abilities of the patient by placing him in a very stable position and asking for free movements of the limbs of a precise nature. The finger to nose test is the classic method of testing co-ordination. In this the inco-ordinate patient either misses the nose altogether or has much tremor before landing and he strikes it rather heavily. This indicates lack of postural fixation of the proximal joints. The patient with sensory loss shows a worsening of symptoms if the eyes are closed.

If the patient succeeds in moving the limbs well when the trunk is in a stable position, it should then be placed in a less stable position so that mechanical proximal fixation is no longer helping the patient.

The movements should be checked for smoothness, ability to stop and start, ability to occur as a whole and not be broken up into joint by joint activities. Later they should be checked as purposeful actions in which the patient's mind is not on the movement but upon the purpose of moving.

Obviously such functions as walking must be involved if the patient is sufficiently able to do so.

Co-ordination between hand and eye can be checked by asking the patient to reach out and take objects of various sizes and shapes and to give them back to the physiotherapist. Objects such as balls can be rolled to the patient for him to take as they arrive, later they can be thrown to him and smaller balls can be used. Shapes and sizes and co-ordination can be tested by asking the patient to put objects of certain shapes through appropriate slots. This requires extremely good hand co-ordination, co-ordination between hand and eye and also sensory perception.

Assessing muscle power

This assessment is most applicable to the lower motor neurone problem as seen in peripheral nerve lesions, peripheral neuritis or in anterior poliomyelitis.

The classic method of assessing muscle power is to relate the ability of the muscle to move the appropriate part of the body against the force of gravity. The Medical Research Council assessment gradings from 0–5 are assigned as follows:

0=No contraction felt or seen.
1=Flicker of activity either felt or seen.
2=The production of a movement with the effect of gravity eliminated.
3=The production of a movement against the force of gravity.
4=The production of a movement against the force of gravity and an additional force.
5=Normal power.

It is usual to start assessing for grade 3 and be prepared to move up or down the scale. Obviously the specific action of the muscle to be tested must be known since positioning the patient must be related to the effect of gravity on the movement to be produced.

It is important to note that a muscle can only give its best performance if its synergists are also participating. For example deltoid is an abductor of the arm and requires a stable shoulder girdle if it is to be successful in this action. It particularly requires the activity of serratus anterior and trapezius as fixators of the scapula to prevent the inferior angle of the scapula from swinging medially as the arm tries to move sideways. Unless these muscles work with deltoid it is unlikely to succeed in producing abduction.

If the physiotherapist is testing a weak deltoid it is important that she checks the abilities of the synergists and fixators to see that the weak muscle gets adequate chance to show its abilities.

If the scapula is not fixed by the patient's own muscles then steps must be taken to fix it manually or mechanically before assessing the power of deltoid. This is, of course, true of all muscles – deltoid has only been taken as one example.

There is not usually much difficulty in coming to conclusions about grades 2, 3 and 4 in this method of assessment. Grade 1 can be difficult and so can grade 5. Before deciding that no flicker is available and therefore scoring 'o' it is wise to try maximum facilitation and see if some activity can be encouraged. In that case grade 1 can be awarded provided it is made clear that it was only achieved with maximum facilitation. Grade 'o' should never be awarded until maximum facilitation has been tried and failed.

For grade 5 the muscle must be compared to the normal side if there is one. It must be remembered that different activities use different levers and that movements against gravity can be done as weight bearing and non-weight bearing activities. Thus, for instance, the hip abductors cannot be graded as 5 unless they can function correctly to prevent a dropping of the pelvis towards the non-weight-bearing side (Trendelenburg's sign) whilst receiving weight in walking, running and jumping (if these last two are applicable to the age of the patient being examined).

These readings can be charted.

Other methods of assessing power include the use of a grip dynometer in which the patient is asked to grip a rubber bulb which is filled with air. The pressure exerted gives a pressure reading which is shown on a scaled dial. This, of course, assesses the power of the finger flexors and the efficiency of their synergists.

Static muscle power can be assessed by using spring balances arranged in series to pulley circuits so that the pull exerted can be recorded.

Dead weights may also be used and increased until the maximum load moved by the patient is found and recorded.

Assessment of speech, tongue movements and swallowing

This is largely the province of the speech therapist but the physiotherapist may need to check some points for herself. The early interrogation will have given some indication of the patient's problems and speech patterns will have been noted.

The physiotherapist also needs to know whether the patient understands the spoken word even if he cannot reply. This can be assessed by asking the patient to make a signal if he understands what is being said. The signal requested must be one of which the patient is capable. It must be appreciated that many patients know what they want to say but can only say one phrase or word which may come out every time they try to speak. Thus they may say 'no' if this is their only word when they mean 'yes' or 'it doesn't hurt' or 'hello'! If this is the case yes/no signals need to be devised and questions worded so that yes or no is the only answer required.

Tongue movements are essential for speech, mastication and deglutition. The physiotherapist can assess the availability of tongue movements by using any of these functions but if they are absent she may need to use a spatula or ice cube to encourage tongue movements whilst urging the patient to co-operate. It must be remembered that the tongue musculature is attached to the hyoid bone and if the synergists which control the position of the hyoid bone are not working control of tongue movements will be difficult. The infra- and suprahyoid muscles are important and may be paralysed. Equally, a patient with poor head control may well have infra- and suprahyoid synergy difficulties.

The ability to swallow involves complicated synergy of tongue, infra- and suprahyoid muscles and pharyngeal activity coupled with the maintenance of the closed mandible and closed lips. The muscles need power and co-ordination to be able to achieve the function.

Swallowing is most easily carried out in an upright position and is much more difficult if the patient is either recumbent or if the neck is extended.

It is important to remember that repetitive swallowing is self-limiting so the patient should not be asked to repeat the activity very often in quick succession.

Respiratory function

This may seem remote from neurology but it must be remembered that respiratory capacity depends not only upon lung field and thoracic mobility but also upon the muscle power and co-ordination of the respiratory muscles which include those of expiration as well as inspiration. Measurements of vital capacity using a spirometer can be graphed and give some idea of the power of the muscles and mobility of the thorax. Consecutive measurements at intervals give an idea of progress or rate of deterioration. A measurement of forced expiratory volume is one method of assessing the power of the expiratory muscles. This group includes the abdominal muscles.

Assessment of functional ability (see Appendix 2, p. 488)

This section has been deliberately held separate from the section on quality of movement since it is important that the two are in no way confused with each other.

When assessing function the physiotherapist is assessing the patient's ability to be independent and this need not, necessarily, be also an assessment of movement quality. In fact many patients with appalling quality of movement may be able to be relatively independent, provided normality of movement is not required.

Such functions as the ability to move about in bed, the ability to transfer from bed to chair, the ability to transfer from chair to toilet seat and to the bath are all included. Dressing, washing and other toilet activities should be assessed. The patient's ability to walk, climb stairs, manage in the home environment, cope with rough surfaces, cross roads, get on buses and even drive a car can be assessed.

If the patient is a wheel chair case then his ability to use his chair must be assessed. His ability to transfer from his wheel chair into a car and out again should be checked.

Functional assessments are best done in conjunction with an occupational therapist since this is also part of her work. In many cases a home visit may be required to relate function to home environment and in some cases a visit to places of employment may be needed. Achievement charts may also be used (p. 194).

Electrical tests

STRENGTH DURATION CURVES

These are done as part of the assessment of a patient suffering from a peripheral nerve lesion. Representative muscles of the affected group are stimulated by stimuli of different durations ranging from 300 ms pulses down to 0.01 ms. As is mentioned in Chapter V, p. 111, denervated muscle is only capable of responding to the longer duration stimuli because the shorter stimuli are too fast for muscle tissue unless very high intensities are used. The shorter stimuli are usually only transmitted via a nerve supply and thus only the innervated muscle can respond to such stimuli.

The term strength duration relates to the duration of the stimulus and the strength of the stimulus applied. More intensity is required for the shorter duration stimuli to produce a contraction even when there is a nerve supply. Thus a characteristic curve can be graphed relating stimulus duration and intensity applied to the contraction obtained (see Fig. IV/2).

It is usual to attempt to obtain a minimal perceptible contraction using a long duration stimulus and then progressively shorten the stimulus duration. If the contraction disappears, the intensity is increased until a contraction of the same degree is obtained, a reading

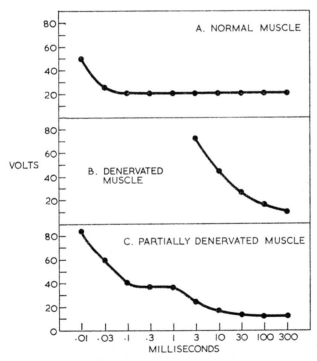

Fig. IV/2 Illustrative strength duration curves

is then taken and recorded. This goes on until the shortest stimulus is reached. However, if the muscle is denervated the long duration stimuli only will be successful and no amount of increase in intensity for the shorter stimuli will produce a contraction. Thus the graph will not be complete for the denervated muscle.

A muscle containing some innervated and some denervated fibres will show a special type of curve with a 'kink' in it. It is a mixture of the short graph for the denervated fibres and the long graph for the innervated group (Fig. IV/2c).

Accurate strength duration curves are only obtainable after 21 days following injury. This is because denervation takes this time to be completed.

Rheobase is a term used to describe the lowest intensity which can produce a muscle contraction when a long duration stimulus is applied. *Chronaxie* is a term used to denote the duration of stimulus which requires an intensity equal to twice the rheobase level, before a contraction is obtained.

As a muscle becomes innervated the chronaxie should gradually be a shorter duration of stimulus and move to the left of the graph.

NERVE CONDUCTIVITY

This is sometimes done to assess whether a nerve which has suffered compression is degenerating or not. The nerve is stimulated directly by a short duration stimulus along its course. When it is stimulated it conveys impulses to the muscles it supplies (provided it has fibres to carry them) and the muscles contract. If this is carried out at intervals from the time of injury the nerve will at first be hypersensitive and require a very low intensity. Later it may require more and, if it is degenerating, it will not conduct after about the fourteenth day. If, however, it does continue to conduct after 21 days the nerve has not degenerated and the injury is only a neurapraxia. In this case voluntary movement may be difficult or absent temporarily but recovery is likely eventually.

The above two tests can be carried out by the physiotherapist.

ELECTROMYOGRAPHY

This is usually the province of the physical medicine consultant. It involves placing needle electrodes into the patient's muscles or using surface electrodes on the skin. These are attached to a highly sensitive piece of apparatus which amplifies and records electrical activities in muscle.

These activities are recorded on a loudspeaker and as line graphs on an oscilloscope.

A muscle is electrically silent when there is no activity in the fibres. This occurs when it is fully relaxed. It creates sound and gives a graph when it is active. The sound and graph give a distinctive pattern.

If a muscle is fasciculating (which it does in certain muscular disorders and at certain stages of denervation), there is a different sound and visual pattern.

Such tests require great accuracy if they are to be valid since it is essential that the needle electrode is exactly in the muscle to be tested. Surface electrodes are not very accurate and there are many factors which can give artefacts in results. A shortwave machine working in the vicinity, for example, can cause interference if it is of unsuitable wavelength.

Other investigations

LUMBAR PUNCTURE

This is a surgical procedure in which a sample of cerebrospinal fluid is extracted from the lumbar region below the termination of the spinal cord. If the needle is connected to a manometer it is possible for the cerebrospinal fluid pressure to be recorded. The sample of fluid can be examined for the presence of blood which could indicate a subarachnoid haemorrhage, for a high protein content, for high cell count, for a Wassermann reaction and sometimes for sugar and chlorides.

Other similar procedures are ventricular punctures and cisternal punctures.

ANGIOGRAM

In this procedure a radio-opaque dye is injected into the circulatory system so that the arteries show up on X-ray. The blood vessels can then be examined for defects such as aneurysms, the presence of constriction or blockage by thrombus formation. Displacement by tumours may also be seen.

ENCEPHALOGRAM

In this case electrical changes in the brain are detected by a sensitive piece of apparatus and graphed upon an oscilloscope screen. Surface electrodes on the scalp are used. Various wave patterns can be detected according to the activity going on at the time and related to abnormalities such as epilepsy.

TESTS FOR MENINGEAL IRRITATION

Neck flexion test. If the patient is recumbent and the head is lifted so that the neck flexes, extensor spasm is produced which prevents flexion. Neck rigidity is said to prevent movement. This together with headache, photophobia and vomiting is indicative of meningeal irritation.

Kernig's sign. The hip is flexed slightly and any attempt then to straighten the knee causes pain and is restricted.

Both of these tests involve flexion of the spine and the rise in pressure in the vertebral canal is likely to be the chief factor in causing pain and muscle spasm.

When the assessment has been made the patient's treatment programme can then be mapped out. It is helpful to have in mind:

1. An immediate aim
2. An ultimate aim

In all cases the immediate aim will change as time progresses. As each aim is achieved a new one has to be made. It may also be necessary periodically to review the ultimate aim as the patient may progress further than originally expected. It is better to set one's sights low and progress, than to aim too high at first only to be disappointed.

If a patient is heavily handicapped it is wise to have a relative present at his final assessment before discharge so that the relative knows how much or how little help the patient needs. It is so easy for good work to be undone by over-helpful relatives who undermine the patient's independence. At the same time it is important that the patient is able to obtain such help as he does need.

CHAPTER V

Principles of Treatment (1)

by HELEN W. ATKINSON, M.C.S.P., DIP.T.P.

Many factors influence the management of patients suffering from neurological disorders. There are many views on appropriate action and treatment, some of which are complementary whilst others may conflict to some extent.

The greatest conflict occurs when the need for urgent independent function is taken as top priority when perhaps a little delay in independence could lead to more adequate adjustment of the patient. There are arguments for both sides. It must be remembered that, whilst early functional independence may decongest hospital wards and outpatient departments, this approach inevitably encourages the development of undesirable abnormalities of movement. These are substitutes for those normal activities which have now been temporarily or may be permanently made unavailable.

If a patient's potential is really quite good, given adequate time to redevelop along more normal lines, it may be quite seriously detrimental to him to allow substitute abnormalities to become a habit. Compromise is not always the answer since the result is often that of 'falling between two stools'.

Thus, the teamwork between consultants, nurses and therapists in addition to other workers is vital. There is nothing more detrimental to the patient than conflicting views between the team members dealing with his own particular case.

The physiotherapist's part in the management will be considered under similar headings to those used in Chapter III so that some correlation between the two chapters may be maintained. Aspects other than physiotherapeutic may be mentioned in passing but will not be discussed in detail.

DISTURBANCE OF AFFERENT INFORMATION

This can complicate the progress of the patient considerably and must always be taken into consideration.

Loss of afferent information

This may be local and specific if the problem is a peripheral one or it may be diffuse if the problem is more centrally placed. In either case there is much in common from the physiotherapist's point of view.

INJURY TO THE AFFECTED AREA

This is an important aspect in the management of such cases since cutaneous loss, in particular, is likely to make the patient vulnerable to cuts, burns from fire and steam, frictional abrasions from contact with harsh surfaces and pressure sores from prolonged contact with a supporting surface.

All patients with this problem should be made aware of this danger and it is the job of all concerned with the patient to ensure that he fully appreciates the dangers.

Obviously avoidance of injuries is to be encouraged and the patient should be told to use substitute measures to enable him to detect hazards. His hands are particularly vulnerable if they are involved since it is hard to avoid injury when the hands are so often used as tools. He must always use his eyes to detect hazards and beware of likely problems ahead of their occurrence so that complications do not arise.

Frictional abrasions and pressure sores can be avoided by adequate padding of areas likely to be subjected to friction and by care over the tying of such things as shoe-laces if there is sensory disturbance in the skin of the lower leg and foot. The application of sheep skin cushions and mattresses for the more heavily disabled is valuable so that the patient is 'cushioned on air' trapped in the wool. Ripple beds and frequent turning are necessary for the severely handicapped patient.

To some extent the patient should be responsible for his own safety. He must be warned to inspect his skin for signs of injury and to take steps to relieve pressure whenever possible. For instance the patient who is confined to a wheel chair should endeavour to lift himself up in the chair by using his arms to relieve the weight and pressure on the buttocks frequently. He will most particularly need to be reminded to do this if he has lost sensation in the buttock region since he will not then receive the uncomfortable stimuli which would normally encourage him to change position.

LOSS OF BODY IMAGE AND REJECTION OF THE AFFECTED AREA

This can be quite a difficult problem and to achieve any measure of success it is important to remember that we develop a knowledge of body image by being able to move, touch and feel objects in close proximity to us and by being able to touch different parts of ourselves. It will be remembered that, as far as the hands are concerned, contact with the face, nose, mouth and hair etc. is important. Thus we may be able to prevent loss of body image and rejection of parts of the body by using passive movements which are directed to simulating some of the more natural activities, e.g. taking the hands to the face and running the fingers through the hair, allowing the affected area to come into contact with more normal parts of the body and *vice versa.*

The patient may be positioned so that he can see the affected part and have his attention drawn to it frequently.

In some problems this aim of treatment is more important than in others. Permanent rejection is unlikely to occur in the localized peripheral problem but it is very common in the more centrally placed lesions.

If rejection and loss of body image has already occurred by the time the patient is receiving physiotherapy then the task is much more difficult to deal with. Sometimes exaggerated application of stimuli helps and heavy compression force repeated with the affected limb in a weight-bearing position may help. Constant handling of the area and helping the patient to simulate normal activities with the affected limb may be of value. Much patience and tolerance is needed in these cases.

The use of mirrors is sometimes of value and of particular importance is the need to encourage the patient who is showing signs of improving.

If the patient is accepting an abnormal position as being normal this must be pointed out to him and explained in such a way that he understands. He must then be allowed to experience the more normal position with the help of the physiotherapist who must, of course, ensure that he is safe and secure in his new normal position.

Mirrors again may be useful as an adjunct since the patient may need to use his eyes as substitutes for defective afferent information regarding general position. Even if the eyes are not needed for this purpose he may need convincing that the new posturing is more normal since it will 'feel' abnormal to him. Once the patient has appreciated the difference he must always be encouraged to adopt the more normal posturing in preference to the abnormal.

In cases of defects of sensory perception of this kind and in cases where loss of ability to move inevitably encourages the immediate adoption of abnormality, the patient must be treated as early as possible to avoid bad habits taking hold. For example, a patient who has had a cerebrovascular accident of such severity that he awakes as a hemiplegic, starts to develop abnormalities *as from that moment*. He substitutes and quickly accepts disability on that side of the body which for a time is virtually useless to him. Very soon it seems 'normal' to carry that half of the body as a passenger and to depend solely upon the non-affected side. This will be perpetuated unless some measures to prevent this occurrence are taken very quickly.

DISORIENTATION DUE TO FAULTY INFORMATION

This can occur if afferent information is not completely cut off so that faulty impressions are being received. For instance, some patients may have diminished touch and pressure sensation. If this occurs in the soles of the feet it gives rise to a 'cotton wool' sensation when the foot contacts a hard surface and very little sensation at all if a soft surface is contacted. This can make life very difficult for the patient. He may develop the type of gait which involves lifting the knee high and forcing the foot down hard onto the floor in order to obtain an exaggerated effect. This method of walking also makes a noise which tells the patient when he has landed. He may also have to look where he is walking all the time.

In this type of problem substitution would have to be encouraged, particularly if the disorder is permanent. Such a patient may have to be advised against wearing cushioned soles and heels since he cannot hear these land on the floor. He may have to wear studded shoes which make more noise than normal when he walks. He would have to be encouraged to use his eyes as substitute sensory organs.

As far as possible his high-stepping, exaggerated weight-bearing should be avoided since this could cause joint injury.

There are special methods of helping the movement problems of such cases. These will be considered under the heading relevant to movement abnormality (page 117).

Vertigo is another problem associated with faulty afferent information. As was stated in the previous chapter the patient may feel giddy and nauseated due to disorientation of the position of the head in space. The fault lies usually in the vestibular pathways or in the vestibular organs themselves. Any movement of the head or even of the eyes may make the patient feel symptoms. Impressions from the eyes and vestibular apparatus are so closely associated with each other that disturbance in one can give problems to the other.

The patient may have to be trained to rely upon the information he is receiving from his joints and skin and from his eyes since these are more reliable than the vestibular impressions. This takes time and whilst help from certain drugs is available to the patient, helping to reduce the feeling of nausea, the patient will still need help in movement activities.

Such patients frequently show a very fixed posture of the head and shoulder girdle because movement of the head is known to trigger off the symptoms.

The more unfortunate patient may well have vertigo in addition to faulty position sense. This makes life very difficult since substitution information is less available. Many patients with multiple sclerosis show these mixed problems and they may also have defective vision to complicate their problem even further.

The method of approach to the movement problem associated with vertigo will be considered under the appropriate heading (page 119).

DISORDERS OF MOVEMENT

The average person has very little appreciation of the complexity of performing an apparently simple function. All the necessary reactions are built in so smoothly that the timing and synchronization of muscle and joint activity escapes notice. Throughout activity movement occurs against a background of malleable postural tone adjusted to maintain the equilibrium of the individual in all eventualities. In this way movement flows in a smooth, co-ordinate and purposeful manner

Even less appreciated is the importance of afferent information. If there is no appreciation of the position in space the necessary steps to alter it cannot be taken. Moreover, if inadequate information is

97

forthcoming during the performance of the movement it can be nothing but crude and wide of the mark since no corrective measures can be taken.

For normal function to occur the nervous system must be in sound order from the receiving, correlative and transmission aspects. There must be adequate mobility available in the joints of both the trunk and the limbs and the muscles must be healthy and able to respond to the activities of the nervous system. It is only under these circumstances that appropriate muscle synergy will be forthcoming giving the common movement patterns associated with normality.

The more common movement patterns incorporate a balanced mixture of the movements seen in the more primitive mass flexion and mass extension patterns. Primitive mass flexion and extension patterns may be seen in the young child but even these are more refined than those seen in the patient whose central nervous system is grossly disordered.

The tiny child does have some control over his reflex mechanisms which gives him the ability to modify these effects to some extent. Although the normal child does show a poor vocabulary of movement when compared with the normal adult, he does have the basic foundations upon which to build the permutations of movement with which we are familiar in the mature individual. Skilled activity is dependent upon mature movement permutations and therefore mature muscle synergy.

Since all human beings are built along essentially the same lines and all require to be able to achieve similar basic functions, certain movement permutations are common to all. During the development of these permutations the child repeats a movement until it can be achieved with ease, thus illustrating the phenomenon of physiological facilitation. Repetitive use of a neuromuscular pathway lowers the threshold of synapses involved and makes it easier for the pathway to be brought into use. Thus the pathway is said to be facilitated.

Since movement involves excitation of some muscle groups and inhibition of others, it is important to remember that we are facilitating both excitation and inhibition when we facilitate a neuromuscular pathway so that a movement occurs. The word 'facilitation' means 'to make easy' and it is in this context that the word will be used throughout this chapter.

The physiotherapist who undertakes the problem of movement re-education in a disabled person is accepting an enormous responsibility. Not only must she be able to detect and assess the degree of, and type of, abnormality presented, but she must have the necessary knowledge and skill to guide the patient towards normality whilst recognizing the limitations set by the nature of the disorder.

THE PROBLEM OF FLACCIDITY

This may be seen when there is disorder in the peripheral system. On referring back to Chapter III it will be noted that such a state of affairs is usually the result of damage to the motoneurone pools of the anterior horns or to fibres passing peripherally from these motoneurones towards the muscles they supply. If all the motoneurones supplying any one muscle or group of muscles are completely destroyed then the muscles concerned will be completely paralysed, become flaccid and show atrophy in which muscle bulk is markedly reduced offering no protection to underlying structures.

If the damage is complete and irreversible, no amount of physiotherapy will restore muscle action. However, if only part of the motoneurone pool is affected, leaving intact those cells which have a higher threshold of stimulation, certain physiological factors may be applied to increase the excitatory effect on the motoneurone pools. In this way the remaining cells and their fibres may be made to convey impulses to the muscle, by the process known as recruitment. Similarly, if the cells or fibres of the motoneurone pools have suffered temporary damage they may eventually regain their ability to conduct impulses to the muscles. This may, at first, be difficult because they may have a raised threshold of activity.

These recovered neurones may also be encouraged to become active more readily by the physiotherapist exploiting her knowledge of physiology so that the use of these pathways is facilitated.

In this instance the physiotherapist has to make use of all the methods she can devise to have an excitatory effect upon the offending motoneurone pool or pools so that each effect can be added together or summated to reach the threshold of excitation.

Methods of excitation which are suitable

THE USE OF NORMAL MOVEMENT PATTERNS
This involves the use of muscles which commonly work with the muscle which is flail. This is of value because the neuromuscular

pathways commonly used are facilitated during the developmental process by repetition. Volitional impulses are conveyed to the motoneurone pools of the whole pattern. Neurones influencing one motoneurone pool in the pattern are thought to branch and also influence the other associated motoneurone pools. By this spreading of effect the motoneurone pool of the weakened muscle will receive maximum volitional stimulation.

USING THE EFFECT OF STRETCH STIMULATION

The stretch stimulus applied to the muscles involved in the whole pattern will, by branching of the afferent nerves, stimulate the motoneurone pools of each other as well as those of their own muscle. The excitatory state of the motoneurone pools including that of the weaker member of the team will be increased for a brief period of time. If to this effect, is added volitional effort (by summation) the excitatory influence may be enough to cause the lower motoneurones to conduct impulses to the muscles showing weakness.

RESISTANCE

This is, in effect, a kind of continuous stretch applied to a working muscle and thus is a facilitatory method. The degree of resistance applied should be as great as the muscle can overcome and *no greater*. In some instances suitable resistance may be appreciably high whereas in other circumstances it may be as little as frictional opposition offered by the joint being moved. The term maximal resistance is often used and this must always be related to the available power in the muscle under treatment.

THE USE OF TRACTION FORCE

Traction is applicable if the movement pattern to be produced is that of flexion. It simulates the natural influences upon such movements which are basically a withdrawal from the pull of gravity. This effect summated to stretch, resistance and volition will further alter the excitatory influence upon the motoneurone pools.

THE USE OF APPROXIMATION, i.e. compression through the joints.

This is a postural stimulus associated with extension and is thus suitable in any situation in which a weight-bearing stimulus could be applied. The extension patterns are most suitably facilitated by the application of approximation. This stimulus, like traction, could be applied to summate with resistance, stretch and volition.

THE USE OF TOUCH

This should be applied over the working muscles and/or to the surface against which the movement is to occur. This supplies skin stimulation which acts as a guidance to the movement and facilitates activity in the motoneurone pools.

THE USE OF VISUAL AND AUDITORY STIMULATION

A well-voiced command facilitates volitional effort. The patient's eyesight is of particular value if sensory information is otherwise a problem.

The timing of the use of stretch, traction or compression and the use of auditory stimulation is of vital importance. These should all be applied together, simultaneously, if they are to offer maximum facilitation to the patient's volitional effort. Use is made of both spatial and temporal summation. Misuse of the timing of the application of various stimuli can lead to a reduction in effect.

THE USE OF COLD

Short duration applications of cold in the form of crushed ice over suitable dermatomes can be used to cause excitatory influences to occur at the appropriate motoneurone pools. A time-lag is usually necessary between the application of the stimulus and expecting a result so, consequently, this is a stimulus which can be applied prior to the other methods and it will then be able to add its effect by summation with the other stimuli.

THE USE OF BRUSHING

This can be applied to encourage excitation if it is carried out briskly over the appropriate dermatome. Usually there is a delay in response of up to 20 minutes, so this can be applied prior to the other stimuli.

THE USE OF RIGHTING AND EQUILIBRIUM REACTIONS

These can be applied if the patient is placed in such a position that balance is rather difficult. The postural and equilibrium mechanisms will influence the motoneurone pools of the muscles concerned in implementing the reaction and if these include the weakened group of muscles the influence applied may well have the necessary excitatory effect.

To use these reactions effectively the physiotherapist must have a knowledge of the most common reactions and which patterns of muscle activity they are likely to stimulate. It is possible to add to this effect by applying approximation through the appropriate limb or limbs and trunk and by commanding the patient to 'hold' whilst counter pressure is applied in different directions.

THE USE OF OTHER PARTS OF THE BODY AS A PRELIMINARY
PROCEDURE

When other parts of the body are used, strongly associated reactions can be seen in those parts not being directly stimulated. This may occur because the nervous pathways controlling the movement influence the motoneurone pools of counterbalancing muscles or other associated groups. This is another form of spreading. Thus, if the affected muscle is in the right leg, it would be quite feasible to work the left leg or either of the upper limbs or even the head and neck or trunk first in order to have an irradiation effect upon the motoneurone pools of the affected limb.

THE USE OF REVERSAL PATTERNS

Sherrington found that the flexor withdrawal reflex was stronger if the extensor thrust reflex preceded it. The phenomenon became known as that of 'successive induction'. This phenomenon also seems to relate to volitional movement. If a movement is preceded by the exact opposite one the final pattern is produced more strongly. Thus it is physiologically sound to precede a flexion pattern by an extensor one in order to obtain a stronger flexion pattern. This method would be reversed if it was desired to use this phenomenon to facilitate extension.

EMPHASIZING THE WEAKER TEAM MEMBERS

When using the above methods to facilitate activity in the weaker members of a muscle team it may be found that the weaker member does show activity. This should then be exploited. One method of doing this is to maintain activity in the muscles concerned in the rest of the pattern by making them hold the pattern strongly. The weaker member of the pattern should then be stimulated, by stretch and command, to participate concentrically, repeatedly through a suitable range. In other words, the total pattern is held in a suitable range and movement is only allowed to pivot about the joints controlled by the weaker member of the team. This approach is often called 'timing for emphasis'.

Let us take an example: the weakened muscle group is that supplied by the musculo-cutaneous nerve of the upper limb. Thus biceps brachii, brachialis and coracobrachialis muscles are involved. The most appropriate movement pattern for involving these muscles is called the flexion, adduction lateral rotation pattern of the upper limb which would be combined with elbow flexion. In this pattern the wrist and finger flexors would be used and flexion would be accompanied by radial deviation. The forearm would supinate, the elbow flex and the shoulder flex, adduct and laterally rotate so that the hand would be carried towards the face and may progress obliquely across. The scapula would protract and laterally rotate carrying the upper limb into elevation across the front of the face.

Let us suppose that the efforts of biceps and brachialis as elbow flexors are to be emphasized. The patient is commanded into the pattern with the physiotherapist using the appropriate grasps, traction and stretch stimuli. The biceps and brachialis may be participating weakly and may need help to produce the elbow flexion. At the point in range where they offer the most activity the patient would be commanded to hold the pattern and pressure would be applied to make the shoulder, wrist and finger muscles hold a strong static contraction whilst stretch stimuli and command to bend the elbow would be repeated again and again to get maximum effort out of biceps and brachialis as elbow flexors. As appropriate, the range of the holding of the pattern may be changed until the two muscles are participating well throughout.

It may, of course, take many treatment sessions to achieve full range participation.

Such an approach may be applied to any muscle group involved in any pattern and may even be used to facilitate a weak pattern of one limb as a whole by making the other limb, limbs or trunk hold appropriate patterns whilst the weaker limb is encouraged to move through some range. This method of approach is exploiting the spreading effect of branching neurones which influence their own specific motoneurone pools and those of associated groups. Thus, volition directed to the weaker groups may be more effective since the excitatory threshold of these motoneurones has been, to some extent, prepared and lowered.

The above methods form an ideal way of: a) initiating activity in the weakened groups of muscles and b) of building on the activity obtained. This second point is very important.

When trying to initiate activity the physiotherapist must be prepared to go to a great deal of trouble to obtain the maximum facilitation and may have to try several methods before a result is achieved.

When activity is seen to occur the physiotherapist must exploit it to the full and try not to lose any ground she has gained. Thus repetition is vital. The more often the volitional impulses are able to cross the synapses and be transmitted the more readily can they effect a crossing. Thus, once activity is seen it must be repeated and repeated again and again until it becomes relatively easy to produce. Progress is then made by reducing facilitation and expecting an equally good action to be produced.

Once the weakened member has been made active, encouragement should be given to getting it involved in as many functions as are appropriate so that it is no longer allowed to become a passenger but has to participate.

These methods are particularly appropriate in the lower motoneurone problem because they make use of strong volitional effort in addition to other stimuli. Since there is nothing wrong with the 'computer' system but only with the external connections strong volition is unlikely to lead to undesirable associated movements. In fact, as has been said before, the associated movements may be highly desirable in this case and can be exploited to good effect.

When the weakened muscles are participating well in pattern with minimal facilitation, muscle strengthening techniques of a standard variety may be used quite effectively. Progressive gravity-free to weight-resistance exercises may be given either in patterns or in a more isolated manner to build up muscle power and endurance. Deep pool therapy may be of particular value. Movement patterns may be quite effectively produced in deep water and the efforts of the patient may be directed to moving the limbs about the stationary body or the body about the limbs.

Pool therapy is of particular value if the patient has large muscle groups involved, when the limbs and trunk may be particularly heavy and unwieldy in a dry land environment. If, however, the muscle weakness is associated with severe reduction in afferent information, as may be the case in polyneuritis, then deep pool therapy may not be so appropriate. Many patients of this type find the weightlessness and lack of sensory information which is associated with immersion in a deep pool, very frightening. They already have sensory loss and do not know their position in space when gravity is being fully effective. If they are then put into a pool where the effect of gravity is minimized then disorientation may be intensified to an alarming level. Each patient must be considered as an individual and assessed and treated to his best advantage.

In this section emphasis has been placed upon the exploitation of physiological factors whilst using movement patterns. The patterns which are most effective are those described by Dr. Kabat, Miss Margaret Knott and Miss Dorothy Voss. They are of a diagonal nature and include rotational components which are of great importance (see bibliography at the end of Chapter VI, p. 145).

The patterns used are described through full range and are most commonly used through full range during certain aspects of treatment. This gives maximum facilitation. Functional daily activities which include these movement patterns through a lesser range are also encouraged in the patient's treatment programme. Eventually, it is hoped that the patient will gain maximum participation of the affected muscles without having to have maximum facilitation on their motoneurone pools.

It is important to note that the use of movement patterns themselves only offers some help to the affected motoneurone pools. Much more is to be gained by exerting the additional physiological influences which can summate with the patient's volitional efforts to produce the movement pattern. In other words the patterns are there to be used, they are not sufficient in themselves.

The techniques described can be applied to straight movements, and even to individual muscle action if the physiotherapist so desires but they are not as effective used in this way because the patient is really using a pattern of muscle synergy which is new and alien to him, and pathways which have therefore not been physiologically facilitated during their early developmental processes.

Following this account it may be helpful to consider one lower motoneurone problem in a little more detail. Let us consider that the patient has had an axillary nerve lesion and that the deltoid muscle is at present not participating at all in any movements although the nerve injury has not been severe enough to completely disrupt the continuity of the nerve fibres. The situation is one of neuropraxia and the nerve fibres are showing a very high threshold of activity.

To deal with this situation satisfactorily the physiotherapist must have a knowledge of the functional significance of the muscle and how it participates in many simple daily living activities.

Deltoid must be recognized as having the following functions.

a. It is an abductor muscle of the upper limb.

b. Its anterior fibres flex and medially rotate the humerus.

c. Its posterior fibres extend and laterally rotate the humerus.

d. It commonly works with trapezius and serratus anterior to elevate the upper limb.

e. It becomes involved in any functional activities in which the arm is taken away from the side of the body.

f. It counters traction force applied by gravity to the upper limb by supporting the humerus up into the glenoid cavity. It is helped in this function by biceps brachii, triceps (long head), coracobrachialis and the smaller rotator cuff muscles in addition to the clavicular portion of pectoralis major.

g. It helps to stabilize the shoulder in weight-bearing activities and is particularly active if weight is being taken on one arm in the prone kneeling position when it acts as a supporter of the shoulder girdle in the same way as the hip abductors support the pelvic girdle when the opposite limb is taken off the ground. It may be seen working strongly in side sitting particularly if the body is being pushed away from the supporting arm. It moves the arm away from the body or the body away from the arm if the hand is fixed.

h. It becomes involved in balance reactions when the body is pushed sideways. One upper limb may move outwards to be placed upon a support at the side of the individual whilst the other may lift sideways in an effort to readjust the overall position of the centre of gravity. In both instances deltoid is involved.

i. It becomes involved in stabilization of the non-weight-bearing arm when hand skills are being carried out. It may be felt and seen to be functioning in many fine skills of the hand as a stabilizer and/or adjuster of the gleno-humeral positioning.

j. It is involved in turning over movements, when moving up and down the bed and from side to side, walking with free swinging arms, carrying the shopping, doing the hair and putting on the hat.

In fact there are so many functions which involve this muscle that a book could be filled with an account of them.

The physiotherapist must have a knowledge of these functions and also a knowledge of the most appropriate movement patterns which may help to facilitate early activity. Probably the most appropriate patterns are the flexion, adduction and lateral rotation pattern and also the extension, abduction and medial rotation pattern.

METHOD OF APPROACH

1. Make the patient aware of the reason for his movement difficulties. This can be done by comparing the activities of the affected limb with those of the normal side.

The patient may also be shown, by using mirrors, the lack of muscle bulk of deltoid and the trick movements which he is inclined to produce due to lack of participation of the muscle.

2. Make the patient as aware of the muscle as possible. This may be done by using simple methods such as handling the muscle and moving it over the underlying bone using a mixture of kneading and picking up massage manipulations whilst talking to the patient about the muscle. This, incidentally, distorts the muscle fibres and may be a start to offering sensory input which may help to bring about excitation of the motoneurone pools. Light clapping over the muscle may also help in awareness and will stimulate the sensory area in the immediate vicinity which may be of value. It is also possible to apply electrical stimulation which will have a similar effect. This will be considered in a later section of this chapter (page 111).

3. Start trying to initiate activity. This may be done in many ways and the physiotherapist should try many before giving up. Some suggestions are as follows:

a. Use the normal limb and have the patient in a lying position. Give strongly resisted flexion, adduction, lateral rotation, reversing with extension, abduction and medial rotation patterns. Whilst doing this watch for associated activity in the affected limb. It is likely to produce a reciprocal extension abduction pattern of the affected limb reversing with flexion adduction. There will not be much movement but a pattern of tone may be noticeable. If this appears to bring about extension abduction and medial rotation of the affected limb then give repeated contractions into the pattern on the normal limb which is getting the desired associated action. This may build up the associated activity. Then, without wasting any time, give flexion adduction lateral rotation as a resisted movement to the affected limb and follow this immediately with a reversal into extension, abduction and medial rotation. If a result is obtained give repeated contractions into this pattern.

b. Another possibility would be as follows: Have the patient in high sitting leaning onto the hand of the affected side or in side sitting with the supporting hand being on the affected side. Stroke over the dermatome of C5 and 6 on the affected side with a piece of ice and then work the normal limb strongly by giving resisted flexion and abduction with repeated contractions into the pattern. The cold will take about thirty seconds to be of value so work the normal limb for about thirty seconds and watch the abnormal deltoid all the time. Action of its motoneurone pools is being facilitated because of the compression force through the shoulder which stimulates stabilizing activity, and because of stimulus of the cold and the effect of spreading from the voluntary activity of the normal limb (Fig. V/1).

If the muscle responds then make the patient hold the normal limb against opposition in flexion and abduction and apply compression

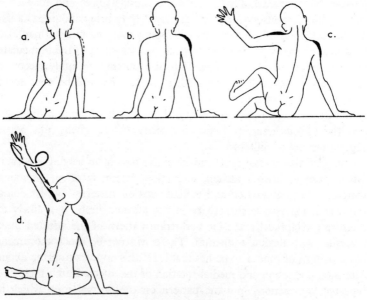

Fig. V/1 Re-education of deltoid

force through the shoulder on the affected side. Sway the patient in many directions and ask him to 'hold' his position. This may further activate the muscle.

There are many other methods which may be used to initiate contraction in this muscle. These approaches are only offered to give a general concept.

4. Follow the contraction which has been initiated into a functional activity. For example in approach (b) the deltoid was used as a stabilizer of the shoulder whilst weight was put through the upper limb. If the muscle has become active in this way it may be worth using lateral displacement of body weight to get a balance reaction and stabilization activity.

Have the patient in high or side sitting. Gently pull the body weight laterally using the affected limb and place it in a supporting position. Repeat this sideways sway several times and allow the limb to receive a little compression force from the body weight each time the limb is in a weight-bearing position.

Gradually take the help of the physiotherapist away and displace the body laterally without helping the arm, watching for deltoid activity. As the body sways laterally gravity will help the arm to move sideways but deltoid is needed to prevent over-shooting when the weight of the body arrives onto the upper limb.

The patient can then be encouraged to push himself back to neutral using the arm as a thrusting tool. If he uses too much trunk substitution resistance can be applied to the trunk to make help from the arm a necessity.

At this stage it may not be possible to get full participation of deltoid in these activities, but it should be encouraged to participate as much and as often as possible.

5. Later progress could involve a short period of maximum facilitation as a 'warm-up' method followed by some further functional activities to encourage easy natural usage. This could then be followed by more specific strengthening techniques.

Functions which are fairly easy include participation in turning over. The patient should be encouraged to lead with the head and lower limbs at first but quite soon should have these parts held back and be encouraged to initiate rolling with the affected upper limb. This can be made easy at first by working from side lying to prone and back but later should come from the fully supine position.

Balance activities in which the upper limbs are involved may be encouraged. Arm swinging when walking is important and a simple stabilization activity for the shoulder when carrying out skills with the hand should be included. An example of this could be tying up the shoe-laces when leaning forward to take the hand down to the foot, rather than doing this with the foot across the other knee. In this case the effect of gravity on the limb is minimal and deltoid only has to stabilize for the hand movements.

Specific strengthening could include repeated contractions with emphasis on deltoid in appropriate patterns through different ranges. It could include the use of pulleys and weights as resistances to the pattern of movement and progressive resistance could be applied.

Strengthening could also involve pool therapy in which the limb is abducted, flexed and extended, using the influence of buoyancy as a support or resistance. On the other hand the limb could be held stable by the physiotherapist and the patient asked to move the body weight away from the limb, the body being supported all the time by the water.

Suspension therapy can be used as a substitute for water and can be made very progressive by some enthusiasts.

6. As the muscle gains enough power to lift against gravity it should require less initial 'warm-up' facilitation and should also be expected to participate in antigravity functions. Such things as prone kneeling, changing to side sitting on alternate sides use deltoid in fairly easy weight-bearing activities. Crawling forwards is more difficult because the weight-bearing arm has to support the shoulder girdle of both sides and the non-weight-bearing arm has to lift forward against gravity.

Balance reactions may be given in which the deltoid is expected to help in lifting the affected limb sideways and forwards in an effort to adjust the overall position of the centre of gravity. Overhead arm and hand activities should be encouraged and light shopping may be carried by the affected limb.

Strengthening techniques should be carried out against the force of gravity and resisted movement patterns may have to be done in the sitting position or some other suitable position so as to involve gravity also. Progressive resistance exercises should include antigravity activity.

7. Eventually the patient should not require any preliminary facilitation methods and should be encouraged to participate in sporting and daily activities which will involve the affected limb totally.

The patient may do some activities as a member of a group in the gymnasium, and have some individual attention but, most important of all, he should be advised on suitable home activities. Eventually he has to manage his own limb entirely. Home activities are always available and should be exploited.

The above outline is *not* intended to be specific. It is used to give a concept and there are many variations to any one theme. The physiotherapist is not a technician. She must have a concept of aim, try to fulfil it and be observant of results so that she can adjust her method. No patient is exactly the same as any other and no patient can, therefore, be treated in exactly the same way as anyone else with the same problem.

Maximum sensory input in these cases will give maximum motor output. This fact must be exploited in the early stages of treatment and modified as the patient progresses.

Electrotherapy in the lower motoneurone problem

If a peripheral nerve has been injured in such a way that the pathways will be disrupted for a prolonged period of time prior to being able to conduct again, it may be advisable to make the muscle contract artificially. This is in order to maintain its mobility against underlying structures and to minimize the rate of atrophy and loss of bulk by promoting the circulation through the muscle itself. In this way the muscle is maintained in a sound condition until such time as the nerve fibres are able to be functional again.

In order to influence as many muscle fibres as possible it is usual to place an electrode at each end of the muscle belly. Modified direct current is used and trapezoidal pulses of long duration (30–300 ms) are given. These pulses are used because they are less likely to stimulate muscles which have a nerve supply, since they rise and fall slowly and the nerves going to the normal muscles will accommodate to them. Muscle does not have such good powers of accommodation and since the electrodes are placed over the muscle which has, at present, no nerve supply this is the muscle most likely to respond. Shorter duration pulses are not suitable as muscle tissue is unable to respond and only those muscles which could receive the stimulus via their nerve supply would be able to contract.

Apart from keeping the muscle in good condition electrical stimulation may also help to keep the patient aware of the muscle and its actions.

Principles of Treatment (1)

It is also possible to use electrotherapy as a re-educative measure. When the nerve has repaired but voluntary effort is still having difficulty in producing a contraction, it may prove helpful to use the faradic type of stimulus to help in the initiation of activity. In this situation a train of short duration pulses are delivered to the muscle via its nerve supply. The electrodes are therefore placed one over the motor point of the muscle and the other over the nerve trunk or nerve roots. Voluntary effort on the part of the patient is requested at the same time as electrical stimulation is given and the patient is asked to maintain the contraction when the electrical stimulation is reduced or ceases. This is a method of re-education and it can be helpful in certain circumstances.

CHAPTER VI

Principles of Treatment (2)

by HELEN W. ATKINSON, M.C.S.P., DIP.T.P.

THE PROBLEMS OF HYPOTONIA AND ATAXIA

Hypotonia and ataxia are so closely allied that they may be considered together. The bias on the stretch receptors is low and there is deficiency of activity of the excitatory extrapyramidal system. This is therefore a central and not a peripheral problem. There is lack of synergy and postural co-contraction of muscles round joints so that precision of movement and stability of posture is lost. Equilibrium and righting reactions are slow in being produced and inclined to over-react when they do occur. Movements are inclined to be slow to start and to be jerky and ill co-ordinated.

The physiotherapist has to attempt to redevelop the patient's movements along more normal lines and to keep him aware of normal movement patterns and normal posture and balance.

It is most advisable to make use of knowledge of developmental sequence in these cases and to encourage the development of postural stability and co-ordinated movements along these lines. The patient should progress from a position in which the centre of gravity is low and the base wide to the use of positions where less stability is offered.

It is very easy to use basic functional positions and movements following the developmental sequence since this inevitably complies with the low centre of gravity and wide base principles of progression.

If approximation is applied in the direction of weight bearing, the stimulus already being applied by gravity will be reinforced. This tends to encourage extrapyramidal activity and gives rise to co-contraction of the muscles supporting the joints over which the weight is being placed.

113

The stimulus of gentle swaying may be applied at the same time to encourage activity in the appropriate patterns. This helps to elicit postural and righting reactions. The patient may be asked to participate volitionally by adding instructions which would be combined with manual pressure in all directions. The instructions would be to 'hold' or 'don't let me move you' as rhythmical stabilizations. These will further encourage co-contraction and combine automatic reactions with volitional effort.

Let us take as an example a patient whose condition is so difficult that she is unable to balance her head in a stable posture over the shoulder girdle because of hypotonia. To start with she would be most suitably positioned into prone lying with her elbows and forearms supported over a small bolster of pillows so that she is in a supported, elbow support prone lying position. If this position is too uncomfortable for the patient because of age and joint stiffness etc. then a supported elbow support sitting could be used as a substitute (Fig. VI/1). In this position all that has to be supported by the patient is her head. The physiotherapist can then help the patient to raise her head and, still assisting, can apply gentle approximation through the head and cervical

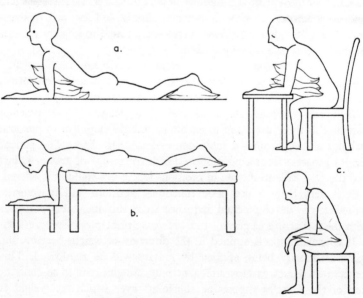

Fig. VI/1 Supported elbow support

spine whilst encouraging the patient to hold the position. She can take her support away and re-apply it in a rhythmical manner to allow gravity to have a frequent momentary influence upon the supporting muscles giving them a repeated small stretch. In this way a co-contraction can be built up encouraging the patient to be responsible for her own head position.

It should be remembered that whilst applying sound mechanical principles here, sound neurodevelopmental physiology is also being applied since control of the head position first shows itself as head lifting from prone lying.

Progress can be made by encouraging the patient to lift the head actively either by using resisted and commanded movement patterns of extension with rotation reversing with flexion with rotation or by making the patient follow moving objects with the eyes in appropriate directions. Holds should be given in various positions so that the patient learns to maintain suitable co-contraction wherever the head happens to be.

As improvement is noticed the patient can be encouraged to be responsible for the stability of the upper trunk and shoulders. The pillow support is taken away so that the patient is in an unsupported elbow support prone lying. The physiotherapist may need to apply quite vigorous and repeated compressions through the shoulder and elbow at first to gain some activity and then may stimulate the action by swaying the patient's weight from side to side and forwards and backwards to encourage excitation of the co-contracting muscles. It may help to use rhythmic stabilizations again here by pressing on the shoulders and commanding 'hold' and 'don't let me move you' etc.

When balance on the elbows is fairly secure the patient may be encouraged to rise from complete prone lying into elbow support prone lying and return down again. This requires a remarkable amount of postural and balance control and can be quite difficult for the patient.

The patient can then be encouraged to bear weight on one elbow whilst using the other limb or pushing on the other hand so that the trunk is rotated towards a more supine position.

Balance activities in this situation can be exploited. The patient periodically is lifted off the almost free hand and pushed down onto it again and made to hold with rhythmic stabilization. In this way the upper trunk rotation components are now being involved and becoming more able to stabilize.

When the patient has reached this stage it is time to start encouraging head control with emphasis on the flexor muscle groups. The patient may be in a supported sitting position with the head in such a situation that gravity would gently pull it backwards into extension. It can then be worked upon as before encouraging a 'hold' and co-contraction round the neck and shoulder girdle region.

Trunk stability is most important in these cases and the rolling activities from side lying are particularly valuable. Spiral trunk rotation should be encouraged and resisted movements of rolling leading with the head and upper trunk and also leading with the legs and lower trunk should be encouraged, provided the patient does not show signs of going into abnormal patterns. Static holds and rhythmic stabilizations can also be of value to give trunk stability.

The natural progression from here is to make the patient stable in side sitting or in an arm forward support sitting prior to expecting her to be able to take up the position for herself.

The continuing progress would take the patient through prone kneeling, kneeling, half kneeling and standing etc. In such case the patient should be encouraged to learn to balance in the position before moving it unaided and before using the position for functional activities.

Patients can be prepared for kneeling by being placed in prone lying with the knees flexed. Co-contraction round the flexed knees can be encouraged by giving compression sharply repeated through the heels and lateral aspects of the foot. In some cases voluntary rhythmical stabilizations may also be used. Half kneeling positions can also be adopted in side lying to accustom the patient to the limb position before being put into a difficult balance situation.

Whilst the above progress is being made it should be remembered that we must also be able to carry out skills with free hands and even free feet and so far the limbs have primarily been used as weight-bearing structures. Thus the patient needs help to move the limbs on the trunk as opposed to moving the trunk over the limbs.

There are many ways of helping the hypotonic patient with this problem. The above approach will help to some extent since it gives the appropriate postural background.

Resisted limb patterns performed against moderate resistance at first quickly and then progressing to slower movements are of value. The emphasis should be placed on smoothness and precision of patterning. Reversals without rest are valuable and starting and stopping with holds in mid-pattern are also useful. At first the trunk should be in a position of supported stability but later progress can be made by making the patient support her own trunk.

The range of the reversals may be gradually reduced and the activity changed to static reversals and eventually to rhythmical stabilizations in different ranges.

It is also possible to train proximal stability for distal movements by using 'timing for emphasis' techniques. The patient is made to 'hold' the proximal part of the patterns whilst moving the distal parts. Resistance in these cases should be light as it is being used primarily as guidance. Gradually the guidance should be removed and the patient left free to move by herself.

It may be of value to use Frenkel's precision exercises in these cases and, in fact, the principles of these can be added to the above account. Movements in pattern may be done to counting in a rhythmical manner and even mat activities such as moving from side sitting to prone kneeling can be done to counting, using markers on the floor as guides.

When the ataxic symptoms are related to sensory loss as well as to hypotonia, the above suggestions are still applicable but more care must be taken to help the patient with afferent stimuli.

Dr. Frenkel's approach may be emphasized more, still using patterns. Mirrors may be a necessity and the patient must be allowed to use the eyes and ears as substitutes for other afferent information. Hard surfaces help this patient more than softly cushioned ones and often the stimuli applied have to be exaggerated to have their effect. Movements carried out to counting or other rhythmical sounds are likely to be more successful than silent performances. All patients showing ataxia have to use cortical control for many of their problems and this can hamper their activities, since movement has to become a conscious activity instead of an automatic one. However, with continuous repetition automaticity can be achieved and automatic balance reactions should be encouraged to occur in a controlled manner.

As the patient gains postural stability he should react in a more controlled manner to gentle, unexpected disturbance of balance. Attempts should be made in all positions to get gentle reactions to body sway, controlled stepping reactions and the use of the hands as a support in standing and sitting only as a last resort. So long as the hands do not have to be used for balance they are free for skills.

It is most important to note that many patients showing hypotonicity may also have an underlying tendency to adopt spastic patterns of movement, mass flexion or mass extension. It is therefore most important to keep a wary eye on the use of volition to see that its excessive use is not encouraging the use of undesirable patterns. If it does, then emphasis on volition should be reduced and more automatic methods adopted to gain the same result.

These patients should not be encouraged to use their upper limbs in 'pulling' functions since this may encourage them to use the arms in a mass flexor manner to pull themselves into standing. They will never gain balance in this way and for this reason such activities should be discouraged. Thus such a patient, if confined to bed, should not be supplied with a monkey bar to help her to move around in bed. It will encourage reflex patterning which is undesirable.

Functional activities

As with the lower motoneurone problem, functions within the capabilities of the patient should be encouraged. Suitable functions should be found relevant to the patient's ability. If good movement re-education is to occur, it is most important that excessive demands are not made upon the patient since abnormalities will inevitably appear which might otherwise be avoidable.

Walking will possibly be a goal and this should be encouraged *after* the patient has the ability to balance in standing. At first some support by the hands may be necessary using walking aids of some kind and only when the patient is secure should she be encouraged to walk without using the upper limbs as balance mechanisms.

It must be borne in mind that perfect functioning is unlikely in these cases and the physiotherapist must be aware of the likely limitations. Occupational therapists and physiotherapists can often work well together with these cases provided each respects the other person's aim for the patient. The goal must be discussed and re-set as progress is observed.

The patient's hopes must not be raised excessively and every step forward must be noted by both the therapist and the patient. Every member of the team should be prepared to meet each problem as it arises and no one should expect too much.

There are other problems with these patients but they will be considered under the appropriate headings since they are common to most neurological patients.

VERTIGO

Patients with this particular sensory problem have to learn to rely upon joint and skin sensation and those sensations from sight rather than those from the vestibular apparatus. As has been mentioned earlier the giddy sensation and sickness are also accompanied by an active inhibition of movement since movement of the head gives rise to increase of the dizziness and nausea. The head and shoulders show rather a fixed posture and the patient is afraid of movement.

Such is the link between eyes and vestibular apparatus that eye movements may even trigger off the symptoms. Thus the patient need not be moving at all but could be watching a moving object and would have symptoms similar to those which would occur if he had been moving.

Re-education of this patient involves giving him confidence in moving and helping him to take notice only of the reliable sensory or afferent information.

He should be treated at first in a fully supported semi-recumbent position so that head movements are unlikely to occur. Relaxation of the head, neck and shoulders should be encouraged and the patient asked to use his eyes only at first. His attention should be drawn to the sensation of complete support that his position offers so that he is aware of the unlikelihood of moving at that moment. He should look at a stationary object which is a comfortable distance away from him and be asked to focus upon it. When he has it in full focus the object should move slowly whilst he follows it with his eyes. If he feels dizzy then he should close his eyes and feel the stationary condition of his body. At first the object should only move as far as his eyes can travel but as he progresses head movements may also be involved, and later still, head movements with closed eyes should be encouraged in order to help him to rely only on joint and position sense.

As he progresses the patient may adopt less stable starting positions and exercise the eyes, head and trunk progressively until he can move fairly freely without suffering from excessive symptoms. Gradually he should progress to using hand/eye activities without losing his balance. Such activities as throwing and catching a ball in all directions are suitable. Standing and walking are advanced activities and the patient must be made accustomed to having objects moving in relationship to him. It is particularly important that stairs are included in his treatment programme, since the sides of a staircase can appear to be moving in the corner of the eye and can give vertigo symptoms in even quite normal people.

As the patient progresses he should be involved in group activities so that people and things are moving about him at the same time as he is moving himself. This does to some extent prepare him for coping with crossing roads and traffic. His treatment is not complete without postural correction and mobility exercises of head, neck and shoulder girdle and at some stage he must be taken in amongst traffic on foot and given the confidence to cross the road.

Exercises as expounded by Dr. Cooksey of King's College Hospital have been found to be most effective in the treatment of these cases.

THE PROBLEM OF HYPERTONICITY

Spasticity

As described in Chapter III the patient will demonstrate at least partial release of certain reflex mechanisms from cortical control and hence difficulty in producing movement patterns other than those produced by the released reflexes. The stretch reflex mechanisms will be extra sensitive particularly in patterns dominated by the released reflexes.

The normal malleable postural background will not be present having given way to stereotyped patterns of a reflex nature. The patient will show poor vocabulary of movement patterns and of quality of control.

There is frequently a lack of synergy, evidence of instability of joint control coupled with lack of righting and equilibrium reactions.

The patient develops a pattern of spasticity related to the dominating reflexes. The reflexes most likely to exert their influence include the tonic labyrinthine, the symmetrical tonic neck reflex and the asymmetrical tonic neck reflex.

These reflex pathways are present in all of us and by the process of maturation of the nervous system their effect becomes integrated into the general control of all our movements. It is only when they are released from integration that they cause disturbance of movement pattern.

A study of these reflexes will show that the position of the head and neck is very important and that if care is taken to control their position and to encourage the patient to control it, excessive domination by the static postural reflexes can, to some extent, be avoided. Careful positioning of the patient can make management easier for the physiotherapist and the nurse and, at the same time, make movement more possible for the patient.

A study of the more dynamic righting reactions is also of extreme value. These reactions enable the individual to obtain the upright position and the spiral movements of the head and neck, trunk and limbs are related to them. It is thought that they may have an inhibitory effect upon the static postural mechanisms. The reduction in spasticity which is seen to accompany trunk and limb rotation may occur for this reason although there is, as yet, no proof that this is so. However, rotation of the trunk and limbs, when trying to reduce spasticity, is a very valuable asset and emphasizes the importance of treating the whole patient instead of dealing only with the offending part.

When treating a patient who shows spasticity it is necessary to carry out three important aims:

a. inhibit excessive tone as far as possible;

b. give the patient a sensation of normal position and normal movement;

c. facilitate normal movement patterns.

INHIBITION OF EXCESSIVE TONE

Earlier in this chapter it was pointed out that inhibition could be facilitated as well as excitation. In cases of spasticity it is important to facilitate the patient's ability to inhibit the undesirable activity of the released reflex mechanisms. As has already been mentioned the position adopted by the patient is important since the head and neck position can elicit strong postural reflex mechanisms. Avoiding these head and neck positions can facilitate the inhibition of the more likely reflexes and if the positions have to be adopted, then help in preventing the rest of the body from going into the reflex pattern thus elicited may be required by the patient. The patient cannot, of course, spend the rest of his life avoiding the positions which encourage dominance by reflex activity but, at first, this may be necessary until the patient has developed some control in the suppression of the effect of the reflex activities. As he develops this control then he can be gradually introduced to the use of positions which make suppression of reflex activity more difficult.

As an early introduction to treatment the side lying position, well supported by pillows, is very convenient since it avoids stimulation of the tonic labyrinthine reflex, and also as the head and trunk are in alignment, the stimulation of the asymmetrical tonic neck reflexes. It makes a good resting position for the patient with spasticity and also is convenient for the application of rhythmical trunk rotations of both a passive and assisted active form. These do help to encourage a reduction in tone.

The scapula is also readily available to be involved in the movements. The upper and lower limb of the uppermost side are also easily accessible for any passive, assisted active or automatic movements which may seem suitable.

Side lying is not always desirable because of respiratory problems in the older patient or because of the need to obtain a greater range of movement. Other attitudes are often very satisfactory such as crook lying or even with the knees as high on the chest as possible. These last two are helpful if there is flexor spasticity. As the trunk is rotated the legs are allowed to lower towards the extended, abducted and laterally rotated position. For older patients trunk rotation may have to be encouraged in sitting.

Limb rotations are also very effective in helping to give a more normal control of muscle tone to the patient.

These facts are of help not only to the physiotherapist but also to the nurse who may be concerned in moving the patient in bed or attempting to position the patient so as to avoid the development of deformities etc.

The important factors in attempting to gain control over muscle tone are:

1. Patterns of movement and posture associated with the released reflex mechanisms must be avoided and discouraged by positioning, guidance and using the inhibitory methods mentioned in this chapter.

2. Conditions which will facilitate control of tone should be given by help in movement and posturing and by giving the stimuli which will encourage normal patterns.

As an example of the above two points let us consider pressure applied to the undersurface of the foot. If it is applied to the ball of the foot it may well stimulate an extensor reflex in which a pathological pattern of extension, adduction and medial rotation of the hip is produced together with plantar flexion of the foot. This would be undesirable in a case of spasticity. If pressure is applied under the heel of the foot then a more useful co-contraction of muscle is likely to occur giving a suitable supporting pattern. The physiotherapist must become familiar with the stereotyped reflex patterning so that she can avoid permitting them to occur.

It is most important that the physiotherapist becomes familiar with the patterning of normal movements and postures so that she can help her patient to move using them in preference to spastic patterns. Help is needed to facilitate the movements by correcting weight distribution, head and shoulder positioning and encouraging suitable rotational balance activities. For example, when walking the right leg cannot be moved forwards unless the left leg is receiving weight correctly and the body is balanced over it. Trunk rotations normally accompany the mature walking patterns as reciprocal balance mechanisms and should be encouraged. Standing from sitting cannot occur unless the head and shoulders are brought well forward so that weight is distributed to the feet. As the patient rises she may extend her neck and trunk too soon and throw her weight back so that she is not successful in reaching a standing position. The timing of neck and trunk extension may need to be assisted. All the necessary automatic adjustments are impoverished in these patients and help may be needed. Sometimes verbal help is needed but more often actual assistance by simply adjusting the movements and waiting for the patient to react may be more helpful. This enables the patient to feel and perhaps see the successful activity. At all times the effect on the whole patient must be observed since it is quite possible to be gaining more normal tone in one part of the patient at the expense of another.

Movement of a normal nature does appear in itself to reduce excessive tone and consequently this should be encouraged in the patient. However, care must be taken if conscious volitional movement is demanded. Due to reflex release, some motoneurone pools are already in an excitatory state and any volitional effort is likely to act as a triggering mechanism to those motoneurone pools giving associated muscle contraction in the spastic pattern. Such patients should not be encouraged to make strong volitional effort since this is inclined to facilitate the production of spastic patterning. Conscious voluntary activity should be kept to a minimum until it is not accompanied by undesirable associated activity. Instead, appropriate stimuli should be given to encourage more normal responses which will automatically help to reduce the patterns of spasticity.

Other methods of reducing spasticity include the application of heat or cold for relatively prolonged periods of time. These can have dramatic effects on some patients provided a large enough area of the patient is included. Total immersion in ice cold water has been recommended for some cases of disseminated sclerosis who show spasticity and the author has seen very impressive temporary results from this approach. The patient who responds to this shows a marked improvement in movement ability for several hours before the process has to be repeated again.

Deep rhythmical massage with pressure over the muscle insertions has proved effective in some cases and many authorities advocate slow, steady and prolonged stretching. This last method does have its dangers since, if the stretching is forced against severe spasticity, the hyperexcitable stretch reflex reacts even more strongly and damage to the periosteum of bone may occur where excessive tension has been applied by the tendons of the stretched muscles.

Rhythmical, slowly performed passive movements through normal patterns may also be helpful and in the more moderate cases the patient may subconsciously join in and by his own activity a reduction in spasticity may occur. Quick movements, abruptly performed, and noisy surroundings are most detrimental as are excitement, anxiety or any form of discomfort.

SENSATION OF NORMAL POSITION AND MOVEMENT

This is of vital importance. A patient who is dominated by reflex patterns never experiences the sensation of normal movement and position unless helped to do so. He is denied normal stimulation and either cannot know or soon forgets the normal. Very quickly the abnormal feels normal and *vice versa*.

A patient showing extensor spasticity of the lower limb will most often hold the limb in hip extension, adduction and medial rotation, knee extension and foot plantar flexion – i.e. mass extensor synergy of the lower limb. Such a patient when standing or sitting may never be able to experience weight-bearing through the heel. When weight is taken through the heel the stimulus encourages a true supporting reaction which gives co-contraction of hip, knee and ankle muscles, flexors as well as extensors, in a malleable co-contraction suitable for normal weight-bearing. Thus there is no hope for the patient who is in extensor synergy unless some method of applying the more appropriate stimulus is found.

If an abnormal position makes a starting point for a movement then an abnormal movement must occur. Because of their spasticity many patients are forced by circumstances to repeat abnormal movement patterns. By repetition the nervous pathways used to cause these movements are facilitated and the abnormal movements therefore occur more and more readily. When this has occurred correction is difficult, if not impossible. Because of this it is important to give early treatment to the whole patient so that, as far as possible, the sensation of normal movement is retained.

Praise for a movement should only be given if it really is good because, having received praise, the patient will try to repeat the same performance. If it was a good movement the second attempt is also likely to be good, but if it was unsatisfactory at first the repeated movement will also be poor and this faulty pathway has been facilitated.

FACILITATION OF NORMAL MOVEMENT PATTERNS

More normal movement patterns can be produced when domination by reflex mechanisms is minimized. Thus, when the patient appears to be relatively free, movement should be encouraged. Movement itself will reduce spasticity if it follows normal patterns. Often automatic adjustment of position is easier to produce than conscious volitional activities. Figs. VI/2 and 3 illustrate some movements and positions which are helpful if encouraged and some which should be discouraged. Rotational movements of the trunk and limbs are important and spiral rolling patterns involving head, shoulder girdle, pelvis and limbs should be encouraged.

In most cases it is helpful to follow a neurodevelopmental approach with these patients. They often have a vocabulary of movement pattern less versatile than that of a newly born child. Thus they are more likely to learn movement control if they are encouraged to follow the sequence of events seen in the movement patterning of a child.

Basic functional movements are the ones to encourage at first. The child does not develop skilled hand movements until the hands are

freed from being props for balance. The same holds good for adults
showing spasticity. One does well if the upper limbs can be trained to
support the patient. The ambition to train skilled hand movements
should be deferred until this is achieved.

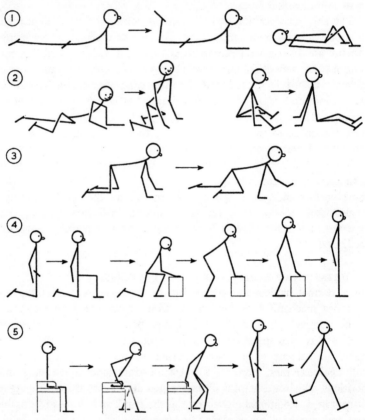

Fig. VI/2 Patterns to encourage

It is important to appreciate that points (a), (b) and (c) (p. 121) are
best dealt with a tone and the same time. In other words one does not
arrange for the patient to fulfil the aim of reducing spasticity and then
proceed to applying appropriate sensation and then re-educate movement. The patient should be placed in an area suitable for seizing the
opportunity of moving as and when a reduction in tone is felt and as a
suitable stimulus has had an effect.

The physiotherapist must constantly observe the effect of her efforts on the whole patient and if an opportunity arises to use a movement which is occurring in a normal manner she should use it without

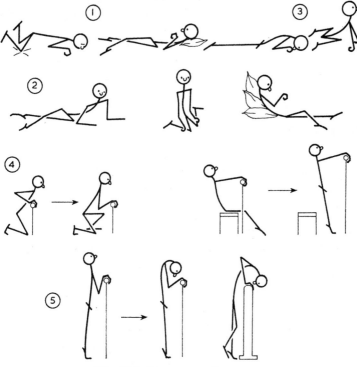

Fig. VI/3 Patterns to discourage

delay. For this reason a sample list of activities is impossible to offer since fixed methods are not applicable.

Functional activities

It is in the field of spasticity that most controversy occurs regarding functions of daily living. If the aim is to normalize movement only those functions which do not produce pattern abnormalities should be encouraged and progress should be made relative to this. The physiotherapist should, in this case, be the person to decide which functions are suitable.

If however, the aim is to gain functional independence at all costs, then movement abnormalities may have to be ignored or even encouraged in order to gain some sort of ambulation. Strictly speaking, the skill of a good physiotherapist should not be used for long if this is the aim, since well-trained aides could fulfil it quite adequately with guidance. It is most important that consultants and therapists exchange views and come to an agreement on which line of approach is to be followed and also when further attempts to help the patient are to be abandoned. Conflicting views can have seriously detrimental effects.

Use of drugs

There are drugs available which will have an inhibitory effect on the stretch reflex. These mainly work by blocking the synaptic functions of internuncial pathways. If they are effective the patient is likely to be hypotonic with underlying movement patterns of the flexor/extensor synergies. Such patients are best treated as hypotonic patients but great care should be given if resisted exercises are used. Free active patterning with some automatic compression stimuli and gentle balance activities are more suitable.

Rigidity

In this situation the patient tends to show excessive postural fixation, axial rotation is non-existent and normal balance reactions do not appear to be available. The patient tends to adopt a fixed head and shoulder positioning and movements which would normally be those of trunk rotation either do not occur at all or occur by the patient moving round as a whole.

The face adopts a mask-like rigidity and the patient appears to be unresponsive to stimuli. A tremor is often present when resting, which disappears when purposeful movement occurs. All these symptoms are seen when the centres concerned with automatic reactions are the site of lesion, so that these reactions do not occur.

Increase in tone causes opposition to all movements, which are therefore slow in being produced and are not readily accompanied by automatic postural adjustments.

As in the case of spasticity the abnormality effectively prevents the patient from experiencing normal sensory information and he quite rapidly 'forgets' the normal and accepts the abnormality as normal.

The physiotherapist can help the patient in several ways, but she must always have the following aims at the back of her mind:

a. To encourage a reduction in the overall sensitivity of the stretch reflex mechanism;

b. To help the patient to experience more normal reactions.

c. To encourage movements to follow normal patterns in as wide a range and as freely as possible.

a. REDUCTION IN OVERALL SENSITIVITY OF THE STRETCH REFLEX MECHANISM

There are several methods available to achieve this aim and the sooner the patient is treated the more effective is treatment likely to be. Methods include: teaching general relaxation in a comfortable, well-supported, recumbent position; the application of rhythmical massage of a sedative nature; and the use of rhythmical passive and/or assisted active movements.

The most effective method is likely to be to give rhythmical passive to active movements with the patient recumbent or semi-recumbent.

The movements which are of most value to the patient are those which are not available to him. Trunk rotations are particularly useful, and may be carried out through a small range at first, gradually increasing the range and speeding up the rate of rhythm of the movement as the rigidity subsides. Such movements can be done passively by the physiotherapist, but she should not discourage the patient from helping if he can. It is not total relaxation that is wanted but only a sufficient reduction in tone to make movement more possible.

Probably the side lying position is a most convenient one for this purpose since trunk rotations can be most easily produced in this position and can also be easily converted into rolling activities when the patient has enough freedom to do so. In addition the patient's scapula is freely available and can be moved prior to encouraging greater range of activity in the whole body.

Since many patients showing rigidity are elderly, the fully recumbent position is not always suitable and rotations may have to be performed in other positions. It is quite possible to help a patient to rotate at the trunk in sitting by moving the upper trunk upon the lower and one can even involve the trunk diagonal patterns of flexion with rotation to one side, followed by extension with rotation to the other.

Limb movements can be encouraged in a similar way involving the diagonal patterns, if possible, and starting with a small range and progressing to a larger range as the movement becomes more available. If the patient assists so much the better.

b. EXPERIENCING MORE NORMAL REACTIONS

Helping the patient experience the more normal reactions is very much linked with the methods suggested under (a). As the patient loosens up when the overall tone of the muscles is reduced, opportunities to react to situations should be given and help to reach and experience the reaction should be offered as needed. For instance if trunk rotation is being encouraged in side lying the patient will gradually loosen up and start to participate. The upper limb should then be encouraged to come forward to receive weight as the trunk comes forward ready for going into prone lying. If the limb does not react automatically the therapist can repeatedly encourage rotation and bring the patient's arm and hand forward into the supporting position. Gradually the patient will appreciate the sensation and will join in until all the physiotherapist need do is gently push the shoulder forward to initiate the reaction. A similar method of encouraging the appropriate lower limb reactions may also be used.

If the trunk rotations are being done in sitting, other balance reactions may be aided. Such reactions as hand support forwards or hand support sideways may be encouraged. Even the lifting reactions of the limbs on the side away from which the patient is shifted can be helped by the skilled physiotherapist in this way, so that the patient experiences the sensation of balance reactions.

By lifting reactions are meant the reactions of the body to displacement of weight sideways or backwards. If the body weight is displaced sideways the upper limb on that side moves sideways to receive some of the weight. The other upper limb lifts sideways to try to pull the body back to its original base. The lower limbs, if free, may also participate by rotating (see Fig. VI/4).

Any sign of regression back into rigidity to an excessive degree should be countered by further rotations. Trunk rotations with rhythmic arm swinging can be very helpful and give the arm swing sensation required when walking. Many physiotherapists encourage this by having the patient in sitting or standing holding one end of a pole in each hand. The physiotherapist is holding the other ends of the poles and using her arm swing, she can encourage the arm swing of the patient.

C. ENCOURAGING MOVEMENTS TO FOLLOW NORMAL PATTERNS IN AS WIDE A RANGE AND AS FREELY AS POSSIBLE

This automatically links with (a) and (b) and has to some extent already been encouraged. Movement patterns may be encouraged with minimal

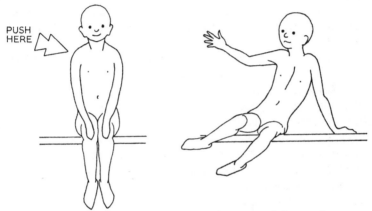

PUSH HERE

Fig. VI/4 Reaction to lateral displacement of the trunk

resistance for guidance. The range should be small at first and slowly encouraged to larger range and faster movement. The patient has to be 'pumped up' to more rapid and fuller range of activity. This also applies to functions such as standing up and sitting down, rolling over and getting started with walking activities.

For the younger patient the author has found the following type of activities most successful:

1. Rhythmical rolling in a spiral manner, first helping the patient and later starting the movement for the patient and allowing him to react by following.

2. Encouraging the adoption of side sitting and moving onto all fours and then sitting on the opposite side. This is started on all fours and the patient sways rhythmically towards the side upon which he will eventually sit before rising back to all fours. At first he does not

sit at all but gradually approaches the sitting position as a fuller range is available. This activity encourages trunk and limb rotation and if rhythmical it will help to keep the overall tone reduced.

3. Rhythmical crawling may also be encouraged by swaying the body weight forwards and backwards and eventually encouraging a step forward reaction of the limbs.

4. Hand support forward half kneeling, changing legs rhythmically, may also help and eventually leads to the adoption of standing.

5. The standing activities should include rhythmical walking, which is best started by rotating the trunk at the shoulders so that an easy arm swing rhythm is started. The patient's body weight is then pushed gently forwards at hip level to encourage a stepping reaction in the lower limbs.

6. The customary stooping position should be avoided and the patient encouraged to maintain as upright a position as possible. Many physiotherapists use poles as mentioned under section (b) to initiate walking and do so by encouraging the patient to step forward with the right leg as the left arm comes forwards.

7. Gradually the walking should include turning and stepping backwards and also across the other leg. These activities may be done as conscious volitional activities but, if possible, should eventually become an automatic response to disturbance of balance.

One cannot do quite such agile activities with the older patient and some of the following suggestions may prove helpful:

1. Sitting: assisted active trunk rotations to encourage a hand support sideways sitting position.

2. Hands supporting to one side: encourage standing up by leaning back to leaning forwards and standing up. Rhythmical swaying may be more suitable at first and then gradually changed to standing up.

3. Standing up to sitting down as before, progressing to standing up again with the hands supporting to alternate sides. This also involves trunk rotations which are so easily lost in these patients.

4. Arm swinging and walking can be encouraged as in the younger person.

In both types of patients limb patterns through full range should be encouraged in addition to functional mat type activities.

Patients' relatives can be taught to help reduce the rigidity at home by encouraging rotational movement and perhaps helping to give the necessary 'pumping up' procedures prior to achieving a particular function. It is most important to keep these patients as functionally independent as possible and relatives must be encouraged to give minimum assistance of an 'educated' nature.

The patient can help himself to a tremendous degree once he receives adequate guidance and provided he receives appropriate encouragement from his relatives. It can be helpful to allow him to have a period of intensive physiotherapy at intervals and to encourage him to be responsible for his own welfare (movement-wise) in the periods when he has no formal treatment. An early morning 'warm up' exercise session involving trunk rotations and rhythmical swinging movements of arms and legs can be very valuable when he is otherwise receiving no treatment.

Odd jobs about the house which require movement are more suitable than those which can be done sitting down. They may take a longer time for the patient to perform but they are a treatment in themselves.

Static activities are undesirable and rhythmical stabilizations do not usually help these patients and so should be avoided if possible.

Drugs are available to reduce rigidity and some surgical procedures have given a measure of relief. The patient may then show variable movement problems and has to be dealt with according to individual peculiarities.

It cannot be emphasized too much that the earlier the patient receives treatment the more effective it will be. When a patient is first suspected of showing rigidity symptoms he is unlikely to show gross abnormality and will not have so much underlying joint stiffness or have 'forgotten' normality to such a degree. He is therefore more able to be receptive to help. This is directed at helping him to help himself. He may then well be able to minimize his symptoms more effectively for longer.

If the patient is very rigid when he first receives help he may also have painful joint stiffness and have mechanical difficulty in addition to physiological problems. Normal movement will be very unusual to him and the likelihood of his being able to help himself adequately is considerably more remote.

THE PROBLEMS OF ATHETOSIS, CHOREA AND BALLISMUS

These three movement abnormalities are grouped together since all show the presence of involuntary activity and fluctuations of tone.

The physiotherapist has to meet problems with these patients when they appear. At one time she may be required to encourage stability in the same way as she would a hypotonic patient and at another time she may have to help in the inhibition of abnormal activities whilst encouraging normal purposeful movement patterns.

Excitement should be avoided at all costs since this increases the symptoms.

Athetoid patients frequently have problems with body image and steps must be taken to improve this by experiences of normal activities and stimuli.

Many athetoids are helped in stability by compression forces being applied through weight-bearing joints. Some children benefit by wearing little leaded caps which add to the weight of the head and give compression force to the vertebral column. This helps to stimulate stabilization. Much of the action advised in preceding sections is useful for these patients and the physiotherapist must use her ingenuity in selecting those activities which help and discarding those which do not. She must receive a constant 'feed-back' from the patient and adjust her stimuli accordingly.

Drugs and surgery have been used to control the symptoms of these disorders and have met with varying success. In such circumstances the patient is still left with movement abnormalities which have to be assessed and treated accordingly.

PROBLEMS OF DEFORMITY

Adaptive shortening of soft tissues is likely to occur when habitual posturing is adopted by patients who have any disease or injury problem. In neurological problems it is particularly likely to occur when no movement is available to the patient and when there is imbalance of muscle pull.

There are many methods of preventing the onset of deformities of this nature. These include:

PASSIVE MOVEMENTS
These were already suggested in an earlier section as being helpful in the maintenance of a knowledge of body image. When used to prevent deformity the physiotherapist must bear two facts in mind:
    i. She must maintain the biological length of the muscles which

work over the joints she is moving. This means that her passive movements must involve elongating the muscle over all its movement components. For example – to maintain the length of gastrocnemius she must dorsiflex the foot and extend the knee and her return movements should be plantar flexion of the foot and flexion of the knee. In that way she has fully lengthened gastrocnemius which pulls over the back of the knee and ankle and she has also put it into its most shortened position.

ii. She must maintain the biological pliability of the ligaments of the joints she is moving. This means that she must be cautious when moving a joint over which a 'two joint' muscle works since it could restrict the range of movement available before the ligaments are fully elongated. For example – ankle dorsiflexion is limited by gastrocnemius if the knee is held extended as the ankle is dorsiflexed. Therefore the ligaments of the joint are not fully elongated by the time movement has stopped. Thus in this case the tension should be taken off gastrocnemius by flexing the knee before dorsiflexing the foot. A greater range will then be found to be available.

CAREFUL POSITIONING OF THE SEVERELY DISABLED PATIENT
This should be done in such a way that constant adoption of one position is avoided. Limbs and trunk should be supported in a variety of positions throughout the day. Extreme positioning of any joint should be avoided.

SPLINTAGE
This is most helpful in patients with peripheral problems as it prevents the flaccid muscle groups from being constantly stretched by normal opposing muscle action. Splints should never be left on permanently but should be used as resting splints when the patient is likely to adopt a prolonged poor position of the joints concerned. Lively splints are very useful since they allow movement to occur and simply return the limbs to a normal position at the end of the movement. They are more functional than the simple rest splints.

Many people use splintage with central nervous system problems but it should only be used in certain well-considered circumstances. Splints applied to such cases effectively prevent normal movement patterns and pressure from the splint may actually increase the spastic patterning. For example a plaster cast applied to the lower leg and foot to keep the foot in dorsiflexion may effectively stimulate (by pressure on the ball of the foot) an extensor response which will take the form of mass extensor synergy. This could be undesirable and worse than no splintage at all. Only in some circumstances is splintage helpful in these disorders.

USE OF BED CRADLES

These are very helpful. They lift the weight of bedclothes off the limbs, which may be paralysed, and therefore the bedclothes do not force the feet into plantar flexion.

The cradle is also useful when hypertonicity is a problem since the constant irritation of bedclothes can stimulate withdrawal reflexes which encourage flexion deformities.

If deformity is already present by the time the patient comes for help, the problem is much greater. The patient may require more help to counter the problem such as traction, manipulation, and surgery. In the latter case tendons may be divided and lengthened or muscles are disattached and left to re-attach in a more suitable position.

The physiotherapist may be able to help in some cases by the application of serial plasters designed to correct deformities gradually.

Some patients, particularly those with lower motoneurone problems, develop adaptive shortening of the muscles antagonistic to those which are paralysed. The physiotherapist can help considerably here to encourage a new resting length for these muscles by using any or all of the following methods:

i. The application of prolonged (about 10–20 minutes) cold packs to the adaptively shortened muscle. The packs must extend over the whole length of the muscle. This method encourages inhibition of the muscle which will relax more, making it possible to lengthen it more easily.

ii. The use of 'hold, relax' techniques in which the adaptively shortened muscle is put into as elongated a position as is comfortable and then made to contract statically – hence the term 'hold'. As the contraction is held for a prolonged time it begins to weaken. When this occurs the patient is instructed to relax whilst the physiotherapist supports the joint or joints involved. When relaxation has occurred the physiotherapist further elongates the muscle passively. If successful she will find that the muscle will allow itself to be elongated more as it has relaxed sufficiently to allow an increase in length.

There are various theories as to why this should work. Some authorities say that the muscle relaxes more because of fatigue and others consider that the golgi tendon organs which lie at the musculotendonous junction are stimulated by the contracting muscle pulling on the tendon. As was stated earlier these organs have an inhibitory influence on the motoneurone pools of their own muscle and may therefore help to induce this excessive relaxation (autogenic inhibition).

Cold packs may be applied at the same time as 'hold, relax' techniques.

'Hold, relax' is most suitable for use when the adaptively shortened group are opposed by completely flail antagonists.

iii. A modification of the above is the 'slow reversal, hold, relax' technique. In this case the procedure is as for 'hold, relax' but after the relaxation stage has occurred the patient is stimulated to use the antagonist to the adaptively shortened muscle concentrically. In other words the adaptively shortened muscle is made to contract statically by a 'hold'. It is then commanded to relax and the reverse movement is brought about by active concentric activity of its antagonist. This technique is most useful when there is some activity available in the antagonist. The phenomenon of reciprocal inhibition is added to the phenomenon of autogenic inhibition in this case.

The above techniques are only of value when movement limitation is due to changes in length of muscle. They do not help if the limitation is due to ligamentous or bony changes.

Some workers claim to have used the above techniques to relax spastic muscle groups. The author does not use this particular technique for fear of facilitating spastic patterning. The student should, however, keep an open mind in all such matters and decide for herself which methods she will use, noting the results and accepting those which give good results whilst rejecting those which do not.

PREVENTION OF INJURY

This has been largely dealt with on p. 94, since much of the damage which can occur in these cases is due to sensory loss.

The patient must be made aware of the dangers, if possible, and if he cannot change his position himself he must be frequently turned. He must be kept scrupulously clean and have his skin toughened and protected against the possibility of pressure sores.

If any area shows signs of breaking down it may be stimulated by ice massage to improve the local circulation, or by heat or mild doses of ultraviolet light. The use of heat has its dangers since sensory loss may make the patient endure a temperature that is too hot for safety. Cold is therefore the method of choice.

The use of ripple mattresses, sheepskins, protective rings and constant changes of position should effectively prevent the onset of sores. If they do develop they are very detrimental to the patient's general condition and must be treated as a serious problem.

CIRCULATORY PROBLEMS

Many patients show disturbances of circulation. Some of these are due to lack of movement and some are due to disturbance in some part of the autonomic system.

In the lower motoneurone problem the loss of 'muscle pump' activity will cause slowing of the circulation through the affected area and, in addition, the peripheral autonomic nerve fibres may also be involved.

These problems can be helped by encouraging activity in other parts of the body. This will speed up circulation generally.

Whirlpool baths for the affected areas may also be used. These will promote circulation to the skin over the affected muscle groups. Contrast baths may also prove valuable. They may stimulate such blood vessel activity as is available.

The central autonomic problem is well described in Chapter VIII. Essentially the patient has to adapt gradually to change of position which puts greater demands upon the problem of maintenance of blood pressure.

In cases of causalgia, in which there is disuse due to pain, similar methods may be used to those advocated for the lower motoneurone problem. Wax baths may also help here, but on the other hand they may cause onset of pain and so should be used with reservation.

Many patients who have hemiplegic symptoms have problems in the posturing of the shoulder girdle. This can cause pressure and kinking of the axillary vessels giving rise to oedema which is further encouraged by lack of use and the dependent position. In this case the weight of the limb may have to be relieved by sling support to reduce pressure on the axillary vessels. This is unfortunate since it discourages movement of the limb. However, the sling need not be retained all the time and other treatments for oedema may be given which involve movement. As soon as the posturing of the patient improves the sling should be discarded.

RESPIRATORY PROBLEMS

Many patients show respiratory problems. These range from those which are due to paralysis of the muscles of respiration to those which are due to restriction of exercise because of the patient's disability.

Patients who have paralysis of the respiratory muscles will obviously need the help of a respirator and will be in an intensive therapy unit. They may also require to have assisted coughing or may even need suction to help to remove secretions.

Only the local peripheral problems will totally escape from respiratory difficulties. The head injury case may well require tracheostomy, suction and the use of a respirator, and the care of such patients is described in Chapter VII.

The patient with a central nervous system disorder of the progressive variety will be inclined to develop respiratory distress as the disease progresses. The muscles supporting the thoracic inlet may be hypotonic and will allow respiratory movements to have a suction effect on the chest wall in this area, thus diminishing the amount of air the thorax can house. Such patients may also have deglutition problems and it is possible for food to be inhaled.

Even the less handicapped patient may show weakness of respiratory movements and will need some help.

Breathing exercises should be incorporated into the treatment of all the heavily handicapped patients. They may be facilitated in lower motoneurone cases by using appropriate arm patterns and by giving repeated contractions to the muscles of inspiration. Both inspiratory and expiratory phases should be emphasized to get maximum respiratory excursion.

The central problem requires a more relaxed approach but respiration must not be forgotten. It is particularly important to the rigidity case and to patients with multiple problems like multiple sclerosis.

The advanced case of multiple sclerosis and also the patient with weakness in the thoracic inlet and deglutition group (omohyoid, mylohyoid, digastricus, thyrohyoid and sternothyroid) may be helped by giving head and neck patterns of a resisted nature, stabilization of the head and neck and combining these with respiration.

PROBLEMS OF SPEECH

These problems are properly left to the speech therapist who is the specialist. The physiotherapist may be able to endorse the work of the speech therapist if the two team members can discuss matters with each other.

It is possible to stimulate movement of the tongue by using a spatula and moving the tongue with it, encouraging the patient to participate. Ice frozen onto the spatula may also help as the cold is a stimulus. As the water forms from the melting ice it acts as a lubricant to the tongue and mouth.

Activity of buccinator can also be encouraged by pressure from the spatula against the inside of the cheek. This may help to train the patient to keep the cheek against the teeth and therefore prevent collection of saliva. This can be very useful when treating facial palsy as the stretch stimulus can be used by pressing the cheek outwards whilst commanding the patient to pull in.

Speech in the severely handicapped is not easily available unless there is control of head position and the physiotherapist may be required to help in this way.

Deglutition is also difficult without head control and may be impossible if the patient is recumbent. The patient who has swallowing difficulties should be fed, if possible, in an upright position.

To speak, we also have to be able to swallow as otherwise we spit as we speak. The swallowing muscles may be stimulated by stroking or brushing over the anterior aspect of the under-surface of the chin and neck and by icing the tongue and lips.

EXERCISE TOLERANCE

This becomes lost if respiration and circulation are impaired but it may also be lost due to disuse. The wheelchair patient never fully uses himself unless encouraged to do so. If possible he should be encouraged to indulge in as active a type of exercise as possible to maintain good exercise tolerance.

Other patients should be given activities in their programme which tax them to their limits so that they maintain good general health. The only exception to this would be, perhaps, the patient who has had a cerebrovascular accident or one with cardiac complications.

Care must be taken to see that the patient and relatives understand that to be overweight is detrimental. The less exercise the patient is able to indulge in, the lighter should be the diet. Overeating is a common problem to the handicapped patient.

PAIN

This, as has been stated before, is a problem most associated with irritative lesions. Relief of the irritation leads to relief of the pain. Pain may also be the result of faulty posturing or of faulty muscle synergy leading to inflamed bursae, etc.

Pain relieving methods include: gentle heat to encourage relaxation; cold, which often helps when heat fails; soothing massage techniques associated with correction of malposturing; and the use of movement activities which help to reduce the discomforts of constant joint positioning.

Many patients who have loss of synergy in the shoulder have severe shoulder pain which spreads down the arm. The hemiplegic patient is particularly prone to this. The pain can often be relieved by the application of a cold pack over the shoulder area incorporating pectoralis major, deltoid and the scapula. If this is followed by rhythmical traction versus compression stimuli the patient frequently reports relief of pain. The explanation for this is obscure but it may be that the cold helps to relax the painful muscle spasm which will be superimposed upon the patients' other symptoms and the compression alternately with traction may stimulate more normal muscle synergy and therefore joint protection.

If the pain is part of a neuritis the position of the vertebral column and shoulder girdle is important.

Cervical traction may be advised as a measure to relieve pressure on the nerve roots and therefore act as a relief to irritation.

The pain of causalgia is another difficult problem and all pain relieving methods may be attempted. Heat is not always successful and may be dangerous if the patient's ability to appreciate degrees of heat is impaired.

Thalamic pain is not very responsive to physiotherapy and drugs may be the only thing to help the patient.

Drug therapy is used widely in the relief of pain which cannot otherwise be helped and even surgical interference may be attempted as a
method of blocking sensory input of a painful nature.

LOSS OF CONSCIOUSNESS

Patients showing loss of consciousness require special care in an
intensive therapy unit. Attention must be paid to the accompanying
respiratory problems and the physiotherapist may be called in to help
in these matters. Chapter VII on head injuries gives a detailed account
of the physiotherapist's part in the care of the unconscious patient and
applies not only to head injury cases but to any other patient showing
this distressing symptom.

As was indicated in Chapter III there are various levels of unconsciousness and much care must be taken to talk to the patient and
not about him in case he is receptive to some stimuli.

EPILEPSY

Fits of this nature are usually held in check by the administration of
phenobarbitone and allied drugs. The physiotherapist must know
whether her patient is prone to these attacks so that she is not completely
unprepared should one occur during a treatment session.

If the fit is of a minor nature it may pass almost unnoticed, but if it
is of a more major type then care must be taken to prevent the patient
from injuring herself and other people. Such patients should not be
left unattended nor should they be treated in areas where they could
come to any severe injury should they have an attack. Pool therapy
may well be unwise for these patients on two counts. *Firstly* there is a
danger of inhalation of water and possible drowning. *Secondly* the
shimmering effect of light on the water may well trigger off an attack.

Epilepsy can be triggered off by light wave bands giving visual
stimulation and for this reason some patients show the onset of an
attack if they sit watching television for long. This is particularly likely
to happen if they are too close to it and in a darkened room.

The flickering light coming through trees and from the road upon
which there are multiple areas of shade and light may also be a con-
tributory factor and patients who are travelling as passengers are
advised to close their eyes when the light fluctuates in this way. Short

wave diathermy has been known to have a similar effect and care should be taken if such treatment is contemplated for any patient known to have epilepsy.

It is as well for the physiotherapist to know this since patients often complain of feeling unwell or of having a mild attack when watching television. The physiotherapist may be able to help by explaining the cause.

INCONTINENCE OF URINE AND BACK PRESSURE

As was explained in Chapter III many of the more severely handicapped patients show these symptoms. Catheterization is the standard method of dealing with this, but unfortunately it often leads to urinary infections which have to be controlled by antibiotics.

Back pressure into the kidneys can be relieved periodically by allowing the patient to adopt the upright position for periods during the day. If the patient is unable to stand he may be supported on a tilting couch which can be wound up into the upright position. The patient may have to be secured by strapping into position, but provided adequate padding is given, there is no danger of skin pressure.

The method of procedure can be useful for the patient suffering from multiple sclerosis who has reached the bedfast stage, and who is in danger not only of having urinary problems but also of going into a flexion position. The weight-bearing stimulus through the feet encourages extension and counteracts the flexion, whilst the urinary complications are minimized.

The patient may be held in this position in the gymnasium (which is a change from the ward) where she may have free use of any movements available in her arms and where she can make social contact with other patients. This may seem to be of small value but values must be related to the situation of the patient. If left, she would be curled up into flexion at this stage, have kidney failure, pressure sores and be unable to make any social contacts. Her remaining weeks would be spent in more discomfort than necessary.

FUNCTIONAL INDEPENDENCE

At some stage in his rehabilitation the patient will require help towards functional independence. Exactly when this is encouraged will depend upon the type of condition and the method of management being used.

To be manageable at home the patient should be able to move himself up and down and about his own bed. He should be able to transfer himself from his bed to a chair of any kind and if he is a wheelchair patient, he should be able to manoeuvre the wheelchair about the house and transfer from wheelchair to toilet seat and into the bath etc. All these things should be possible with minimal assistance from relatives. In some cases special hoists have to be supplied to patients to help them to be independent and aids have to be given to make some functions possible. It is, however, most important that aids are only supplied as a last resort or as an intermediate measure from which the patient will progress.

The physiotherapist and occupational therapist are involved in functional independence and should work in close conjunction with each other.

Such activities as dressing and washing must be related to the patient's ability to balance in various positions and to carry out fine movements of the hands. Although the occupational therapist is very involved with this aspect the physiotherapist must also take an interest since she is probably responsible for the balance training and will know when the patient can be expected to use hand skills.

For the housewife kitchen training is dealt with as a rule by the occupational therapist who is concerned with any adaptation required for the patient's own kitchen. However, the physiotherapist may well be able to help by giving the patient the necessary skills of movement to use her kitchen either as it is or with its adaptations.

Home visits may be necessary and should be made ideally by the occupational therapist and the physiotherapist together. Much of the patient's treatment programme can be adjusted to suit the particular home problems and the physiotherapist gains much by seeing the difficulties likely to be faced by the patient.

In some cases functional independence cannot be achieved without some kind of aid such as a weight-relieving or weight-bearing caliper, a pair of sticks, elbow crutches, or a wheelchair. The patient must be correctly assessed for these appliances and must also be adequately instructed in their use.

The education of relatives is important. When the patient is sent home the relatives have an all-powerful position and can make or break the patient's progress. They need help to understand the problems faced by the patient and to know how best they can help him. If they smother him with help they may make him relinquish his independence and then he will be wholly dependent and become a burden. If they offer too little help life may become too difficult for the patient and he will give up trying. Thus the relatives have a considerable responsibility when the patient finally goes home.

Finally, the need to get out and to see other people is very great and relatives and patient alike must appreciate that confinement to four walls eventually imprisons the mind. Herein lies a great problem. Handicapped people often rely upon others to help them to get out and if they do not get away from home they become fractious and difficult since their horizons become narrowed. The opening of day centres for severely handicapped patients helps a great deal. Patients who have been away from home for a day meet their relatives in the evening with refreshed minds and have something to offer as a social contact. Naturally it is hoped that most patients will be able to work but those who cannot must not be forgotten and it is for these patients that day centres are of most value.

REFERENCES

Bobath, B. *Adult Hemiplegia: Evaluation and Treatment* (Heinemann). 1970.

Bobath, B. 'The Very Early Treatment of Cerebral Palsy'. Developmental Medicine and Child Neurology, Vol. 9, No. 4, 1967.

Bobath, K. *The Motor Deficit in Patients with Cerebral Palsy* (Heinemann). 1966.

Buller, A. J. 'Spinal Reflex Action'. Physiotherapy, Vol. 54, No. 6, 1968.

Campbell, E. J. M., Dickinson, C. J. and Slater, J. D. H. *Clinical Physiology* (Blackwell). 3rd ed. 1968.

Gesell, A. *The First Five Years of Life* (Harper & Row). 1940.

Goff, B. 'Appropriate Afferent Stimulation'. Physiotherapy, Vol. 55, No. 1, 1969.

Haymaker, W. and Woodhall, B. *Peripheral Nerve Injuries* (W. B. Saunders). 1953.

Illingworth, R. S. 'Sequence of Development in the Child'. Physiotherapy, Vol. 51, No. 6, 1965.

Knox, J A. C. 'Neuromuscular Transmission'. Physiotherapy, Vol. 54, No. 6, 1968.

Knott, M. and Voss, D. E. *Proprioceptive Neuromuscular Facilitation* (Hoeber). 1956.

Lance, J. *A Physiological Approach to Clinical Neurology* (Butterworth). 1974.

Lane, R. 'Physiotherapy in the Treatment of Balance Problems'. Physiotherapy, Vol. 55, No. 10, 1969.

Matthews, P. B. 'Receptors in Muscle'. Physiotherapy, Vol. 54, No. 6, 1968.

McGraw, M. B. *The Neuromuscular Maturation of the Human Infant* (Hofner). 1943.

Rosenbloom, L. and Horton, M.E. 'The Maturation of Fine Prehension in Young Children'. Developmental Medicine and Child Neurology, Vol. 13, 3–8.

Ruch, Patten and Woodbury, *Neurophysiology* (W. B. Saunders).

CHAPTER VII

Head Injuries

by ELIZABETH L. RENFREW, M.C.S.P.

The physiotherapist will meet and will have to treat patients suffering from the effects of varying degrees of head injury, not only in the neurosurgical units but also in the general hospital wards. Many such patients who previously would have died now survive their injuries due to the improved methods of resuscitation and care employed in the 'Intensive Care' type of unit.

There are two distinct phases of general care and treatment:

1. The *early phase*, when the patient is unconscious and needs intensive care and therapy. This phase may last for an hour, or for weeks, months and even years.

2. The '*recovery phase*', when the residual disability may be relatively mild or extremely severe.

A knowledge of the mechanism of brain injury and the pathological changes caused will help in understanding the complexity of the disability, and the clinical syndromes presented in the two phases, which must influence the physiotherapeutic care.

TYPES OF INJURY

Head injuries can be classified most simply as those caused by:

1. Blunt injury
2. Penetrating injury
3. Compression injury

Blunt injuries

These, the most common form of head injury, occur in two ways:

147

a. When the head comes into forcible contact with a fixed object, as when the head hits the road, in a road traffic accident.

b. When the stationary head is suddenly accelerated in space after being struck by a blunt moving object.

As a result of blunt injuries the skull may be fractured at the site of impact. This fracture may be linear, depressed or compound with risk of infection.

Brain damage may occur at the site of the impact even when there is no fracture present. It may also occur on the surface of the brain immediately opposite the site of impact. This is caused by movement of the brain against the opposite side of the skull, the so-called 'contre-coup' injury.

The movement of the brain within the skull may cause diffuse neuronal damage, with resultant loss of consciousness; or shearing of the nerve fibres within the brain. These forms of damage occur particularly when the head is suddenly accelerated or decelerated in space. Because of this they are often referred to as 'acceleration – deceleration injuries'.

From what has just been said it is clear that in these injuries the most critical brain damage occurs, not at the site of the impact but at the point where greatest associated movement of the brain takes place.

Penetrating injuries

This form of injury is seen most frequently in war-time and results in local damage along the path which the penetrating agent has travelled. There is no diffuse neuronal damage and therefore often no loss of consciousness.

Compression injuries

These occur when the head is slowly crushed, producing multiple fracturing, but often with no loss of consciousness.

BRAIN DAMAGE SECONDARY TO THE INITIAL LESION

Certain secondary lesions may be produced by any type of head injury, and they may be caused by:

a. Intracranial haemorrhage and formation of haematoma.

b. Intracranial infection through a compound fracture.

c. Brain swelling caused by oedema and venous congestion.

d. Hypoxia which may result from any of the above three factors; from a drop in blood pressure due to shock and possible bleeding from associated injuries; or from chest injuries and depression of the respiratory centres, producing inadequate ventilation.

ASSOCIATED INJURIES

One-third of patients with head injuries also have associated injuries (Jennett 1970). These injuries may be relatively minor ones or may be as critical and as urgent as the head injury itself. Such injuries include fracture-dislocation of the cervical spine, fractures of the long bones, ribs, pelvis or face, and damage to the lungs or abdominal viscera. Immediate operation may be needed to deal with these serious complications and to prevent further brain damage resulting from poor ventilation caused by lung injury or severe shock. The surgeon will have to decide on priorities, and treatment of both the head and associated injuries may have to be delayed until the general condition of the patient has improved.

SEVERITY OF HEAD INJURY

The severity of head injury is classified on an assessment of the length of post-traumatic amnesia (P.T.A.) which can be defined as the 'lapse of time between the injury and the return of conscious memory' (Jennett 1970). This includes the time after regaining consciousness, when the patient is still confused and disorientated and suffering from cerebral irritation, up to the time when he recognizes his relatives and is aware of his surroundings.

Using this classification the degrees of head injury may be described as:
Slight head injury having a P.T.A. of less than one hour.
Moderate head injury having a P.T.A. of one to twenty-four hours.
Severe head injury having a P.T.A. of one to seven days.
Very severe head injury having a P.T.A. of more than seven days.

CLINICAL FEATURES SEEN IN THE HEAD INJURY

It is only when the patient begins to regain consciousness and attempts to regain his former state that the full extent of any residual neurological dysfunction will become obvious and the clinical signs of that dysfunction will become apparent. It is however important that the physiotherapist should know the complications that may occur from the earliest stage, the signs and symptoms they present and the way in which they may influence the patient's rehabilitation.

When the patient is first admitted the chief features may be:

i. Respiratory complications.
ii. Unconsciousness.
iii. Associated injuries, such as those previously mentioned.

RESPIRATORY COMPLICATIONS

Respiratory distress and therefore inadequate ventilation may be caused by:

OBSTRUCTION OF THE AIRWAY

The unconscious patient may inhale nasal secretions, vomit, or blood from fractures of the jaws, face and base of the skull, or from lacerations around the mouth. These may partially or completely block the airway resulting in inadequate ventilation.

DEPRESSION OF THE RESPIRATORY CENTRE

Situated in the brain stem this vital centre may be damaged, thus affecting control of the rate and rhythm of respiration. When this happens the patient will require mechanical assistance to maintain respiration.

ASSOCIATED INJURIES OF THE CHEST

There may be injury to the chest wall and damage to the lungs and pleurae, interfering with the mechanics of respiration.

General care

Where any of the above factors produce respiratory difficulties measures will be taken to maintain an airway and if necessary to provide mechanical assistance.

Maintenance of the airway means ensuring that there is an adequate passage for oxygen to get to the lungs.

If the patient is not suffering respiratory distress and the upper respiratory tract is clear, he will have an airway passed only when routine suction of the chest is required, at two-hourly intervals. He will be nursed in the prone and semi-prone position to prevent inhalation of secretions.

If the patient requires frequent suction, mechanical assistance to breathe or immediate anaesthesia, a cuffed endotracheal tube will be passed, and the cuff inflated. Suction may be applied and if assisted respiration is required the ventilator will be connected to this tube.

If after twenty-four hours the patient shows no sign of regaining coughing and swallowing reflexes, or requires continued ventilation, a tracheostomy will be performed. Suction and ventilation will then be carried out through the tracheostomy tube.

When the patient cannot maintain his own ventilation satisfactorily the lungs will be inflated with air by a ventilator. This will produce intermittent positive pressure, inflating the lungs, and expiration will then occur passively. Some machines may also have a negative phase of suction which removes the air in the expiratory phase. Each intensive care unit may use varying types of ventilators and the physiotherapist should have the mechanics of an unfamiliar one explained to her.

The air supplied by the ventilator may be humidified as a substitution for the work of the nasal passages which have been by-passed.

UNCONSCIOUSNESS

The arousal and maintenance of the conscious state in man is thought to be due to the actions of the *reticular activating system*. This is the name given to certain of the centres of the reticular formation and their corresponding projection fibres through the brain, and in particular to the cerebral cortex.

This system may be inactivated or depressed by shearing strain on the brain stem or diffuse neuronal damage to the cerebral cortex leading to loss of consciousness. This may be transient, lasting only a few minutes, or as previously mentioned it can last for weeks, months and even years.

The damage to the brain stem may completely inactivate the reticular activating system, the respiratory centre, and other vital centres, and then is incompatible with life.

If the head injury is less severe causing only a short period of unconsciousness (e.g. less than one hour) there may be little or no sign of neurological dysfunction. The patient may however show what is sometimes described as 'post-concussional syndrome', characterized by headache, dizziness, irritability, hypersensitivity to noise, and lack of concentration.

CLINICAL FEATURES APPARENT THROUGHOUT THE VARIOUS STAGES OF CARE

Most of the clinical features to be described will only be seen as consciousness returns, but some features of the neurological dysfunction, notably spasticity, will be evident while the patient is still unconscious.

1. *Disturbed Neuromuscular Function and Impaired Inhibition.*
   a. Increase of muscle tone and release of primitive and infantile reflexes and reactions.
   b. Tremor.
   c. Decrease in muscle tone.
   d. Ataxia.
   e. Disturbed righting and equilibrium reactions.
2. *Sensory Disturbance.*
   a. Effect on motor function.
   b. Perceptual problems.
3. *Disorders of Speech, Communication and Hearing.*
4. *Changes of Personality, Control of Emotion, and Impairment of Intellect.*
5. *Visual Disorders.*
6. *Epilepsy.*
7. *Incontinence.*
8. *Complications of Prolonged Immobilization.*
   a. Pressure sores.
   b. Deformities of joints.
   c. Myositis ossificans.
   d. General reduction in muscle tone and disuse atrophy.

Disturbed neuromuscular function and impaired inhibition

INCREASE IN MUSCLE TONE AND RELEASE OF REFLEX ACTIVITY
Damage to the higher centres of the brain responsible for the control and inhibition of excess muscle tone, and for the integration of neuro-

muscular reflexes, will cause hypertonus (spasticity). This may show in several ways:

i. as a dominance of sustained muscle activity in one pattern, either of flexion or extension. Examples are the flexion of the fingers, wrist, elbow and shoulder; or the plantar flexion of the foot, extension of the knee and adduction of the hip.

ii. as the recurrent response pattern of primitive neuromuscular reflexes, such as the tonic neck and labyrinthine reflexes centred in the brain stem; as the response pattern in the infantile neurological reactions, such as the grasp reflex in the hand, crossed extension reflex in the legs; or as the total extensor reaction of the trunk described as 'extensor thrust'. In the normal infant these primitive responses are fleeting, but in the patient with head injury the response is often sustained, and the more the reaction is stimulated the stronger it becomes (e.g. by touching the back of the head in the case of extensor thrust).

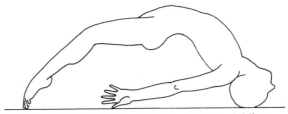

Fig. VII/1 Opisthotonus in decerebrate rigidity

iii. as 'decerebrate rigidity' in the patient with gross brain damage. When damage to the cerebral cortex is severe and widespread the brain stem takes over complete control, producing a primitive and total response with violent hypertonus. The patient lies in opisthotonus (see Fig. VII/1) with the arms extended and internally rotated, the legs fully extended and the feet plantarflexed. If decerebrate rigidity occurs after the initial phase of the injury, it should be reported at once, as it may indicate that further damage is occurring. It is often seen in fatal injuries when the higher centres of the brain have been completely cut off from the rest of the nervous system.

TREMOR

This may occur in two forms:

i. Continuous tremor is seen where there is damage to the extrapyramidal system, in particular to the basal ganglia. It is characterized by fluctuating tone in opposing muscle groups, causing continuous tremor.

ii. Intention tremor is seen when the cerebellum or cerebellar tracts have been damaged, and only when the patient attempts voluntary movements.

HYPOTONUS

True flaccidity is only seen when the head injury is accompanied by a cervical cord transection, or as local flaccidity where there is a peripheral nerve lesion accompanying a limb fracture.

Damage to the cerebellum and other centres may cause disturbance of postural tone, so that in the stage of recovery there is poor head control, poor general postural tone in the trunk and at the shoulder and pelvic girdles, giving a general impression of 'floppiness' and total dependence.

ATAXIA

Ataxia of general movement and of gait may arise as a result of damage to the cerebellum or its tracts. This damage interferes with the normal sequence and organization of movement patterns which become inco-ordinated and clumsy.

Another type of ataxia, namely sensory ataxia, is caused by damage to the postcentral gyrus of the cortex, to the gracile and cuneate tubercles and to the ascending tracts in the brain, or to the thalamus. When this happens exteroceptive and proprioceptive sensations are imperfectly perceived, or not perceived at all. This means that the initiating centres of movement have little or no sensation of the body's position and external condition, and this in turn leads to the imperfect organization of postural tone and co-ordinated movement.

DISTURBED RIGHTING AND EQUILIBRIUM REACTIONS

Damage to the centres in the brain stem concerned with the righting reflexes will lead to the patient's inability to adopt and maintain an upright position against gravity.

In the same way equilibrium reactions may be disturbed, with impairment of the normal mechanisms required to maintain balance against gravity and changes of position, such as forwards, sideways and backwards protective extension, stepping reactions and general postural adjustments. In some patients these may be latent and will be stimulated into activity by treatment, but in others these reactions may be completely inhibited by the dominance of primitive neurological activity.

Sensory disturbance

Damage to the sensory area of the cerebral cortex, and the posterior column tracts in the brain may lead to lack of appreciation of sensory stimuli, as described earlier under ataxia. There may be loss of sensation in the soles of the feet. Sometimes this is due to the effect of prolonged recumbency and not bearing any weight and corrects when weight-bearing is resumed. If there is true loss of sensation it will cause a sensory ataxia of gait.

PERCEPTUAL PROBLEMS

Although perceptual disorders can be seen where there is seemingly full sensory function, many of the perceptual problems which follow head injury are due to a sensory deficiency.

Testing for and treatment of perceptual problems is the field of the occupational therapist, but the physiotherapist must recognize that these problems may be present and complicate her treatment. This is particularly so where there is a disturbance of proprioceptive sensation or misinterpretation of it and the patient is unaware of parts of his body or their position in space. An example of this may be seen in hemiplegia resulting from head injury when the patient is unaware of his affected side.

Some patients may appear to have forgotten how to carry out specific acts although they have the motor ability to do so. This type of problem is described as apraxia and there are several types.

Another feature sometimes seen in the head-injured patient is an unawareness of his disability and sometimes the patient will deny the presence of a severe disability. This is known as *anosagnosia*.

The head-injured patient may also have spatial problems, finding it difficult to relate objects to each other and to himself. This can take many forms, but will affect the physiotherapist if the patient fails to appreciate the idea of going 'through' a door, or 'round' an object.

For the full details of perception and spatial problems appropriate textbooks should be consulted. In the treatment of patients with such problems the physiotherapist should co-operate with the occupational therapist.

Disorders of speech, communication and hearing

Again this is not the province of the physiotherapist but she should realize that these problems may be present, and may require a special approach, often in combination with the speech therapist. For example the speech therapist may want to know the best position to obtain relaxation of the chest and shoulder girdle in a patient with severe hypertonus, while she could advise the physiotherapist on the best method of communication with the patient, especially if there is loss of hearing.

The patient with loss of hearing or a speech defect may appear at first to be unreceptive and unintelligent and this requires special care in management. Care must be taken not to discuss the patient, even when he is unconscious, within earshot. It is not unusual for a patient who has recovered to recount things said in front of him, when he appeared too 'deep' to hear anything.

It is important, too, that the semi-conscious, partially hearing or speech defective patient should always be spoken to as a normal person, not as a child or as someone mentally defective.

Changes of personality, control of emotion and impairment of intellect

Changes of personality occur frequently after a head injury. Patience and encouragement of both the patient and his near relatives are required to enable them to accept the change, which is not always a pleasant one.

The patient may have difficulty in controlling his emotions, and sudden changes in mood may occur, varying from elation to depression. In some instances these changes are diminished with the passage of time, but in others may continue for many years or be permanent.

Impairment of intellect may vary from a mild confusion, or a poor retentive memory and attention span in those with a moderate injury to severe mental defect requiring institutional care.

In all patients with personality or intellectual changes the staff, and the relatives, should adopt a patient and kindly, though when necessary, firm attitude towards the problems. In severe cases the help of a psychiatrist may be needed.

Visual disorders

These may vary from nystagmus and double vision to loss of sight, either partial or complete.

Epilepsy

Epilepsy is a frequent sequel to head injury. It may occur in the first week after injury as a single fit. This may never recur, or it may be the beginning of a permanent condition, calling for drugs to control it.

In some cases the first fit may not occur until quite a few years after the injury, and in others there may be occasional fits separated by intervals of years.

Incontinence

The unconscious patient will require catheterization for bladder drainage, which always carries with it the risk of urinary tract infection. As consciousness returns the catheter may be gradually discarded, but in some more severely damaged patients incontinence persists after recovery.

Complications of prolonged immobilization

PRESSURE SORES
These may be prevented by routine and adequate care of the skin and frequent turning of the patient. Special care is needed when traction, splints or plaster are applied, particularly where muscle spasm is present.

DEFORMITIES OF JOINTS
These may be caused by faulty positioning, and failure to maintain mobility in the presence of hypertonus, thus allowing shortening of muscles and contracture to occur. They may also occur in the cases where limb fracture has been associated with the head injury and difficulties in management have arisen.

MYOSITIS OSSIFICANS
This is a common complication of head injury. Calcification and bone formation appears in muscles and around joints leading to stiffness

of the joints. It may be precipitated by overzealous stretching of hypertonic muscles, but in other cases no obvious cause can be found.

GENERAL REDUCTION IN MUSCLE TONE AND DISUSE ATROPHY
This may occur in prolonged recumbency.

THE PHYSIOTHERAPIST'S APPROACH
TO TREATMENT OF THE HEAD INJURY

1. The mild head injury.
2. The moderate and severe head injury.

The mild head injury

If a patient regains consciousness within twenty-four hours and there are no signs of complications, the usual procedure is to nurse him flat in bed until all signs of headache have disappeared. He is then allowed to sit up, and then stand out of bed, and progress to walking and increasing activity if the headache does not recur.

Some of these patients suffer from dizziness and impaired balance. For these a scheme of head and neck exercises combined with general movement, such as are used for vertigo will be found useful in helping the patient to accommodate to, and overcome the dizziness. The aim should be to progress gradually to normal activities.

A sympathetic and encouraging approach is called for from the physiotherapist. A head injury, even though relatively mild can be a frightening episode, especially if it is accompanied by a period of unconsciousness.

Moderate and severe head injuries

The treatment described here applies principally to the severe and very severe head injuries, but will apply in the same way to the moderate injury except that the period of treatment in the unconscious phase will be shorter. The disability arising may also be considerably less complex in some cases.

Treatment is divided into the following sections:

Acute stage – The care of the unconscious patient.

Sub-acute stage – The care of the conscious but dependent patient.

Stage of rehabilitation – The patient is rehabilitated to the highest level possible with the residual disability.

THE CARE OF THE UNCONSCIOUS PATIENT

General care

The unconscious patient will be nursed where some form of intensive care is available. This may vary from a purpose-built unit to the side room of a general or orthopaedic ward. In either case precautions to avoid introducing infection should be taken, and the physiotherapist will be expected to wear cap, mask and sterile gown and to change her footwear on entering the unit.

The patient is usually nursed naked between sheets in the prone and semi-prone positions, to prevent inhalation of secretions. Turning is carried out at two-hourly intervals to prevent chest complications and pressure sores. Problems may arise with positioning and turning where associated injuries require some form of splintage, such as padded plasters or traction. If a fracture-dislocation of the cervical spine is present the patient may be nursed on a turning frame.

If, as is frequently the case with head injuries, a high temperature persists, the patient will be cooled by electric fans, ice packs or in a specially ventilated room, to reduce the temperature as much as possible.

When unconsciousness persists for more than twenty-four hours, the patient will be fed six-hourly with water and a fluid, high protein diet through a nasogastric tube.

As well as the usual recording of temperature, pulse and respiration other vital functions will require constant recording. The level of consciousness and response to stimuli will be recorded from admission until the patient is fully conscious.

In some units the patient may be connected to multi-monitoring units for recording pressure of cerebrospinal fluid and the level of CO_2 in the blood; for producing electro-encephalograms, electro-cardiograms and for giving immediate warning of apnoea and cardiac arrest. The physiotherapist may find this type of equipment bewildering at first and should have it explained to her by a member of the medical staff.

Before outlining the aims of treatment relevant to the physiotherapist, the importance of co-operation between the nursing and therapy staffs must be stressed. The care of the unconscious patient, whether as a result of head injuries or any other cause, must be a combined effort. There is no place for the attitude that one member of the team is more important than the other. Very often care overlaps and the nurse and physiotherapist may have to fit in with each other's routine. Thus the physiotherapist may carry out her chest regime at the same time as the routine turning.

Aims of physiotherapeutic care

1. To maintain a clear airway and prevent lung collapse.
2. To maintain mobility, inhibit primitive motor activity, and prevent contracture and deformity.
3. To maintain circulation and prevent thrombosis.
4. To assist in the care of the skin and treatment of any pressure sores.
5. To stimulate the patient generally.

Maintenance of a clear airway and the prevention of lung collapse

To prevent secretions gathering in the chest, partial or complete lung collapse, and inhalation of secretions from the upper respiratory tracts the following measures are employed:

  (a) Mechanical suction to clear secretions.
  (b) Routine chest vibrations on expiration and the frequent change of position to help clear the secretions and maintain full expansion.

MECHANICAL SUCTION
Suction will be required throughout the unconscious phase. An electrically operated suction machine is used, except in modern units where suction apparatus may be incorporated in a wall unit along with the oxygen supply. A soft sterile catheter of suitable size is introduced through the endotracheal tube, the tracheostomy tube, or the oro-pharyngeal airway. If the patient is being artificially ventilated the tube to the machine will be *momentarily* disconnected from the tracheal or endotracheal tube.

One contra-indication to suction through the nasal passages is the presence of rhinorrhoea. This may indicate a leak of cerebrospinal fluid with consequent risk of ascending infection. For this reason in some units nasopharyngeal suction is not used in head injuries.

In some units suction is the duty of the nursing staff, in others the duty of the physiotherapist. The student should refer to the suggested further reading on p. 171 for details of the technique of suction.

ROUTINE CHEST PHYSIOTHERAPY

This should be carried out before suction and as far as possible timed to coincide with the turning of the patient.

The chest should be vibrated on the expiratory phase of breathing or ventilation, with slight overpressure at the end of expiration, to stretch the intercostals and stimulate full expansion. This should be carried out over the lateral and posterior costal areas and then over the apical region. The chest should then be sucked out, the patient turned and the procedure repeated. If this does not clear the secretions adequately the postural drainage positions in elevation are sometimes used, provided the medical staff see no contra-indications to this. The physiotherapist should always consult the medical staff before carrying out full drainage positions in this phase.

The frequency of suction and the chest regime will depend on the individual patient. Some may require it every two hours or even more frequently. In some the suction will be carried out each time the patient is turned, but physiotherapy will be needed only in the morning, afternoon and late evening. In every unconscious patient it is essential to carry out vibrations in each position, at least every morning and afternoon, to prevent lung collapse.

Routine chest physiotherapy should be modified where there are chest injuries.

Maintenance of mobility, inhibition of primitive motor activity, and prevention of contractures

When treating the head injury it is essential for the physiotherapist to treat the patient as an organic whole, not as a series of isolated joints. With experience the physiotherapist learns to handle and move the patient in the best way to preserve mobility, employing and combining different techniques to do so, and to prevent contracture. Sometimes however joint stiffness may occur, but even so while giving local treatment to that joint the physiotherapist must still continue the general physical treatment of the patient as a whole, as described below.

GENERAL HANDLING AND POSITIONING

The aim should not be only to maintain mobility but also to inhibit any released primitive neuromuscular activity, such as reflex patterns.

Rolling the patient from side to side, into prone and into supine positions is an important part of the general handling and can be done when the patient is due to be turned routinely. When rolling, trunk rotation should be promoted and passive counter-rotation of the shoulder and pelvis carried out. This has the effect of reducing excessive muscle tone in the trunk, particularly in the presence of a tonic labyrinthine reflex and an extensor thrust. It has the secondary effect of preventing shortening of the trunk muscles.

Certain precautions must be observed when handling the patient, because of the possible presence of the primitive reflexes mentioned in the section on clinical features, page 152. It is easy by injudicious handling to make these reflexes more active and dominant, and this must be guarded against.

If these reflexes are dominant the first stage of handling should be to inhibit them. Some examples of dominance are given below.

a. A patient with an active asymmetrical tonic neck reflex (see page 35) if rolled over suddenly so that the head rotates will imediately adopt the attitude characteristic of that reflex. If left in this position it will be maintained until such time as the patient is moved again, or stimulated in some way.

b. A patient with a dominant tonic labyrinthine reflex (see page 34) may be totally extended in supine lying and when suddenly pushed into side lying, may assume and remain in a position of total flexion.

c. A patient who is suddenly pulled up into sitting may adopt the response typical of asymmetrical tonic neck reflex, with extended head and arms and flexed legs. If the head falls forward the arms will be flexed and the legs extended with no achievement of the sitting position.

The appearance of these reflexes varies from one patient to another, and the physiotherapist must learn to anticipate the appearance of these primitive responses and know how to avoid provoking them. In many cases the reflexes will be present in a very mild form, and showing only as moderate spasms of one limb. Even so this spasm should be suspected as being part of a primitive reflex pattern, and it will often be found that by keeping the head in the midline during all phases of handling the spasm will be diminished.

In some milder head injuries hypertonicity may be seen only in the calf muscles. By changing the total position from supine to side-lying, tone in the calf muscle may be sufficiently reduced to allow full movement at the ankle joint, preventing contracture.

A knowledge of the patient's responses in the unconscious phase will help the physiotherapist to anticipate primitive reflex activity in the conscious phase and to plan her scheme of handling to prevent the patient using them functionally and thereby increasing their dominance.

To sum up this stage of treatment: the physiotherapist should roll the patient from the hips, using counter-rotation on the shoulder; sit the patient up over the edge of the bed, or if this is not possible flex the knees up with one arm under the thighs and with the other round the shoulder girdle sit him forward over his knees; roll the patient into the prone position ensuring that the arms are not flexed under the patient, or lying one in flexion, one in extension.

Positioning the patient in the unconscious phase is as important as moving him. He should not be left lying in the position of a primitive response, or one of violent hypertonus. If this happens the increased tone will become dominant and will eventually cause shortening. If for instance a patient is left lying in the asymmetrical tonic neck response particularly of one side, contracture of flexors on one side and extensors on the other will eventually occur.

The physiotherapist should co-operate with the nursing staff, advising them on the positions best suited to the patient's disability. It must always be remembered however that factors other than the abnormal reflex patterns may have to be considered – such as feeding, use of the ventilator and tracheostomy, the treatment of associated injuries and of pressure areas. Special care will be needed with chest injuries and fracture-dislocation of the cervical spine, and the scheme of handling will require modification.

Correct handling of the unconscious head injury may appear complex and onerous to the physiotherapist, but she will find that this is the basis of her future work. Careful attention to correct handling at this stage will reduce considerably the complications of prolonged recumbency described earlier.

PASSIVE MOVEMENTS

In the treatment of the head injury there is only limited scope for passive movements of isolated joints. Certainly all joints must be put through a range of movement as often as possible, but this should be done as part of the total pattern of movement of the whole limb. This gives a more normal pattern of joint movement, as joints do not usually move in isolation but as part of a total pattern. Only when one joint has become, or is becoming, stiff should isolated passive movement of that joint be carried out, or when plaster fixation or traction prevents total movement of the limb.

The physiotherapist has been warned about the danger of myositis ossificans and the formation of ectopic bone in muscles and should beware of stretching severely hypertonic muscles. If hypertonus is present round a joint and is limiting movement the physiotherapist should not try to force movement. Rather she should reduce the spasm by general positioning of the patient and by using rotational movements at the proximal joint of the affected limb. If for example there is spasm of the biceps brachii, leading to stiffness of the elbow joint, the spasm can be diminished by rotation of the shoulder joint and pro-traction-retraction of the shoulder girdle. Other measures to reduce local hypertonus are described in the next section.

The reptilian-amphibian patterns of movement described by Temple Fay (Fig. VII/2) (see also Chapter XII, p. 276) and the patterns used in proprioceptive neuromuscular facilitation are the patterns of movement through which the limbs should be taken. The rotation combined in these patterns will be found useful as a means of reducing excessive tone.

LOCAL MEASURES TO REDUCE SPASM AND MUSCLE SHORTENING

The application of ice over the hypertonic group of muscles may reduce spasm and this can be followed by the application of well-moulded and padded splints, with careful watch for pressure sores.

Sometimes correction of shortening by manipulation is carried out and a 'plaster' applied to maintain the correction. Some units will use full plasters as opposed to splints and in some cases traction may be applied to the lower limbs where there is strong flexor spasm. In other units these measures will not be favoured and more conservative methods used.

Muscle-relaxant drugs are often used to reduce spasm. They may be given routinely or administered some time before physiotherapy to facilitate movement of the patient. One of the drugs most commonly used, and often very successfully, is diazepam.

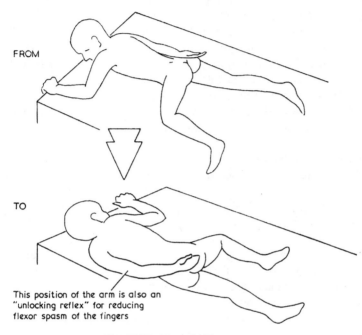

This position of the arm is also an "unlocking reflex" for reducing flexor spasm of the fingers

Fig. VII/2 Temple Fay patterns

CORRECTION OF ESTABLISHED SHORTENING AND CONTRACTURE

When contractures become established and conservative methods of treatment fail, operation is usually undertaken. This, as a rule, is not done until the patient has regained consciousness.

Serial manipulation of joints and the application of plaster may give correction, or a tenotomy, open or closed, of the shortened tendon followed by plaster fixation is performed.

Maintenance of peripheral circulation

The use of the handling techniques described earlier will stimulate the circulation and aid the prevention of deep venous thrombosis.

Assistance in the care of the skin

With constant pressure, frequent incontinence, perspiration, lack of awareness, violent restlessness or long spells of immobility, pressure sores readily develop in these patients, and the pressure areas should be repeatedly treated by the usual nursing procedures. The physiotherapist may assist the nurse in the care of the skin by increasing the circulation locally in the areas which seem likely to, or are about to, break down. This can be done with local infra-red or ultraviolet rays. Great care should be taken with infra-red in the unconscious patient, and the Kromayer lamp should be used to give a local first degree erythema. One of the simplest and most effective ways to produce a local erythema is to rub the skin with a *wet* ice cube and a little pressure for about two minutes. A wet ice cube as opposed to a dry one should be used, since dry ice can give a superficial burn.

If the skin does break down and the initial abrasion is clean and not sloughing, a local dose of infra-red for ten minutes and at a mild heat may initiate the healing process; a local dose of ultraviolet calculated to produce a second degree erythema, if given to unbroken skin, should be given to the abrased area; some crushed ice in a damp cloth, applied directly to the sore is often extremely quick in stimulating the healing process. This form of ice should be applied for the first time for two minutes and increased by two minutes each day until a maximum of ten minutes is reached.

The use of splints, plaster or traction in the treatment of associated injuries will demand careful attention to the areas of pressure, and instant treatment of any threatening areas. It may be necessary to remove a splint or a plaster to prevent a sore becoming worse.

Finally in positioning the patient before leaving him after treatment the physiotherapist should check on all pressure areas and leave him in the optimum position with regard to these areas.

GENERAL ATTITUDE TO THE UNCONSCIOUS PATIENT

The handling of the unconscious patient should never be carried out in silence, or even worse, while chatting to other members of staff over the patient. Talking to the unconscious patient, using his Christian name, telling him what you are going to do, asking him to do it with you, even shouting at him – all this may, in the early stages, seem futile and not a little embarrassing. It does however provide constant stimulation along with the handling and movement. As consciousness begins to return the patient finds himself in a very bewildering situation and it is good to hear someone speaking *to* him, calling him by his name, instead of discussing him in an off hand sort of way – 'He does seem a bit brighter today, poor soul,' as so often happens.

Sub-acute phase

As the patient's level of consciousness rises and he shows some response to stimuli, the amount of handling and general stimulation should be increased.

If the general condition permits, supported sitting and standing should be introduced. This is aimed at increasing the sensory input, and may stimulate general postural tone. The help of two or more assistants may be required as the patient will still be fully dependent. These manoeuvres may provoke strong abnormal responses, violent increase in tone or tremor, and in that event the handling should be combined with, or preceded by inhibitory measures.

At this stage in recovery measures to maintain mobility may be carried out on a mat rather than in bed. This gives more scope for activity and sensory stimulation. Rolling and head raising, first in prone, then in supine should be initiated passively and when maintained by the patient, should be reinforced using stabilization techniques. Care should be taken when doing this not to elicit the tonic neck and labyrinthine reflexes.

The chest regime outlined earlier should continue until the patient can cough, clear his own secretions and maintain his own respiration without distress. If the patient is still on assisted ventilation the handling measures will have to be modified, and the patient will be gradually weaned off the ventilator.

When the swallowing reflex returns the patient will be encouraged to take sips of fluid by mouth, the quantities being gradually increased.

Bladder drainage may not be discontinued until the patient is fully conscious. At first this is for short periods until control is established.

Stage of rehabilitation

This covers the period from recovery of consciousness to the time when the patient is discharged home or to further care. During this period active co-operation with all other disciplines is needed to get the best results. The general approach to the patient will have to be varied considerably according to his emotional state, difficulties in communication, and his adjustment to his disability. The physiotherapist's approach may need to vary from day to day to match her patient's moods.

When deciding on the approach to treatment at this stage, the physiotherapist should try and see her patient's problem as a whole, relating the residual disability to the total pattern of the brain damage. Local deformity or hypertonus should be seen as part of a pattern of disability related to the whole body. It should not be regarded as being a local or isolated disability, to be treated by purely local measures.

The aim of the physiotherapist in rehabilitation is to restore as much function as possible, and then teach the patient how to cope physically with the disability and impaired function that remains, and to do this in as normal a way as possible. Many of these severe head injuries will make remarkable progress in the first eighteen months. After that progress can still be made and some follow-up studies show that improvement may go on for up to ten years.

Physical re-education

The physiotherapist should use the sequence of development of motor function in the infant as the basis for the re-education of movement, stability, co-ordination and balance. The achievement of motor skills is then occurring in the most normal sequence.

INHIBITION
In brain-damaged patients the physiotherapist must anticipate and take necessary measures to inhibit as much as possible any abnormal neuromuscular activity such as hypertonus, released reflexes and tremor, before trying to facilitate the return of motor function. From her knowledge of the patient in the unconscious phase the physiotherapist will have gained some idea of the abnormal activity that is likely to persist.

There are many different methods and techniques available in the neurophysiological approaches to treatment and they have been described elsewhere in this book. As well as the methods described by Bobath, Knott, Kabat, Rood and others the physiotherapist may find useful some of Temple Fay's patterns and 'unlocking reflexes' (see Fig. VII/2, p. 165, and Chapter XII). In many cases the inhibitory techniques can be combined with the facilitatory measures, as for example when using rotation in the movement patterns of proprioceptive neuromuscular facilitation and in using the Temple Fay patterns it will be found that this diminishes hypertonus while at the same time facilitating movement. In the same way, the use of 'slow reversals' to improve co-ordination often seems to reduce tremor.

FACILITATION

There are many varied methods of facilitating postural stability, movement, co-ordination and balance. In the different facilitation techniques use is made of cutaneous stimulation, proprioceptive stimulation such as resistance to mass movement patterns, joint traction and compression, stretch and the use of the rotational elements of movement. Careful handling is of the utmost importance in facilitating postural reaction and movement.

The physiotherapist may find that one particular technique is more suited to one patient than to another, and she must adapt her methods accordingly. It is wrong to use one method exclusively and expect every patient to fit into it. It is essential to understand the theory that is the basis for a particular technique and relate that theory to the brain damage that is causing the disability. For example, a patient who has dominant tonic neck reflexes should not be subjected to a method of treatment that does not take into account the abnormal reflex activity, inhibiting the reflexes before attempting to increase voluntary movement by facilitatory techniques. 'Movement at all costs no matter what kind of movement', is not a good maxim for the physiotherapist working with the head injury. If this were the case she would make her patient function using the abnormal reflex mechanisms, such as the tonic neck reflexes.

The patient's progress should be kept under constant review and any hold-up in that progress should be assessed to see if any change in the approach and method of treatment on the physiotherapist's part is needed.

In spite of continuous treatment deformities may develop and corrective and orthopaedic measures may be needed. The physiotherapist should not look upon this as being a reflection on her treatment, or as an interference with that treatment. Judicious operations, such as those measures described earlier, can be a great help to the physiotherapist and she must co-operate in post-operative treatment by whatever methods are needed. These will have the aim of maintaining correction of deformities, and helping the patient to make the most of the improved function that the surgical treatment has restored. Tenotomy has been mentioned as one operative method often used. The other operative measure that the physiotherapist may encounter is the removal of ectopic bone from muscles and around joints. This, however, is not carried out until the bone deposited is mature and the process is complete.

GENERAL ATTITUDE TO THE PATIENT

This must be one of constant encouragement, with understanding during moods of depression which may be frequent if the patient is severely disabled and can no longer lead the kind of life that he has been used to.

If the disability is minimal the patient should be assisted back to as near normal a life as possible. In rehabilitating the head injury the physiotherapist may see one patient go to an industrial rehabilitation unit and then see him resettled in employment of some kind. She may see another patient who is so disabled that his only future will be one of permanent care in a residential institution.

The physiotherapist who chooses to work with head injuries will find the task of rehabilitating them an intensely interesting but always challenging one. In many cases the prognosis may be poor but will often prove to be too pessimistic. Little can compare with the satisfaction of seeing a previously unconscious and dependent patient regain awareness and gradually function fully again.

REFERENCES

Bobath, B. (1965). *Abnormal Postural Reflex Activity in Brain Lesions*. William Heinemann Medical Books Ltd.
Fay, T. (1954). 'The Use of Patterns and Reflexes in the Treatment of the Spastic'. British Council for the Welfare of Spastics, London.

Gleave, J. R. W. (1971). 'Clinico-pathological Syndromes in Head Injury'. Occupational Therapy, **34,** 2, 17.

Jennett, W. B. (1970). *An Introduction to Neurosurgery*. William Heinemann Medical Books Ltd.

Jennett, W. B. (1971). Personal Communication.

Knott, M. (1968). *On the Treatment of Spastic Pareses*. Sjukgymnasten, Stockholm.

Lance, J. W. (1970). *A Physiological Approach to Clinical Neurology*. Butterworth, London.

Levitt, S. (1968). *On the Treatment of Spastic Pareses*. Sjukgymnasten, Stockholm.

London, P. S. (1971). Personal Communication.

Marshall, R. S. (1971). 'Cold Therapy in the Treatment of Pressure Sores'. Physiotherapy, **57,** 372.

Miller, H. and Stern, G. (1965). 'The Long Term Prognosis of Severe Head Injury'. Lancet, **1,** 225.

Renfrew, E. L. (1971). 'An Approach to the Severe Head Injury'. Physiotherapy, **57,** 50.

Treip, C. S. (1971). 'Pathology of Head Injury'. Occupational Therapy, **34,** 2, 11.

Williams, M. (1970). *Brain Damage and the Mind*. Penguin Books Ltd, London.

FURTHER READING

1. *The Nervous System*. Peter Nathan (1969). Penguin Books Ltd., London.
2. *A Physiological Approach to Clinical Neurology*. James W. Lance (1970). Butterworth, London, Chapter 9.
3. *An Introduction to Neurosurgery*. W. Bryan Jennett (1970). Wm. Heinemann Medical Books Ltd., London, Chapter III.
4. *Management of Head Injuries*. Walpole Lewin (1966). Baillière, Tindall and Cassell, London.
5. *Management of the Unconscious Patient*. E. R. Hitchcock and A. H. B. Masson (1970). Blackwell Scientific Publications, Oxford and Edinburgh, Chapter 5.
6. *Brain Damage and the Mind*. Moyra Williams (1970). Penguin Books Ltd., London.

Articles Published in Journals

7. 'Rehabilitation after Severe Head Injuries'. Injury – the British Journal of Accident Surgery, October 1969.
8. 'The Rehabilitation of Patients Recovering from Severe Head Injuries'. The lectures given at a study course. Occupational Therapy, Vol. 34, Nos. 2 & 3 (1971).

9. 'The Role of the Physiotherapist in the Intensive Care Unit'. A. E. Holderness and R. J. Cooper. Physiotherapy, March 1968.
10. 'A Survey of Recent Developments in Cold Therapy'. J. Haines. Physiotherapy, July 1967.
11. 'Rehabilitation of Patients with Head Injuries'. A. McC. Symons. Physiotherapy, September 1967.
12. 'An Approach to the Severe Head Injury'. E. L. Renfrew. Physiotherapy, February 1971.

CHAPTER VIII

Spinal Cord Lesions

by BARBARA GOFF, o.n.c., m.c.s.p., dip.t.p.

In the developing embryo up to the third month of fetal life the spinal cord occupies the whole length of the neural canal. However, the rate of growth of the vertebral column is greater than that of the spinal cord so that at birth the lower end of the cord lies opposite the third lumbar vertebra. The growth rate of the vertebral column continues to exceed that of the cord so that finally the lowest limit of the cord in the adult lies opposite the disc between the first and second lumbar vertebrae. One consequence of the disparity of bone and cord levels is that when injury to vertebrae causes cord damage this is at a lower segmental level than is the bone damage. For example, at thoracic ten vertebral level, cord damage would be to the first, second, third and fourth lumbar cord segments (see Fig. VIII/1). Damage to bone below lumbar two would cause damage to nerve roots within the neural canal but not to the spinal cord. Such damage is known as a cauda-equina lesion.

TABLE I

Examples of anatomical relationships of spinal cord and bony spinous processes in adults

Cord Segments	Vertebral Bodies	Spinous processes
C8	Lower C6 Upper C7	C6
T6	Lower T3 Upper T4	T3
T12 L1	T9	T8
L5	T11	T10
Sacral Segments	T12 and L1	T12 L1

With minor exceptions each pair of spinal nerves supplies an area of skin with cutaneous nerves and autonomic motor nerves, certain muscles or parts of muscles and certain portions of bones.

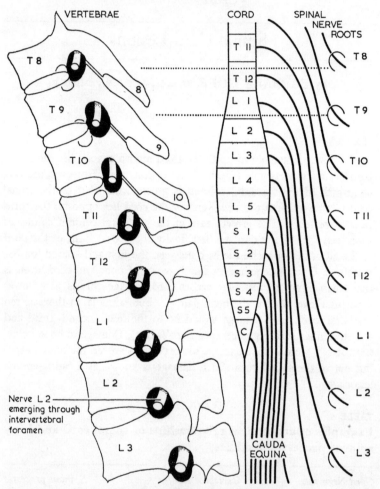

Fig. VIII/1 Scheme to show relative nerve root, cord and bone levels of the lower segments of the spinal cord

The term *myotome* is used to indicate the muscles supplied by one pair of spinal nerves via the anterior root. The motor fibres arise from the anterior horn cells of one portion or segment of the cord, hence the term 'segmental innervation' (see below).

TABLE II

Simplified summary of motor segmental control of limb movements (Myotomes)

Lower Limb

Hip	Adduction	L2	
	Flexion	L3	L2 to L5
	Abduction	L4	
	Extension	L5	

Knee	Extension	L3 and L4	L3 to S1
	Flexion	L5 and S1	

Ankle	Dorsiflexion	L4 and L5	L4 to S2
	Plantar flexion	S1 and S2	

Foot	Inversion	L4
	Eversion	L5 and S1

Note that four segments of the cord control the hip movements overlapping with four segments which control the knee movements, the latter being one segment lower. Drop one segment and the next four segments control ankle movements.

Upper Limb

Shoulder	Abduction	C5
	Extension	
	Adduction	C6
	Flexion	C7

Elbow	Flexion	C5 and C6
	Extension	C7 and C8

Forearm	Supination	C6
	Pronation	C6

Wrist	Flexion	C6 and C7
	Extension	C6 and C7

Fingers

Proximal interphalangeal	Flexion	C7
Metacarpophalangeal	Extension	C8
Distal interphalangeal	Flexion	C8
Metacarpophalangeal	Abduction Flexion Adduction	
Interphalangeal	Extension	T1
Thumb	Opposition	

A *dermatome* is the term used to describe the area of skin whose sensory fibres pass to one segment of the cord via one sensory nerve root (see Figs. VIII/2 and VIII/3). Similarly the term sclerotome is used for the area of the skeleton supplied via one spinal nerve root (see Fig. VIII/4).

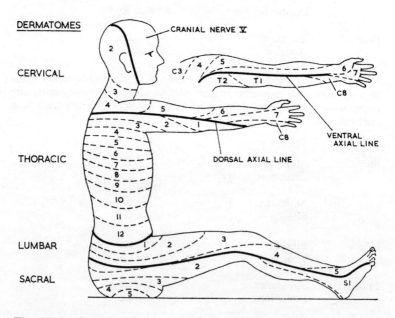

Fig. VIII/2 Plan of dermatomes of the body and segmental cutaneous distribution of upper limb

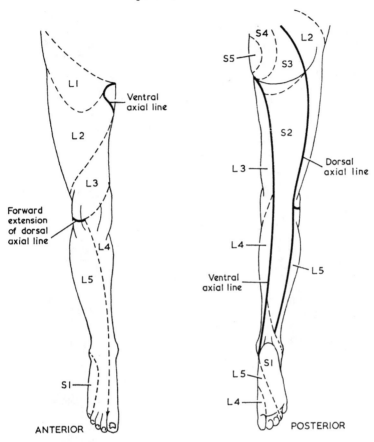

Fig. VIII/3 Plan of dermatomes of lower limb

Causes of cord lesions

The spinal cord can fail to develop normally as in spina bifida and diastematomyelia. It may be crushed or lacerated in fractures or fracture dislocations of the vertebral column (Plate VIII/1). It can be compressed as a result of bone disease, gross deformity of the vertebral column, oedema and inflammatory exudate, and by neoplasia.

The spinal cord is occasionally involved in inflammatory and degenerative lesions such as in rheumatoid and osteoarthrosis. Circulatory

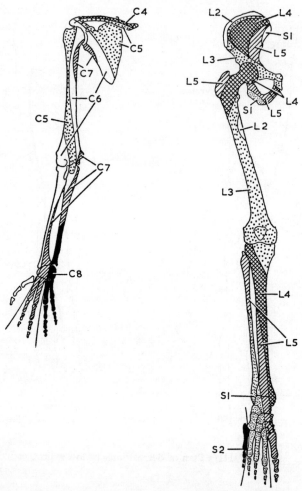

Fig. VIII/4 Anterior view of bones of the right arm and leg to show
the segmental nerve supply

defects resulting in an inadequate blood supply or haemorrhage will
also damage it.

Trauma is most common in the cervical and the dorso-lumbar
regions where mobility is greatest.

The causes of spinal cord lesions as listed above produce various
types of lesion. Sometimes the cord is completely destroyed for several

centimetres, the damage may extend centrally to higher and lower segments, so-called 'coning', and possibly involve one or more nerve roots also. The cord may be only partially affected at one or more segments, the distribution being very variable but examples include a half lesion of one segment mainly affecting right or left halves of the cord, or certain tracts or cells. Accordingly the signs will vary not only with the level at which damage occurs but also depending upon its extent, severity and completeness.

Signs and symptoms of cord lesions (see Plate VIII/1)

The result of complete or partial destruction of a portion of the spinal cord can be considered in three parts.

Firstly loss of function will occur of the cells destroyed at the level of the lesion.

Secondly there is loss of function of the fibres conveying impulses to the brain from below the level of the lesion. These are interrupted by the damage to the cord.

Thirdly tracts from cells in motor centres in the cerebrum, basal ganglia, cerebellum and brain stem are interrupted at the lesion causing loss of their modifying influence on spinal reflexes. The release symptoms of unmodified, exaggerated spinal reflexes only apply to the activity of undamaged segments of the cord caudal to the lesion. It should also be noted that some nerve roots may be permanently damaged within the neural canal or as they emerge from the intervertebral foramina.

A variety of signs, symptoms, and functional disabilities result. The mode of onset, whether this is sudden or gradual influences the signs, as does the age of the patient. Treatment will accordingly vary with these factors.

SIGNS RESULTING FROM CELL DESTRUCTION

At the level of the lesion grey matter is destroyed. Destruction of lower motor neurone cells in the anterior horn results in permanent flaccid paralysis of the muscles they supply. Some muscles, partially innervated by spared motor neurones, will be weakened.

Cells in the posterior horn are interneurones and second order sensory cells. When these are destroyed incoming impulses at the level will fail to be transmitted further. Not only does this result in loss of sensation but interrupts the afferent arm of reflex arcs so it results in loss of reflex activity at the affected site. A similar result follows the destruction of cells in the posterior root ganglia of any spinal nerves involved in the lesion.

In the thoracic and upper two lumbar segments the cells in the lateral horn are preganglionic sympathetic motor cells. Destruction of these results in vasomotor disturbance leading to impaired circulation and nutrition. Also as a result there is failure of regulation of blood pressure and body temperature.

Similarly in sacral segments the cells in the lateral horn are preganglionic parasympathetic motor cells. Destruction of these, in low level lesions, destroys or impairs reflex control of the tone in the walls and sphincter of the urinary bladder. Automatic bladder control is thus almost impossible to train as a flaccid or spastic bladder persists after the initial stages.

SIGNS RESULTING FROM INTERRUPTION OF WHITE FIBRE TRACTS
Although there is no definite evidence to confirm this, it is thought that when white fibres are destroyed within the central nervous system they do not regenerate, so permanent interruption of nerve conduction occurs.

The ascending tracts convey impulses to the sensorium and also to many other centres in the brain. Interruption of these not only results in loss of all modes of sensation below the level of destruction but also produces a profound effect on centres controlling automatic postural reactions.

The descending tracts convey impulses from the pyramidal, extrapyramidal and cerebellar upper motor systems mainly via the cortico-spinal, reticulo-spinal, rubro-spinal and vestibulo-spinal tracts. Interruption of these tracts produces release symptoms because the undamaged motor cells below the level of the lesion are now free to respond, with no modification, to all incoming afferent stimuli. Spinal reflex action is apparent once spinal shock has worn off.

Stimuli which will produce flexor withdrawal, or crossed extensor reflexes include not only potentially harmful ones such as a pin-prick but also a sudden change in temperature, a pressure sore, bladder infection, sudden noise, or even the movement of bedclothes. All muscles respond to stretch so, after a flexor withdrawal has occurred and gravity tends to pull the limb down again, a second flexor spasm sometimes occurs elicited by the resulting stretch as the flexors relax. In some cases flexor spasticity is very difficult to prevent and every care must be taken to try to avoid reinforcement and exaggeration of this by such factors as are listed above.

SIGNS RESULTING FROM CELL AND FIBRE IRRITATION
Some cells and fibres may not be completely destroyed but inflammatory reaction and later scar tissue sometimes cause irritation which, especially in the case of sensory cells and fibres, is very troublesome. 'Girdle' pains and 'phantom limbs' are examples of this.

SIGNS RESULTING FROM INVOLVEMENT OF NERVE ROOTS
In most cases several nerve roots at the level of cord damage are also involved. This adds to the severity of the signs from damage at the level of the lesion.

In a minority of cases it appears that many nerve roots are damaged even below the bone damage, possibly from traction on the whole spinal cord at the time of the injury. This may explain the absence of spinal reflex activity which persists permanently in a minority of cases.

VISCERAL SIGNS
In complete lesions and in some partial ones control of external sphincters of bowel and bladder is lost so double incontinence occurs. There is also loss of sexual function.

FUNCTION LOSS
Control of active movement is impossible in complete lesions. In partial lesions spasticity is usually present so even if some control of limb movement is spared this is of a mass primitive type. Control of postural stability is absent or so masked by flexor or extensor mass patterns of movements that normal use of the limbs, for stance, locomotion or manipulative skills, is impossible.

Postural and equilibrium reactions are lost and absence of protective pain makes joint and skin damage a serious possibility.

Respiratory function and removal of secretions from the respiratory tract are impaired in all high level lesions.

Secondary complications

CHEST COMPLICATIONS
Vital capacity and ventilation are reduced in high level lesions in which the intercostal muscles are paralysed and paralysis of the abdominal muscles makes coughing ineffective or impossible. Secretions collect in the lungs and cannot be removed by the patient's own efforts.

VISCERAL COMPLICATIONS
Bladder infection, retention or a high residual urine are likely complications.

CIRCULATORY COMPLICATIONS
Vasomotor paralysis, loss of movement and use of the affected parts all impair circulation. Deep vein thrombosis occurs in trunk or leg vessels of some patients.

Oedema and trophic changes frequently occur in the hands of tetraplegic patients. Because of interruption of nerve pathways from the vasomotor centre in the medulla oblongata the regulation of peripheral resistance and therefore of blood pressure is not adequate. Sudden changes of position from horizontal to vertical result in pooling of blood in the abdomen and legs so syncope and vertigo are frequent complications. This is most severe and persistent in the high level lesions.

LOSS OF JOINT RANGE AND SOFT TISSUE RANGE
Joint range becomes limited and soft tissue contractures soon prevent good functional positioning unless treatment is vigilantly carried out regularly.

DEFORMITY
This may be defined as a malalignment of body segments which impairs or prevents function. It is related to loss of joint and soft tissue range. Impaired circulation, deposition of calcium salts in soft tissue around joints, persistent pull of spastic muscles or unopposed pull of spared muscles whose antagonists are flaccid all contribute to the risk of deformity. Certain muscle groups are stronger than their antagonists or more likely to be involved in spastic reflex actions and the force of gravity mitigates against some joint positions.

JOINT AND SKIN DAMAGE

Unrelieved pressure quickly impairs the circulation on weight-bearing surfaces. The loss of protective pain is devastating in its effect and the patient does not move to relieve pressure as he is unaware of it. Sunburn, extremes of temperature, scratches and strain on ligaments can all readily cause skin or joint damage. Prominent nails in shoes and failure to dry skin carefully after washing are other examples of how easily skin damage can occur. Poor circulation reduces the resistance to infection so abrasions or small pressure sores easily become infected. Careless handling of paralysed and insensitive parts unfortunately can also contribute to joint or soft tissue damage or risk of fractures.

CALCIFICATION OF SOFT TISSUE

In some cases calcium salts are laid down in soft tissue around joints. The reasons for this are not fully understood but some disturbance of local circulation or trauma are possible causes (Plate VIII/2).

SPASTICITY

The uncontrolled activity of lower motor neurones in undamaged segments of the spinal cord below the level of the lesion produces a number of problems. The result may be severe flexor spasticity which predisposes to pressure sores, contractures, deformity and greatly reduced function. Even in partial lesions, with some control of movement of the trunk and limbs, spasticity prevents normal postural reactions and normal use of the part.

PSYCHOLOGICAL FACTORS

This is discussed finally not because it is least important but because all other signs, symptoms and complications revolve around the degree of acceptance by the patient of his disability. The sudden complete loss of function, dependence on others and uncertainty about the future inevitably have a profound effect on the mental and emotional state of the patient. Even for patients whose lesion is at a low cord level or where the onset is gradual many psychological problems arise.

In the case of some tetraplegic patients the dependence, which lasts for many weeks and may be permanent, includes not only total care of bladder and bowel function, turning and all personal hygiene but also feeding with fluids and solid food.

Concern about dependants, relatives and friends, future occupation and indeed all domestic and social affairs causes great distress to all but the youngest patients.

The emotional state fluctuates. After an initial depression a period of reactionary optimism usually occurs followed later by the most difficult period of more penetrating realization of the predicament.

The psychological complications are frequently aggravated by a well-meaning but unhelpful attitude of relatives and friends.

The influence of mode of onset

The rate and mode of onset influences the type of signs and symptoms which develop. *A sudden interruption of the spinal cord,* by violent trauma, haemorrhage or acute infection results not only in loss of function of the damaged segments but also, temporarily, of all function of the undamaged segments below the level of injury. This is known as 'spinal shock' and presumably is caused by lack of excitatory impulses from the brain since the segments above the lesion do not suffer in the same way (Fulton and McCouch). The signs are of complete loss of function of neurones and tracts. Thus there is complete loss of all forms of sensation of parts supplied from the level of the lesion and below it, together with flaccid paralysis of all skeletal muscles at and below the level of the cord injury. All reflex activity is lost. Visceral signs are of retention of urine and faeces and unless the patient is catheterized back pressure will occur and the kidneys will be damaged.

This state of complete non-function of the cord below the level of injury wears off gradually. Visceral signs change to overflow incontinence in a matter of days as some tone returns to the bladder wall. Spinal reflex activity returns gradually to the undamaged portion below the injured segments. The stretch reflex becomes apparent in muscles supplied from this portion of the cord presenting as spasticity of muscles. The time for this to develop is very variable as is the severity of flexor or extensor spasticity. In a minority of cases the flaccidity of all muscles below the level of the lesion remains permanent. The reason for this is not fully understood but one theory is that so many nerve roots are damaged at the time of the injury that conduction of nerve impulses along them is permanently interrupted.

Some injuries, being less severe than those described above, do not

184

cause spinal shock. The signs are then similar to those described above as appearing when the spinal shock gradually wears off.

Cord lesions caused by pressure from the results of deformity or neoplasia and by degenerative lesions such as disseminated sclerosis or syringomyelia also show no spinal shock. Instead a *gradual development of impaired function* presents as a variety of symptoms and signs. Loss of sensation is partial and may only include cutaneous or kinaesthetic sensation because interrupted impulses resulting in such loss normally travel in different tracts in the cord.

The motor signs are very variable but the most common sign is that caused by interruption of some fibres of the corticospinal tracts. This produces a spastic state of muscles similar to that in the leg of a patient with spastic hemiplegia.

The plantar response is extensor, ankle clonus occurs on slight stretch of the calf and gradually control of learned patterns of movement with selective control of individual joints is lost. Instead of the limbs taking part automatically in postural reactions to changing stimuli, only limited patterns of total movement are available.

Normal function such as rising from sitting and normal gait are difficult or impossible. At first the extensor thrust pattern predominates, there being a combination of extension, adduction and medial rotation at hip, extension at knee, plantar flexion at ankle and inversion at the subtalar joint. Later, as the control from the brain is further reduced by more extensive cord involvement, the predominant pattern is of total flexor withdrawal of the leg or legs. The predominant pattern is now of flexion, abduction and lateral rotation at hip, flexion at knee, dorsiflexion and inversion of the foot. It should be noted that these two patterns are produced by superficial muscles passing over two joints and the postural reactions of deeper muscles passing over only one joint are not elicited.

The reasons for this failure of normal postural reaction are complex. The spastic total patterns prevent normal stimuli occurring in the deep pressure-bearing area of the heel or in the structures composing joints, thus abnormal afferent input elicits mass movement of withdrawal or thrust instead of postural stability for weight-bearing. There may also be interruption of some tracts of the spinal cord from the extrapyramidal and cerebellar centres, thus further reducing modification of spinal reflexes. If existing nerve pathways for postural reflexes are not used, synaptic resistance increases and the normal responses become less and less easy to elicit. Expressed differently this means that if spasticity is not relieved or reduced it becomes more severe. The flexor withdrawal reflex being the most primitive protective reflex is the most persistent and vicious reflex, once it is released from modification.

Circulatory disturbance occurs, which aggravates the sensory and motor disability. Secondary complications also produce further loss of function unless prevented by adequate treatment. Examples of this are contractures of soft tissue especially of the strong flexors of the hip and knee, the adductors of the hip and the calf muscles.

PRINCIPLES OF TREATMENT COMMON TO ALL SPINAL CORD LESIONS

Early stage in cases with sudden onset

The first principle is to save the patient's life. This is endangered from respiratory complications especially where the lesion is high in the cord. Secretions cannot be removed by coughing so internal secretional obstruction threatens to reduce further the vital capacity and ventilation already lowered by paralysis of intercostal and abdominal muscles. Intensive care is essential, a tracheostomy may be needed as may artificial respiration by the use of intermittent positive pressure respiration apparatus. Secretions are removed by appropriate physiotherapy and by the use of suction apparatus if necessary.

Another basic need is to prevent any further damage to the spinal cord whilst the vertebral column remains unstable. Means to achieve this include careful positioning and its maintenance by use of pillows or special beds and also, in cervical spine injuries, the use of skull traction.

The development of pressure sores, the loss of range of joints and soft tissue and circulatory complications are discouraged by careful nursing procedures, turning and moving the patient at regular intervals.

Physiotherapy techniques play an important part by passive movements and careful handling.

Another principle which must be observed right from the commencement of treatment and continued throughout the whole rehabilitation programme is to help the patient to accept his disability. A positive attitude must be encouraged and every means taken to help him achieve as much independence as possible. It should be pointed out that many occupations and sporting activities can be enjoyed. A paraplegic woman can run a home, bear children and bring them up. Insemination is possible by some males with spinal cord injuries; medical advice should be sought on this subject if required.

Stage when weight-bearing through the spine is permitted

A work habit of regular hours five or six days a week is established once weight-bearing through the spine is permitted, usually at eight to twelve weeks after a spinal injury. Social activities during the evenings, at weekends and in competitive meetings such as paraplegic sporting contests all help to give a cheerful atmosphere to a spinal injuries unit.

Once weight is allowed through the spine emphasis is on activity to gain independence. This is achieved by nursing, physiotherapy and occupational therapy techniques. Adjustment to sitting and standing positions in wheelchairs and in splintage must be acquired. Balance and posture training are taught. Care of their own skin and joints in insensitive areas must be trained by example and instruction.

Safe transfers from bed to chair, chair to lavatory, chair to floor and back must be taught. Locomotion is achieved in a wheelchair or in some cases by the use of leg calipers and crutches. Resettlement at home and in a suitable occupation is the most important and all-pervading essential. The efforts of the patient, the whole medical and para-medical team together with the local welfare authorities and the patient's relatives must be co-ordinated to this end. The medical director of a specialized spinal injuries unit has an inspiring example of how to achieve such an objective in the person of Sir Ludwig Guttmann, lately Director of Stoke Mandeville Spinal Injuries Unit.

A final principle of increasing importance as more patients are successfully resettled out of hospital care is that of follow-up and after-care. Bringing patients back into hospital for regular review only partly achieves continued support. A system of domiciliary visiting by a specially trained nurse or therapist is helpful and this is now established for the wide area covered by the Midland Spinal Injuries Unit.

TEAM WORK

As is evident from the foregoing section, team work is essential. Consultation among and co-operation of the activities of all members of the team are imperative. All personnel concerned in any way with treatment and resettlement must understand the objectives at all stages. Each must have some knowledge of the role of the other members of the team. Often treatment involves nurses and therapists working together and the timing of turns and other procedures needs careful co-ordinating. This is necessary not only to avoid overlap but also to avoid too much disturbance of the patient or disruption of the programme of one or other team members. Ideally patients with spinal injuries should be treated in special centres with facilities for their total care at all stages of rehabilitation. In some instances it is also helpful if cases of progressive lesions of the spinal cord can be accommodated in a spinal injuries unit.

A list of the personnel concerned in the care of such patients is given below. It should be noted that the ambulance or first-aid team head the list as unskilled handling of a person with a suspected spinal cord injury can cause increased neurological damage.

Team members

The team includes the following:
Ambulance and first aid personnel.
Medical personnel including physicians, neurologists, orthopaedic surgeons, urologists, plastic surgeons, and radiologists. The medical director of a spinal injuries unit not only heads the team of consultants and registrars but co-ordinates the efforts of all personnel concerned in the well-being of the patients. Prognosis is his responsibility, as is the difficult task of deciding when to explain this to the patient and his relatives. When the patient is ready to go home the general practitioner plays a part in the ultimate stages of patient care.
Nursing personnel include the chief nursing officer, nurses at all levels of seniority and nursing aides and orderlies.
Occupational therapists and physiotherapists whose efforts are often combined both have a vital role in rehabilitation of paraplegic and tetraplegic patients.
Splint fitters and makers play an important part in preparing patients for standing and ambulation.
Welfare personnel include the medical social worker who provides an essential link between home and hospital. Her responsibility includes the arrangement of necessary social adjustments such as arranging

for financial benefits and for alterations to the house. Local Authorities and the Disablement Resettlement Officer (the D.R.O.) of the Department of Health and Social Security are contacted by the medical social worker. Physiotherapists, occupational therapists, nurses and the medical social worker usually co-operate in selecting and ordering such aids as splintage, urinals, wheelchairs, motorized vehicles, and also in advising on alterations to the home.

The D.R.O. contacts employers and attempts to re-establish in suitable employment all patients who were wage earners previous to their illness or injury.

Personnel in Training Centres and Industrial Rehabilitation Centres must be also included among those concerned with resettlement.

RELATIVES AND THE PATIENT

Lastly, but of vital importance, the relatives must be included as theirs is the task of support at all times. Eventually it is they and the patient himself who share the responsibility for the success or otherwise of restoring him to an independent life in the community. In the case of the most severely disabled patients the relatives may be able to undertake nursing care at home after suitable instruction and with the necessary equipment as for example a turning bed. The services of *district nurses and health visitors* may also be needed.

PROCEDURES

Surgery, nursing, physiotherapy and occupational therapy for patients varies in detail with the diversity of symptoms and signs at the different levels of cord injury. They also differ in accordance with the severity of interruption of cord activity. For this reason details of therapy will be discussed in several sub-sections. However, certain procedures are needed in all cases and these will now be discussed briefly. Further details can be studied in other textbooks, a list of which is given later.

Surgery

Some surgeons favour open reduction of the fracture dislocation for a very few cases. Indications for surgery include severe pain associated with massive haematoma, displacement of vertebrae which is unlikely to reduce spontaneously, and a history and X-ray evidence suggesting that surgery would relieve pressure and might thereby reverse some neurological signs. A further indication for surgery is the need to obtain stability of the vertebral column in cases where the paralysis of muscles and excessive weight of the patient cause mechanical difficulty. Surgery merely to attempt to relieve cord pressure is useless if there are signs of complete destruction of several segments of the cord. Such destruction is permanent and relief of pressure cannot obtain any improvement of neurological function. Thus contra-indications to surgery include signs of irreversible cord damage to a complete cross-section of the cord, sepsis, expectation of respiratory complications following general anaesthesia, and weakening of spared back muscles by surgical incisions.

Positioning

The objective of careful positioning is to hold the spine still in such a position that further cord damage is prevented. This principle should be observed by the personnel who convey the patient from the scene of the accident to a hospital. It should continue to govern the subsequent procedures until the spine is considered sufficiently stable to allow trunk movement and weight to be taken through it in a vertical position. This is not usually until eight to twelve weeks after injury. Thus positions must be maintained during all X-ray examinations, throughout all nursing and therapeutic procedures such as washing, attendance to bowel and bladder function, clearing secretions from the chest and necessary change in position or passive movements of the limbs.

Secondary objectives of careful positioning are to prevent circulatory complications, prevent deformity and damage to skin, joints, or soft tissue. Prevention of compression of veins especially in the calf and prevention of pressure on bony prominences help to achieve these aims.

Details of positions and methods to maintain them vary according to several factors. The level of the lesion is one factor; skull traction and support for the neck by sandbags, a cervical collar or special head rest is used for patients with cervical cord lesions. In the case of patients with dorsal or lumbar vertebral level of lesion support for the neck is not essential but the lower parts of the spine must be prevented from moving and the lumbar lordosis maintained. This is usually achieved by the placing of pillows. It is vital for all team members to be meticulous about positioning and in each case they must know which method is used and why it has been selected.

Another consideration in choosing a method of positioning is the number of persons available to turn the patient at regular intervals. A method proved to be effective is the use of firm pillows and small mattress sections carefully placed under head, trunk and legs and to separate the legs and support the feet. However, a minimum of three trained persons is needed to execute each turn to a different position whilst maintaining the immobility of the spine. Details of this method, the position of trunk and limbs, the various limb positions and how to place the pillows is given in detail in books on orthopaedic nursing. (See list at end of chapter.)

Special beds are manufactured having been designed to achieve maintenance of appropriate positions and to allow automatic and/or continual turning. The 'rota-rest' bed is an example, its mechanism, electrically operated, turns the bed slowly through one hundred and thirty degrees, thus pressure on any point is never prolonged. A beneficial effect is also obtained on the lungs and possibly the kidneys. When the motor is switched off the bed remains stationary in any desired position so that nursing or physiotherapy procedures can be attended to. One great advantage of this type of bed is that a team is not needed for turning, therefore it is suitable for use both where there is a staff shortage and for use in the home for tetraplegic patients who cannot turn themselves even in the chronic stage.

Turning

Turning the patient in rotation from right side lying to supine, to left side lying and back to supine position is necessary during the early stage of bed-rest. At first the turns are at two-hourly intervals throughout each twenty-four hours but gradually this may be reduced to three- or four-hourly turns providing there are no signs of threatened skin breakdown on pressure-bearing points such as the sacrum or the femoral trochanters. During the turn the position of the spine must be maintained and special instruction and training must be given to all personnel on the ward who at any time help to form the turning team. The senior nurse present must direct the team and ensure that the turn is correctly done, she also gives commands so that the timing of the turn is co-ordinated. During the turn, if necessary, linen is changed, the undersheet is straightened and meticulous care is taken to ensure that no crumbs or other abrasive material are left in the bed. The skin must be inspected to detect any signs of threatening pressure sores. Care must be taken not to disturb the catheter, if present, or to pinch or compress this. If the patient has other intubation such as a naso-oesophageal tube or tracheostomy tube similar care of these must be observed. Further details of care of a tracheostomy tube and treatment for respiratory complications will be discussed later but it should be noted that physiotherapy techniques to help clear secretions and to assist coughing are frequently needed just before and after turning.

The nursing and physiotherapy staff work in close co-operation at all times but in the early stages of care of the cervical cord cases this is particularly necessary, not only to avoid too many disturbances for the patient, and to make the contribution of each team member more effective, but also because they often act as a substitute for each other. Physiotherapists frequently act as members of the turning or lifting team and all personnel working on a spinal unit are taught how to, and do, make the patient cough to help clear secretions.

Another important feature of the turn is that the limbs are repositioned at each turn. This not only ensures relief of pressure on bony points but helps maintenance of circulation and joint and soft tissue mobility. It is a disadvantage of the use of the automatically turning bed that the limb joints are not moved as it turns. Physiotherapy care for patients on these beds needs to be more frequent for this reason.

Chest care

Respiratory complications occur in patients with spinal cord lesions for many reasons, for example, pre-existing chronic respiratory disorder, lowered resistance to infection, paralysis of muscles of inspiration or those needed for effective coughing. An added factor is paradoxical respiration caused by paralysis of intercostal muscles. Details of physiotherapy will be given later in the sub-section on tetraplegia but any case of spinal cord injury or dysfunction from other causes may require treatment to prevent internal secretional obstruction and to improve the ventilation of the lungs. All cases should have respiratory function tests carried out regularly and the results should be recorded. Vital capacity measurements with a spirometer, peak flow measurements by a Wright's peak flow meter or the use of a Vitalograph machine are routine procedures in most spinal injuries units.

Care of urinary bladder and of excretion of urine and faeces

As the paraplegic or tetraplegic patient has double incontinence the care of the kidneys, urinary bladder and excretion of urine and faeces is as urgent and essential as care of the chest, skin and circulation. Ultimate responsibility for this is borne by the medical director but the task of catheterization in the early days of spinal shock and later of training an automatic bladder function, falls to the medical and nursing staff. The physiotherapist must however be fully aware of the need for care to avoid retention of urine, or infection of the bladder and also how to avoid damage to urinals by careless handling, positioning or application of splintage.

In later stages of treatment the activities of the patient are largely carried out by or in the presence of the therapist and she must realize that the insensitivity of the patient's skin prevents his awareness of the leakage of urine or faeces, or the twisting and trapping of any part of his urinal, therefore she must teach him by the example of her careful handling and observation and by instruction how to avoid such accidents. Tact is needed to help the patient accept the distressing complication of double incontinence, to be responsible ultimately for his own care of bladder and bowel function and to help him to realize how vital is such care not only to his social acceptability but to his general well-being.

Retention of urine or bladder infection not only have a direct effect on kidneys and general health but also greatly increase the severity of spasticity of the limbs. Obviously the care of these matters is even more difficult or impossible manually by tetraplegic patients but the responsibility can still be the patient's as he can request attention if needed and should be encouraged to take such responsibility for himself.

Transfers

Whether the patient can achieve these independently in the later stages of rehabilitation or has to depend on others to lift him from place to place, certain fundamental points apply. All members of the team concerned in any way with patient care should know how to lift patients alone or with help, and how he should lift himself, if possible, without damage to skin or joints. The physiotherapist can help instruct other personnel such as orderlies and nursing aides in this important procedure. Details will be given later of how to lift and how to teach the paraplegics to lift themselves.

Assessment and documentation of records

The capabilities of the patient, his control of movement, the extent of motor and sensory loss and also later his ability to compensate for motor loss must be assessed at regular intervals. Joint range and the presence of any deformity likely to impair function should also be considered. The examination of the patient and tests for functional ability including the respiratory function tests are carried out by several members of the team. The doctors, physiotherapists and occupational therapists all share this responsibility. Charts of function achievement specially prepared for paraplegic and tetraplegic patients are helpful.

ACHIEVEMENT CHART   PHYSIOTHERAPY AND OCCUPATIONAL THERAPY

NAME   CLINICAL DIAGNOSIS

AGE   CORD LEVEL

Weight and Pulley (Shoulder Extensors and Adductors)	........lbs.	........lbs.	........lbs.	........lbs.
Springs fixed to bed head (Triceps)	........lbs.	........lbs.	........lbs.	........lbs.

		A	Date	Ach	Date	Comments
Balance	i. Long sitting ii. High sitting					
Wheelchair management	i. Propulsion ii. Brakes iii. Pressure relief					
Transfers	Bed........Chair Toilet......Chair Floor.......Chair Bath........Chair Easy Chair..Chair Car........Chair					
Turning	i. Mat ii. Bed					

	A	Date	Ach	Date	Comments
A.D.L. i. Feeding **(Women)** ii. Drinking iii. Teeth iv. Washing and Drying v. Make-up vi. Hair					
Housecraft i. Kitchen ii. Housework iii. Laundry iv. Ironing					
Standing a. Bars **Walking** i. 4pt. ii. Swing-to iii. Swing-thro' b. Crutches i. 4pt. ii. Swing-to iii. Swing-thro'					
With crutches i. Transfers ii. Stairs iii. Kerbs iv. Uneven surfaces					
Dressing and i. Top half **undressing** ii. Bottom half iii. Shoes & Stockings					
A.D.L. i. Feeding ii. Drinking iii. Teeth iv. Washing & Drying v. Shaving vi. Hair vii. Emptying Urinal					
Communication i. Writing ii. Typing					
Sport i. Archery ii. Table Tennis iii. Swimming iv. Others					
Transport i. Normal ii. Hand Controls iii. Noddy					

A = Attempted   Ach = Achieve

Nurses measure and chart such things as body temperature, pulse and respiratory rate, arterial blood pressure, fluid intake and output.

All records must be carefully dated and filed and be freely available to other team members.

Regular consultation between all team members at case conferences are needed and are greatly enhanced by well kept records.

For references and further reading see end of Chapter X, p. 234.

CHAPTER IX

Physiotherapy in Spinal Cord Lesions (1)

by BARBARA GOFF, O.N.C., M.C.S.P., DIP.T.P.

Both the degree of potential independence a patient can achieve and the necessary physiotherapy vary according to the level and severity of damage to the spinal cord. Details of treatment will be discussed in several sections.

COMPLETE LOW PARAPLEGIA

If a fracture of the ninth thoracic vertebra causes damage to the spinal cord the segments involved will be in the region of the twelfth thoracic and first and second lumbar cord segments. The roots of the twelfth thoracic and first lumbar nerves may also be damaged as may nerve roots of thoracic nine, ten and eleven as they also lie within the neural canal at the level of the fracture (see Fig. VIII/1, p. 174).

Severe damage to the cord at this level is a frequent consequence of fracture-dislocation of the spine and results in permanent neurological dysfunction. This level of lesion has been selected as typical of a complete low level paraplegia. 'Complete' is taken to mean a lesion in which no voluntary control of muscles returns and in which the complete sensory loss is permanent. In some such cases there is clinical evidence that motor centres in the mid-brain may have some influence over the spinal reflex activity of the undamaged cord segments below the lesion. This implies that there may be nerve conduction via some upper motor pathways although those necessary for willed movement are interrupted.

As onset is sudden, spinal shock occurs and persists for several weeks. Medical and nursing care is as described in the previous chapter.

197

Physiotherapy will now be described, giving details of the most important techniques at various stages of rehabilitation.

Treatment in the early stage

The aims of physiotherapy are to help prevent the complication of deep vein thrombosis; to help maintain a good circulation to the lower limbs, thus lessening the risk of pressure sores and to maintain range of joints and soft tissue. As soon as is allowed strengthening exercises are given for the upper limbs. The exact time after injury depends on the stability or otherwise of the spine and whether there are any fractures of the clavicle or ribs. Activity also helps to achieve another aim which is to aid the patient's psychological adjustment to his disability.

Only cases with pre-existing chronic chest disorders or trauma to the chest at the time of injury are likely to need intensive physiotherapy to maintain or improve respiratory function.

During all treatments the principle of preserving the correct position of the spine and its immobility must be observed. Care is taken not to disturb the catheter. Vigilant observation of skin colour and temperature is necessary and signs of any circulatory abnormality such as oedema must be noted and reported, as should any sign of return of muscle tone to the leg muscles.

METHODS

Passive movements to the legs are done at least twice daily in the first three to six weeks and possibly reduced to once a day later if good circulation and range are being maintained. As hip extension to neutral is not possible in the lowermost limb with the patient in side lying it may be necessary to visit the patient several times so that each leg can be treated when it is uppermost.

Sensitive handling is needed because damage can occur to soft tissue around joints especially during the stage of spinal shock. It is also necessary later to guard against eliciting spinal reflexes. The physiotherapist must learn to feel when the limit of joint and soft tissue range is approached. Movements should be in normal patterns, performed slowly and eventually in full range at least twice at each handling. During the first few weeks pain at the site of the lesion may limit slightly the range obtained on passive movement.

Maintenance of the length of some structures which pass over more than one joint is especially important to prevent deformity which would later hamper good function such as long-sitting, standing, or crutch walking. Overstretching of soft tissue is harmful but functional length must be maintained in the following structures: muscles, tendons, ligaments, and fascia. For long-sitting length is needed in the hamstrings. Requirements necessary for standing are full hip extension, full knee extension and length of calf and fascia sufficient to allow at least 90° at the ankle with knee straight and the foot flat on the floor. Toes should not be allowed to curl or claw so that shoes can be put on easily and do not cause pressure sores.

To improve circulation passive leg movements are repeated for at least three minutes to each leg and for this purpose need not be in full range. The legs are moved one at a time and care is taken not to allow sufficient hip flexion to cause movement of the lumbar spine. If there is any sign of oedema careful measurement of girth of the calf is made, recorded and subsequently repeated for comparison. The prothrombin time is taken and the leg movements stopped until the doctor's instructions are obtained to recommence these.

After treatment the pillows supporting the legs and feet are replaced correctly.

The exact number of treatments needed each day depends upon such factors as the method of nursing and turning the patient, his age and the probability of circulatory complications. For example, when the automatic turning bed is used limb movements by physiotherapists are needed more frequently than for patients who are turned manually as in the latter case leg positions are changed at each two, three or four-hourly turn.

When spinal shock wears off, muscle tone returns to the leg muscles and very careful nursing and handling during physiotherapy are needed to prevent reinforcement of spasticity. The physiotherapist's hands should be smooth and warm and care taken not to elicit either a flexor withdrawal or an extensor thrust. Pressure through the heel and the long axis of the limb together with slow smooth movements tend to elicit a postural response of all deep muscles acting on the knee and ankle. These then work in combination to stabilize the joint as they do in normal weight-bearing and total spastic movements are inhibited (Plate IX/1).

Exercises. Six to eight weeks after onset some increasing activity of upper limbs is usually allowed. Exercises are given to strengthen the arm and upper trunk muscles and to maintain full range of movement in preparation for transfers, use of wheelchair and crutch walking. Any suitable method of graded resisted exercises is used and progressed as the muscles strengthen. Strong grip, elbow extension, shoulder adduction and extension and depression of the shoulder girdle are needed for activities.

Instability of the spine or pain in the back may delay the start of greater activity but at eight to twelve weeks after injury the patient is usually allowed to commence taking weight vertically through the spine. During the rest period a wheelchair is ordered and it is ready by the time the patient gets up. Full length band-topped calipers, hinged at the knee, are measured for and supplied, either at the end of the bed stage or early in the weight-bearing stage.

Residual neurological defects are now apparent and must be assessed and recorded. The level of cutaneous and kinaesthetic loss is from thoracic eleven or twelve downwards including the skin of the lower trunk, buttocks and legs and joint sensation of pelvis and legs. The lower portions of the trunk muscles, the hip flexors and adductors are often found to remain flaccid when spinal shock wears off. This is because the lower motor neurone cells at thoracic twelve and lumbar one and two cord segmental levels are destroyed by the damage to the cord.

The nerve roots of thoracic nine to twelve spinal nerves are also likely to be damaged at the level of the spinal injury where they lie within the neural canal.

The remainder of the leg muscles usually show spasticity because the lower part of the cord is not damaged but is partially or completely isolated from the influence of the brain and shows only spinal reflex activity.

The severity of spasticity varies with the efficiency of early treatment, with the position of the patient and in response to incoming stimuli from the skin, deep structures of the legs and from the urinary bladder. If involuntary spasms occur the risk of pressure sores is increased. Sores, bladder infection, and contractures in soft tissue all increase stimuli likely to elicit spasms and aggravate spasticity. A vicious cycle may result as increased spasticity and uncontrolled spasms predispose to a greater risk of contractures, sores, bladder dysfunction and later, when the patient is allowed up, to poor posture and function (see Fig. IX/1). It is affected by psychological stress and is much more troublesome in some patients than in others. Although so many factors influence spasticity an attempt should be made to evaluate its severity. Techniques to try to relieve spasticity and to prevent its reinforcement will be discussed in the next section of this chapter. It must be remembered that there is a great risk of dominance by the flexor withdrawal

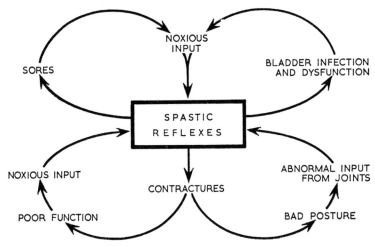

Fig. IX/1 Vicious cycles

reflex in complete cord lesions unless adequate treatment is given to prevent this.

Stage when weight-bearing through the spine is permitted

Treatment is rapidly progressed to increasing activity by the patient. The nursing staff are usually responsible for sitting the patient up in bed with the back supported by a back rest. Physiotherapy is given with the patient sitting up in bed to commence balance training and lifts to relieve pressure.

When the patient is allowed to sit out in a wheelchair the aims of treatment are as follows:

Firstly readjustment of postural sense and equilibrium reactions. The patient must learn to retain a good posture and to maintain balance in many positions without the support of a back rest or his arms (see Fig. IX/2, overleaf). The physiotherapist must try to understand that until the patient sits up for the first time with no support or contact with a supporting surface for his head, trunk or arms he cannot fully

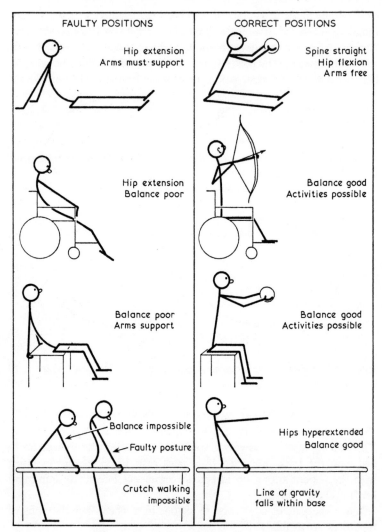

Fig. IX/2 Correct and faulty positions

realize the consequence of the sensory loss in the lower part of his body.

Posture correction and balance is trained with the patient sitting on a pillow on a low plinth. The feet should be supported on the floor or a low platform so that the thighs are fully supported and the hips, knees and ankles are at a right angle. The physiotherapist should take great care that the patient does not fall or damage his buttocks or legs.

The patient is lifted to the plinth by two people until he is strong and has learned to transfer himself safely. Use of a mirror may be helpful at first and any suitable method of balance training is used. Arm movements are given when balance is good and activities including ball games are added as soon as possible.

Balance is also practised in the wheelchair. Use of the chair, negotiation of slopes, curbs and picking up objects from the floor are all taught (see Plate IX/2).

Secondly, care of skin and joints must be taught by example of careful handling and by instruction. All insensitive parts are protected by vigilant observation, avoidance of extremes of temperature, careful positioning and inspection. A hand mirror is used by the patient to inspect the skin over the sacrum and ischial tuberosities. He is instructed to report to the nursing staff immediately he suspects that there is any sign of skin damage.

There should be a firm base to the bed to prevent a sagging mattress which causes creases in the sheet. During long periods of sitting in a wheelchair the skin over the ischial tuberosities must be protected by using a wooden-based, sheepskin-covered, firm sorbo cushion. Regular lifts performed by the patient himself, relieve pressure and allow return of circulation to the skin. The lifts must be maintained for fifteen to thirty seconds and are needed every fifteen minutes when the patient first sits up. Some patients eventually need to lift at less frequent intervals but the relief of pressure soon becomes an automatic action.

The patient can turn himself in bed and a habit of doing so is established. Regular reminders by the night staff may be needed until turning is automatic. The patient is taught to use the prone lying position to eliminate sacral pressure.

The length of time that the patient is allowed up is gradually increased. He must be taught to observe the position of his legs and to lift them carefully when moving.

Thirdly the patient learns self-care. He must be able to wash, dress, attend to his own urinal, maintain joint range in the legs by doing his own passive movements and apply his calipers. These activities are taught by several members of the team but balance in the long-sitting position must be achieved to facilitate good function.

Activities such as transfers (see Plates IX/3 to IX/8) are taught from and to the wheelchair and the bed, plinth, bath, lavatory seat, motorized vehicle etc. Also taught, is safe transfer from and to a mat for treatment sessions. Various methods are tried out and the best for the individual is finally selected.

In teaching safe transfers the principles include correct positioning of the chair, ensuring that the brakes are fully on and lifting the legs with the hands onto the plinth, bed or floor from the footplates of the chair. During these manoeuvres care must be taken not to knock the legs or drag them along a hard surface. When the legs are positioned correctly the trunk is lifted so that the buttocks are clear of the support and will not be dragged or knocked as the transfer is completed.

In transferring from a wheelchair to a plinth the approach can be from the side or one end. In the former case the chair is placed slightly obliquely alongside the plinth, the arm of the chair on the near side is removed and if necessary a pillow placed over the top of the large wheel of the chair; the brakes are applied securely. Next the legs are lifted and placed on the plinth, the far leg is sometimes crossed over the other. Then the near-side hand is placed on the plinth sufficiently centrally to allow room for the buttocks to be placed on the plinth also, the other hand is placed on the far side-arm of the chair. A good high lift of the trunk follows and it is swung over onto the plinth and the long-sitting position is thus obtained.

Alternatively the chair can be placed about fourteen inches from one end of the plinth, the brakes applied and the legs lifted one at a time and placed on the plinth in front of the chair. The brakes are then released, the chair wheeled close up to the plinth and the brakes reapplied securely. As the chair approaches the plinth the legs move along the plinth but care must be taken to see that they slide smoothly with no possible risk of abrasion. The hands are placed on the front of the chair arms and a high lift of the trunk given with a thrust forward carrying the patient's buttocks well onto the plinth. Care is needed to see that the skin is not knocked or dragged along. Once in the new position the patient must lean forward quickly to keep the line of gravity through the trunk falling well within the base provided by the legs and buttocks. The knees are then slightly flexed by the patient's hands and a further lift forward completes the transfer well onto the plinth.

In both methods of transfer there is a risk of the chair moving if the tyres are worn or the floor slippery. The patient soon learns to be cautious and to position the chair correctly to avoid slipping between the chair and the plinth. (Plates IX/3 to IX/8 illustrate some stages of transfers.)

A programme of resisted exercises is arranged for all spared muscles. Mat work (see Plate IX/10 and IX/11), transfers, use of weight and pulley circuits (see Plate IX/12), including the use of a Westminster pulley circuit and also proprioceptive neuromuscular facilitation techniques of manually resisted trunk and limb patterns of movement are all useful.

Sport is now included, for example, swimming, team ball games in wheelchairs, archery and field events. These achieve many objectives, for example, they provide strong exercise, balance training, stimulation of increased exercise tolerance and an opportunity for social activities in the evenings and at weekends in competition with other patients.

Stance and gait are trained as soon as sitting balance is good. Standing balance in leg calipers is taught in parallel bars (see Plate IX/9 (a) and (b)). The posture is very important as the weight must be over the feet to keep upright without the control of muscular power in gluteal muscles and hamstrings. The patient must learn to pay attention to sensation in the upper trunk and compensate for loss of equilibrium reactions in the legs and lower trunk. The hips must be slightly hyperextended and the dorsal spine straight. Many patients can maintain good balance for short periods without the support of both arms. This skill is essential for a good 'swing-to' or 'swing-through' gait (see Plate IX/15).

To get to standing from the wheelchair the patient first extends the knees passively and locks the knee hinges in extension. Some patients need to place the leg on a support to achieve this, others manage by a 'high kick' type of lift or by extending the leg out in front of the chair with the foot on the floor. When both knees are locked in extension, and the chair correctly placed with the brakes on, the buttocks are lifted forward to the front of the chair seat, the hands grip the parallel bars or wall bars and a lift up and forward takes the body into the standing position. Care is needed to see that the feet do not slip forwards (see Plate IX/13).

In the early stages of training, weak patients, or those with short arms, may need assistance and the physiotherapist stands in front of the patient, between the bars, placing her feet in front of the patient's shoes and if necessary gripping the top of trousers or slacks to assist the action of standing.

Gait is trained at first in parallel bars progressing to one crutch and one bar as the patient gains confidence and proficiency. Finally two crutches are used and steps, slopes, curbs, rough surfaces and stairs are negotiated if possible. The four-point gait is the most elegant and takes least room in a crowded place. However the swing-to or swing-through gait is quicker and most young patients with strong arms can achieve this method of crutch walking. Elbow crutches with swivel tops are used so that the patient can stand and rest his forearm on the upturned arm support and have his hand free to open doors etc.

When the patient is proficient in crutch walking he learns to get up from the chair to standing, place the crutches correctly for use, turn and walk away from the chair. This activity needs careful planning, strong arms and upper trunk and good equilibrium reactions to gain balance once upright. The exact method is usually worked out by each patient to suit his or her particular abilities. The physiotherapist uses her experience to help each patient learn this activity. A demonstration by a more experienced patient, such as one back in hospital for review, can be most helpful.

One method of standing up from the wheelchair with no other support than the chair will be described. The turn can be to either side to suit the individual's abilities but will be described as for turning to the left. The chair is placed with the back against a wall or firm support and the brakes secured. The calipers are locked in extension and the right leg lifted across the left. The shoulders and trunk are twisted to the left so that the left hand is placed behind the patient's trunk on the right chair arm and the right across in front of the trunk onto the left arm of the chair. A good high lift follows with a twist of the pelvis to bring the patient to standing facing the chair. He then achieves balance in standing so that he can release one arm to reach and place his crutches ready to back away from the chair and walk.

Other methods may be possible, each patient should be encouraged to find the most suitable method for his ability. The crutches must be placed near or leaning against the chair so that they are within reach once stance is achieved. Patients should be encouraged to discuss their achievements and difficulties during treatment sessions, and group activities are of great psychological value.

Overcoming physical difficulties can be a source of great fun and the sense of achievement is similar to that of learning any new skill. To create a happy atmosphere but one of hard work should be the objective of every physiotherapist working in a spinal unit.

Transport in a petrol-driven car is encouraged in either one supplied by the Department of Health and Social Security to a disabled driver or in a specially adapted car of his own. Transfers to and from these and lifting a transit chair into and out of the car must be taught and arrangements made for driving instruction.

Another principle is to assess fully the patient's ability and function charts are useful to record this. Regular reassessments are helpful, not only to note progress but to stimulate the patient's interest and to help to wean him from dependence on physiotherapy or nursing staff. Detailed sensory charts are completed by the medical staff or may be the responsibility of physiotherapists. Tests of voluntary power are only appropriate for muscles completely or partially denervated by loss of lower motor neurones at the level of the lesion. Power in spastic muscles cannot be graded on a voluntary power scale but the severity of spasticity should be evaluated and recorded.

During the time of increasing activity the *medical social worker* and the *occupational therapist* will discuss possible occupational training which may be needed, also any necessary alterations to the home.

Every encouragement should be given to include *relatives in the rehabilitation* of patients from an early stage. For example they are shown by the physiotherapist how to help the patient care for his skin and how to maintain full joint and soft tissue range.

As can be seen by the variety and extent of the new skills the patient must learn, there should be very little time for inactivity. A full day's programme five or six days a week is helpful in maintaining a work habit and is of immense psychological value. He should be responsible for his own timekeeping as this helps to restore self-respect and wean him from depending on nursing staff and physiotherapists.

Before the patient is finally discharged he is usually allowed home for weekends. This allows for a gradual adjustment to his new situation and on his return any problems encountered can be discussed. Time spent at home is eventually increased to periods of a week or longer before final discharge.

Follow-up after discharge by frequent reviews is needed to provide continuing support when the patient returns to the community.

At review the following must be checked: the range of joints and soft tissue, the health of the bladder and of the skin, also the state of splints, crutches and the wheelchair. Any problems which have occurred can be discussed and all help given to maintain full independence.

INCOMPLETE LOW PARAPLEGIA

A lesion at the same level as that discussed above but less severe may only partially damage the cord. Such damage results in an incomplete paraplegia. Spinal shock may not occur, or if it does, lasts only a few days or weeks. Muscle tone returns very quickly to those muscles supplied from the undamaged segments of the cord below the lesion. The reflex activity in the legs, elicited by handling the legs during nursing procedures or even spontaneously by contact with the bed clothes is often mistaken for return of voluntary power in leg muscles. This situation can raise false hope in the patient and his relatives who must be warned not to mistake reflex movement for recovery. No psychological harm is done from the caution if subsequently the patient does gain some control of movement.

Various syndromes result from a partial cord lesion at the twelfth thoracic and first and second lumbar cord segments. Posterior sensory tracts may be the most severely damaged tissue of the cord with the result that loss of kinaesthetic sense may be the main disability factor. Cutaneous sensation may be partially spared or almost complete cutaneous anaesthesia result.

Autonomic motor function may be disrupted producing circulatory defects in the legs. Usually reflex and voluntary control of the bladder reflexes and control of micturition are disturbed, the degree of dysfunction being variable. The bladder wall may be flaccid or spastic and each contribute to complications such as retention of urine or infection of the urinary tract. The external sphincter is usually flaccid so there is incontinence of urine.

The motor signs also vary considerably from case to case. The hip flexors and adductors and lower parts of the abdominal muscles are usually flaccid because the lower motor neurones in the anterior horn of grey matter are destroyed at the level of the lesion. All the other leg muscles are usually spastic but there may be some control of movement in total spastic patterns of flexor withdrawal or extensor thrust. The lack of control of isolated movements and the release of primitive spinal reflex mass movement is caused by interruption of some fibres in the cortico-spinal tracts.

The hypertonicity is of the spastic type similar to that in the stage of residual signs of spastic hemiplegia caused by a cerebrovascular accident (see also Chapter XIII). The extensor thrust pattern usually predominates unless the patient is inactive, or gets severe bladder complications or pressure sores in which circumstances a flexor withdrawal reflex becomes dominant. If the hip flexors and abdominal muscles are weakened or denervated completely the flexor withdrawal is not as strong as it is if these muscles are innervated and therefore play a part in the withdrawal reflex. Sometimes upper motor tracts from the basal ganglia, reticular formation and the vestibular nuclei are still partially intact and so release of tonic reflexes influences the spinal reflexes. An example of this is observable if the patient has a much stronger extensor thrust in the supine position than in side lying or prone lying which indicates some release of the tonic labyrinthine reflexes.

As stated above a vicious cycle can develop if spasticity is allowed to increase the risk of sores and contractures (see Fig. IX/1, p. 201).

Treatment in the early stage

The aims and methods of treatment are as described for a complete lesion. As muscle tone returns very quickly positioning in bed may become difficult to maintain and if flexor spasms occur the trunk position is disturbed. Should this occur the instability of the spine may allow further displacement at the fracture site endangering the cord anew. For this reason surgery may be contemplated to ensure stability and possibly also with the hope of relieving some pressure on the cord with relief of neurological damage.

Because the cord lesion is only partial the neurological signs may change rapidly as inflammation subsides. The physiotherapist must be especially observant as she performs passive movements to the legs. Any change in muscle tone, sign of voluntary control of movement or of return of sensation should be recorded and reported to the medical director. Prognosis depends on the extent and rate of recovery of neurological function in the first weeks after onset.

If there is sensory sparing the patient should be encouraged to think of the movements of the legs as the physiotherapist performs these. Similarly if some voluntary control of movement returns at this stage he is encouraged to try to assist leg movements as the physiotherapist performs them.

An explanation of spasticity should be attempted by the physiotherapist to the patient. This often proves difficult and the difficulty in controlling a spastic limb with imperfect voluntary movement is more frustrating to some patients than is the acceptance of a completely paralysed one.

Even during the early stage of bed rest the physiotherapist must try to elicit a postural response of support and stability rather than a mass movement of the leg. Quick movements must be avoided and the placing of skin contacts selected with great care. Methods of handling suitable for a spastic paralysis are discussed in Chapter VI. These should be used and those found most effective selected (see Plate IX/1).

Another important consideration is that strong muscle work in the unaffected parts may cause overflow to the lower segments of the cord. This may elicit spasms or reinforce spasticity so the programme of muscle strengthening for the arms may have to be modified.

The time needed for healing of the spinal injury is as for a complete lesion.

Stage when weight-bearing through the spine is permitted

This is similar to that described for a complete low paraplegia so only the difference of treatment which may be needed will be discussed.

If not previously completed a *full assessment of sensory loss and motor ability must* now be carried out. Some attempt must be made to grade the severity and distribution of spasticity. This is not easy as the factors influencing spasticity are many and vary from time to time. The testing position influences the dominance of flexor or extensor reflexes as will the combinations of position or movement requested or imposed by the examiner. Most favourable and least favourable conditions should be estimated and noted as a guide to planning treatment and for comparison with subsequent findings.

In estimating joint range and range of soft tissues the influence of spasticity must not be overlooked as this can so easily mask true joint and soft tissue range. An example of this is the apparent tightness in the calf and apparent lack of control and power in the dorsiflexors of the ankle if the movement of dorsiflexion or control of this movement by the patient is attempted whilst the knee is held passively extended.

If the spasticity of the calf is reduced by appropriate procedures the foot can usually be brought to a right angle with the knee straight and the patient may even be able to control this combination of positions of knee and ankle voluntarily.

The patient must learn *self-care, postural control* and must practise all activities needed in preparation for *transfers, stance* and *gait*. The principles involved are those discussed for a complete paraplegia and methods are similar. However, modifications must be made in teaching activities according to the individual differences of each patient's abilities, symptoms and signs.

Where sensory loss is complete, care of skin, joints, and teaching postural adjustments are tackled in the ways described above. Even when some control of movement is spared, spasticity usually complicates all activities. The methods used to reduce spasticity and teach transfers, stance and gait must be selected with great care and frequent adjustments made to achieve the best possible function. The physiotherapist must learn from experience to be aware which positions, stimuli and techniques are helpful and which elicit an undesirable result. Reinforcement of spasticity by strong resisted arm and trunk exercises must be avoided and yet the patient must be encouraged to be active. The patient must be aware that in his efforts to gain independence he must learn to manage his spastic limbs in such a way that he does not elicit spasms so defeating the purpose.

It is impossible to give techniques suitable for each case and every physiotherapist must use the techniques she can use successfully. However, certain basic principles should be considered and these will be discussed briefly.

The flexor withdrawal and the extensor thrust are both mass movements, neither is suitable to support the weight of the body or useful for activities, such as standing from sitting, standing or walking.

Every consideration must be given to providing afferent stimuli which produce a stabilizing co-contraction of the deep muscles whose activity results in providing a mobile but stable postural background. If this can be achieved the patient will be able to realize his potential for independence.

Preparation must be planned for good postures of sitting, prone kneeling, kneeling and standing (see Fig. IX/2, p. 202). The patient must learn to elicit a postural response rather than a spastic total movement. For example the spasticity of the calf is often a great nuisance, prevents a good stance and makes walking almost impossible. The length of the soleus is the key to the situation and a slow maintained lengthening must be achieved by the physiotherapist and by the patient before standing is attempted. Even if long leg calipers are needed and even if an attempt is made to control the extensor thrust by ankle control on the caliper a reduction of spasticity prior to standing will be of great benefit. If no caliper is needed the patient should sit in a good position with the heels firmly on the floor and some weight through the tibiae should be provided by pressure on the knees. The pressure should be maintained for five minutes or until the calf relaxes.

Insufficient hip flexion to get the weight of the trunk well over the feet is another fault of sitting posture. This is likely if the extensor thrust is strong and is also contributed to by too much decline in the angle of the back of the chair (see Fig. IX/2, p. 202). The patient must learn to lean well forward, keeping the spine straight and head posture good.

When the correct starting position is achieved the patient is instructed and helped if necessary to stand, pushing the heels down, the hips forward and the shoulders up and back. The physiotherapist should help to keep the patient stable by pressure down through the legs by pressure on the iliac crests. Once a good standing position is achieved the trunk should be moved, keeping an upright posture, so that the weight is transferred from side to side, from before backwards and in a turning motion rocking over the feet. At all times the aim is to keep good pressure on the heels and avoid a sudden stretch of the ball of the foot which elicits a thrust pattern.

When the patient is sitting in a wheelchair or on a stool and in long-sitting the correct posture must always be attempted. Line drawings are given in Fig. IX/2 to illustrate good and bad postures.

A position which has been found useful for patients with spasticity is a modified cross-sitting. The hips are flexed, laterally rotated and abducted, the knees flexed and the soles of the feet are in contact. This must be accompanied by a posture of erect spine, not a rounded spine and only in a sitting position so that it is not a flexor-withdrawal pattern of legs and trunk.

Standing with or without calipers with the support of parallel bars or a standing frame is helpful to reduce spasticity providing a good normal alignment of feet, legs and trunk can be achieved (see Fig. IX/2 and Plate IX/13 and 14). Some patients may not need long calipers but may find a below knee splint useful to control the ankle position.

The patient must be aware that a sudden stretch on the ball of the foot may elicit an extensor thrust and throw him backwards off balance.

Most patients with incomplete low paraplegia can walk well eventually but need the use of crutches, sticks or a 'fender' aid. They learn to negotiate stairs and obstacles but many need a wheelchair for long distances.

Resettlement problems are similar to those of patients with complete lesions and all the members of the team assist in solving difficulties. *Follow-up* is essential for these patients and at review a careful reassessment must be made especially of the spasticity and problems it may create. Length of soft tissues must be assessed to ensure that contractures are not developing. Good function, once achieved, is the best way to prevent deterioration.

LOW CORD LESIONS NOT CAUSED BY TRAUMA

Vascular accidents, neurofibromas, transverse myelitis, disease of bone such as tuberculosis and degenerative lesions, for example multiple sclerosis are among other causes of cord lesions. When these involve the upper lumbar cord segments the neurological symptoms are similar to those in an incomplete traumatic cord lesion.

Some lesions, for example transverse myelitis, occur suddenly and show signs of spinal shock. Other lesions are usually of gradual onset. The former are treated almost identically to patients with traumatic lesions except for the medical care which will include measures such as chemotherapy to control infection, or surgery to decompress lesions caused by abscesses or neurofibromata.

Other lesions may necessitate rest in bed to control bone disease in which case the treatment is similar to that for traumatic cases. Where the onset is very gradual the patient will probably not require in-patient treatment.

Physiotherapy in all cases follows the principles discussed for traumatic lesions of the spinal cord. A careful assessment must be made of the abilities of each patient and the causes of disability must be considered in planning suitable treatment. The precise regime is decided by the nature and extent of the signs and symptoms.

For references and further reading see end of Chapter X.

CHAPTER X

Physiotherapy in Spinal Cord Lesions (2)

by BARBARA GOFF, o.n.c., m.c.s.p., dip.t.p.

COMPLETE HIGH PARAPLEGIA

A cord lesion in the upper thoracic segments occurs with severe bone damage of the upper thoracic vertebrae, the cord level being one or two segments lower than the bone level. A cord lesion at thoracic three and four segments is taken to illustrate a case of typical high complete paraplegia.

The sensory loss will be from about the nipple line downwards so only the upper back and shoulders, the head and upper limbs will have normal sensation. Autonomic involvement will include extensive vasomotor paralysis leading to hypotension, which is a great problem when the patient first sits upright. The motor involvement includes a lower motor neurone lesion with flaccid paralysis of several pairs of intercostal muscles and spastic paralysis of the lower trunk muscles, the abdominals and all leg muscles. The spasticity is of the type found in complete cord lesions, there being only spinal reflex activity. The spasticity gradually becomes apparent as spinal shock disappears several weeks or months after onset.

In some cases there is evidence of some sparing of influence of the motor centres in the brain stem. This presents as released tonic reflexes. In other cases the trunk muscles remain flaccid when spinal shock wears off. The reason for this is not determined but one theory is that many nerve roots are permanently damaged at the time of the injury so a sensory and lower motor nerve lesion persists at several segments below the actual cord damage.

All bladder reflexes are absent at first but as tone returns in the wall and sphincters of the bladder it is often possible to establish a good automatic bladder emptying. The reflex centres of control of bladder and bowel are in the lumbar and sacral cord segments so these escape destruction. There is no voluntary control of the external sphincters so double incontinence occurs.

If, when the spinal shock wears off, the abdominal muscles are spastic, a severe type of flexor withdrawal spasm may be elicited by noxious stimuli from skin, bladder, the gut or from external stimuli such as a sudden loud noise. Both legs may be flexed simultaneously and the lumbar spine flex at the same time. These strong spasms are often painful and are easily reinforced as they instigate a vicious cycle of movement, rubbing of skin as the movement occurs, stretch of spastic muscles as the spasm fades, sores, contractures and visceral complications (see Fig. IX/1, p. 201).

Treatment in the early stage

This is exactly as described for a low lesion of the cord. The aims and methods of physiotherapy are the same as for low paraplegias and the only difference of detail is that a greater range of hip movement is usually permitted whilst the movements of the arms and head must be restrained if it produces pain or risk of movement at the unstable region of the spine.

An additional problem may be *chest complications*, the intercostals being flaccid at least in the early stage of spinal shock. Paradoxical movements of the thoracic cage occur, further reducing the ventilation already affected by inactivity of inspiratory intercostal muscles. In the early stages the abdominal muscles may not show rhythmical reciprocal action with the diaphragmatic excursions although when tone returns to muscles supplied from undamaged segments of the cord this automatic action may recover. Reflex coughing may also recover later but in the early stages will be absent making the removal of secretions from the lungs impossible by the patient's own efforts.

If secretions collect in the lungs physiotherapy will be needed at four-hourly intervals, or more frequently, throughout the day and may have to be continued during the night if any chest infection complicates the situation. Localized breathing should be attempted but is often impossible as the patient relies solely on diaphragmatic breathing. Vibrations and gentle shaking can be used if this does not cause pain or move the unstable spine. In a very few cases suction apparatus may be necessary for use with an endotracheal tube to help clear secretions from the upper respiratory tract. Inhalations and chemotherapy may also help relieve respiratory complications and smoking must be discouraged..

The combined resources of medical, nursing and physiotherapy personnel are needed if serious respiratory complications develop. Once secretions have collected in the upper respiratory tract the physiotherapist is able to assist coughing by careful placing of her hands or hands and one forearm and by giving firm pressure on the upper abdomen and lower parts of the chest in time with the patient's effort to give a forced expiration. This procedure needs experienced care both to be effective and to avoid damaging the chest cage or the contents of the abdominal cavity. Plate X/1 (a) and (b) shows the position of the hands for assisted coughing.

Auscultation and chest X-rays are used to locate areas especially involved in the collection of secretions or atelectasis but the physiotherapist learns from experience to palpate the chest to locate abnormalities of air entry.

Respiratory function tests are carried out each week or daily if thought necessary. Vital capacity is estimated by the use of a spirometer and the effective force of expiration by estimating the peak flow in litres per minute by the use of a peak flow meter.

Co-operation with nursing staff is essential for good treatment of respiratory complications. Secretions collect in the lower side of the chest and after each change of position these must be cleared. Timing must coincide with turns and the nurse and physiotherapist often work together to use chest care and suction techniques.

Treatment when weight-bearing through the spine is permitted

This follows the principles and methods described for low lesions. An added problem is that of postural hypotension which often occurs when the patient first sits up against the support of a backrest in bed. Instruction to take several deep breaths may relieve the symptom. In some cases an abdominal binder or belt of some kind may be needed to prevent syncope if the upright posture is taken too suddenly or maintained for too long. Later the tone returns to blood vessel walls but there remains a risk of a sudden fall in blood pressure when the patient stands or sits up from lying.

The same methods are used to *teach self-care, postural adjustment* and *activities* such as transfers as those described previously. Progress is slower than for low paraplegia and the ability of the patient is hampered by lack of postural stability and automatic postural adjustment of the spine. Arm movements are less effective lacking the fixator action of trunk muscles. Exercise tolerance is reduced by weakness of respiratory muscles and lack of control of the abdominal muscles. Patience and perseverance are needed by both patient and physiotherapist and encouragement must be given by all team members to help the patient overcome his disabilities and achieve good independence. As each activity and function is successfully tackled it is noted on the patient's functional activity chart, thus providing a record of his achievement and an incentive to further efforts.

Weaning the patient from dependence on others should be an objective of the medical team. This particularly applies to the physiotherapist who, whilst taking a pride in her patient's success, must not make him feel that her continuing help is essential.

Posture training is essential and balance in the wheelchair must be practised to allow good use of the chair without depending for support on the back and arms.

One useful method of safely reaching the footplates or floor with one arm is to hook the other arm behind the handle of the chair back thus preventing a fall should the line of gravity fall too far forwards.

Standing in overlapping plaster of Paris shells for the legs or in long calipers is practised. At first a tilting bed may be used so that the risk of collapse from hypotension is avoided. Another method is to use a standing frame, the tray in front of the patient prevents him falling forwards, a cushion is placed on this and the patient can lean forwards over it if he feels faint or giddy. Sheepskin-covered straps support the buttocks, keep the knees extended and prevent the heels from slipping back. A board slotted into a holder can be adjusted to a suitable position to prevent the toes slipping forward (see Plate IX/14).

Standing is encouraged even if crutch walking is thought to be of little use or impossible for the patient. The upright position helps to maintain good range of movement, health of leg bones, stimulates good kidney function, helps to reduce spasticity and is of psychological value also.

Fixed parallel bars or a standing frame can be supplied to the patient for use when he goes home so that he may continue to stand for periods of up to an hour several times a day.

Spasticity may become a problem and care must be taken to try to prevent its reinforcement. Sometimes all attempts to control flexor spasticity fail, in which case surgery may be needed to release tight structures. Permanent interruption of spinal reflex arcs may be attempted by neurosurgical means or by alcohol blocks introduced by subdural injections at the level of cord segments responsible for the severe flexor spasms.

Even in less severe cases sudden flexor spasms may endanger the stability of the patient whilst standing or sitting without the support of the arms.

If complications of bladder infection, pressure sores and contractures can be avoided the risk of troublesome spasms is greatly reduced. Good function, possible if no spasms occur, helps to maintain health of skin and bladder etc. Conversely a vicious cycle is set up if poor function or any complication arises. R. A. Kuhn states that 'Alteration in dominance of postural and protective reflexes may occur but extensor spasms are the natural outcome of complete transection of the cord in man if complications can be avoided.' (See References at end of this Chapter.)

Resettlement can be difficult for high level paraplegics, very few being able to return to a former occupation. The use of a wheelchair is essential for locomotion because crutch walking is only possible over short distances under ideal conditions. However, every effort should be made to return the patient to the community. As a famous lady, herself a paraplegic, says 'They do not want pity but opportunity'. (Baroness Masham; see References at end of this Chapter.)

INCOMPLETE HIGH PARAPLEGIA

Most high level paraplegias with bone lesions in the upper thoracic part of the spine are complete lesions but occasionally a crush fracture of the body of a thoracic vertebra results in a partial cord lesion. As discussed above in the section on incomplete low paraplegia the signs will vary considerably from mainly sensory involvement to mainly spastic paralysis.

Treatment in the early stage

This follows the principles and method for all traumatic cord lesions. Spinal shock occurs involving respiratory function, bladder reflexes and motor and sensory loss from the upper thoracic segments downwards. Nursing care and regular physiotherapy for chest care and passive movements are needed.

Spinal shock wears off rapidly and the residual signs become apparent. As with low level incomplete paralysis some control of movement may recover but reflex activity also returns early so may be mistaken for voluntary control of the limbs.

The exact methods of treatment are governed by the symptoms and treatment is planned accordingly. Should voluntary control return whilst the spine is still unstable the patient is encouraged to assist leg movements performed passively by the physiotherapist. The correct position of the legs must be maintained, however, and the patient must be instructed to try to maintain a good position in bed.

As with a partial low paraplegia there is a risk of dominance by spinal reflex movements of the legs and very careful handling and nursing are essential to try to prevent reinforcement of spasticity.

Stage when weight-bearing through the spine is permitted

The principles of treatment are similar to those for complete high lesions and for incomplete low lesions as discussed above.

A full assessment must be made and treatment planned to help each patient overcome his particular problems.

Even when some voluntary control of movement returns there is a likelihood of troublesome flexor spasms involving the abdominal muscles and hip flexors.

Treatment follows that described for a low partial lesion but even greater care is needed to avoid stimuli which may trigger off spasms which throw the patient off balance.

Hypotension may be a problem and the trunk instability may persist creating problems of poor posture, poor respiratory function and inadequate fixation for arm muscles.

These patients need encouragement and individual attention to help them realize their potential for independence.

Should flexor spasticity be very severe the solution by a spinal block is not considered if sensation is spared or some control of micturition has recovered.

Resettlement needs careful attention unless residual disability is minimal in which case the patient can usually return to his former occupation.

Follow-up is needed with reassessment to ensure that good function is being maintained.

COMPLETE TETRAPLEGIA

A cord lesion above the first thoracic cord segment involves some paralysis of the hand and arm muscles, sensory loss in the hands and possibly the arms and impaired circulation to the arms. As all four limbs are involved as well as the trunk such cases are known as tetraplegic patients.

The precise level of the lesion decides the degree of involvement of the arms and a physiotherapist working in a spinal injuries unit must be familiar with the segmental innervation of skin and muscles of the arm. The distribution of paralysis is not always symmetrical; one hand, wrist or elbow may be spared more control than the other. The principal nerve roots and cord segments which control each joint movement are summarized in Table II, Chapter VIII, p. 175.

It should be noted that a cord lesion at cervical seven or just below this leaves some control of elbow extension and wrist extension. One just below this leaves some control of flexion of the proximal interphalangeal joints of the fingers and some control of the thumb may be spared also. A higher level of lesion destroying the seventh and eighth cervical cord segments leaves elbow flexion intact but no elbow extension. High cord lesions occur with little or no control of any arm movement except some abduction, extension, and lateral rotation at the shoulder joint if the fifth cervical cord segment is spared.

The function possible when the patient is allowed up in a chair varies enormously according to the precise muscle power which is spared. Lower motor neurones in the injured segments are destroyed so a flaccid paralysis occurs of the muscles supplied by these segments. The loss of function is aggravated by loss of cutaneous and kinaesthetic sensation in the hands. Even when sensation and muscle power exist in the upper part of the arm an insensitive, powerless hand at the distal end of the limb makes motivation and use of the limb very unlikely.

An added problem is the loss of autonomic motor supply to the blood vessels, sweat glands and hair follicles of the denervated dermatomes. Trophic changes occur, the skin of the hand becoming dry and scaly and in severe cases changes in circulation and in bone health occur, similar to those in Sudeck's atrophy.

In very high cervical cord lesions the spinal cord segments supplying the lower part of the arm and hand may be intact but isolated from the high centres in the brain. A spastic paralysis can be observed in some patients with this type of lesion after the spinal shock wears off.

Paralysis of intercostal muscles and abdominal muscles produces effects on respiration similar to those already described as obtaining in high thoracic cord lesions and in very high levels of lesion the diaphragm may be weakened also.

The patient with a fracture dislocation of the cervical spine needs extremely careful handling and the attention available at the time of injury may have a profound influence on the final outcome. Whilst the neck is still unstable slight movement may increase cord damage. The patient should not be lifted from the stretcher except under the supervision of the surgeon. X-ray examination is carried out with the patient still on the stretcher unless the surgeon is present to direct the lift to an X-ray table. When the X-ray is available the surgeon will decide on the type of support needed. Skull traction is frequently used and special head and neck support also.

Treatment in early stages

The principles of nursing care and physiotherapy are observed. Intensive therapy is an urgent necessity to save the patient's life. Unless there is pre-existing chronic chest disease or an infection of the respiratory tract occurs a tracheostomy should not be necessary. The secretions are cleared from the chest by regular physiotherapy consisting of gentle vibrations and shaking, timed to follow immediately before and after a turn to change the patient's position. Co-operation with nursing staff is essential, the nurse usually clearing secretions from the throat by the use of suction apparatus and an endotracheal tube. Sips of a drink made from diluted unsweetened fresh lemon juice are helpful, as are inhalations or the introduction of a small quantity of fluid into the endotracheal tube, for example a solution of bicarbonate of soda. The aim of this is to reduce the viscosity of secretions.

Assisted coughing is attempted but in the early stages must be very gently and cautiously performed to avoid any damage to the ribs or abdominal contents. Whilst spinal shock is present there is no tone at all in the abdominal muscles and similarly the tone is low in the walls of the gut. In these circumstances a firm compression of the abdominal wall is likely to cause damage to the gut and so produce further complications. The risk of a paralyticus ileus must not be overlooked.

Respiratory function tests are carried out as described for high paraplegics. *Passive movements* must be performed as described for paraplegia and movements to the upper limbs must be included. The length of biceps must be maintained so that the hand can be brought flat on a supporting surface with the forearm pronated, the elbow extended and the shoulder adducted and extended. This combination of positions of the segments of the arm is necessary to prop up the trunk during certain activities when the patient is allowed up. It is also needed for self-care and feeding. Similarly a functional length must be maintained in the long finger flexors. However, these must not be overstretched because if wrist extension is actively possible the hand may be able to grip objects by a 'tenodesis' action. This is a passive flexion of the joints of the fingers produced by active hyperextension of the wrist. If the long finger flexor tendons are overstretched such an action is not possible.

Circulation to the hand is frequently very poor and the maintenance of range in the joints of the hands is then very difficult. A roll of sorbo rubber is placed in the hand to try to preserve a good position. One method of trying to control oedema in the hand is the use of inflatable plastic splints. These are placed around the hands and forearms, care being taken to see that the whole hand is encircled, then the splints are inflated until a comfortable gentle squeeze is experienced on the fingers of the physiotherapist when she places them within the grip of the splint. These splints are left on for up to twenty minutes once or twice a day. Ideally a pump should be connected to the valve of the splint so that an intermittent pumping action is obtained. Care is needed to ensure that the pressure is not too high, for the patient cannot guard against this as the hands have no sensation.

The length of soft tissue must be preserved. Elbow extension is difficult to maintain if the elbow flexors are active and the extensors flaccid or very weak. The patient bends his arms and cannot then extend them. A splint or padded board to which the extended arm is bandaged is useful but must be carefully applied and removed to allow repeated rapid passive movements to be given to help maintain the circulation to the hand.

In a very high cervical lesion the biceps may be spastic which also causes a problem and often contractures at the elbow. The posterior fibres of deltoid become tight unless full length is maintained by passive movement.

During all treatment the *stability of the neck* must be maintained. If the patient is on skull traction this must be maintained during the turns. Whilst the patient must have treatment for the chest and arms great care is needed to give adequate treatment, whilst preserving the correct neck posture. Vigorous shoulder or shoulder girdle movements must be avoided. Careless handling or neglect of arm movements may cause a periarthritis.

Some patients suffer pain which may arise in the neck or in the shoulder joint. The exact cause of this is debatable but one theory is that it is caused by irritation of nerve roots from the cervical segments of the cord. Every possible means should be used to maintain as good a range of movement as is feasible and the health of the skin, bone, ligaments, muscles etc. in the forearm and hand. Thus whatever muscle power is spared the best possible use can be made of it.

The psychological problems for the patient and relatives are very great. A realistic outlook must be taken by the physiotherapist who must not get emotionally involved in the patient's problems. It is cruel to raise false hope but equally so to offer no hope at all. Whilst the patient is in bed the long hours of inactivity are almost overwhelming for some, but the realization of the extent and permanence of their disability is gradual. Once the patient is allowed to sit up in a chair as much activity as is possible and tolerable will help him to have a more positive and objective outlook.

Stage when weight-bearing is permitted through the spine

As for other levels of cord lesion the degree of stability of the vertebral column decides when weight may be taken through it. In the case of cervical cord lesions a sorbo collar to support the neck is sometimes needed when the patient is first propped up against the support of a back rest.

Postural hypotension is an almost inevitable complication of cervical cord lesions although as tone returns to trunk and leg muscles some adjustment occurs. The use of an abdominal binder or support of some kind assists the control of this problem and also allows a measure of stability to the trunk.

A semi-reclining chair with a high back is used for patients with a high cervical lesion. Later the patient may be able to tolerate a more vertical trunk position in sitting and a lower chair back.

A tilting table of some kind is very useful, especially one with a mechanical device to tilt it. The patient is lifted onto the table which is covered with a suitable soft mattress or foam rubber pad, a pillow is placed under the head and one over the hips. Straps secure the patient to the table at the knee and the hip and it is then raised at the head end until it is almost vertical. Two attendants must be present to help to keep the patient firmly and correctly positioned and to ensure that the table can be swiftly lowered to the horizontal position should the patient suffer from syncope. The upright position is only maintained for a very short period at first; just for a few minutes. The time is gradually increased as the patient's tolerance of the vertical position improves. Later still the patient can be supported in a standing frame or in parallel bars if leg splints of some kind are used.

Chest physiotherapy can be more vigorous than in the early stages. If necessary more vigorous assistance can be given whilst the patient is breathing out. This is done when the patient is in supine or side lying. One positioning of the hands and forearm for assisted coughing for a tetraplegic patient is shown in Plate X/1. Correct timing is essential to achieve a good result. A specimen of sputum should be collected for pathological examination if a chest infection occurs, and regular treatment given as often as is necessary.

Adjustment of posture and balance must be taught. Extreme patience and encouragement are needed on the part of the physiotherapist and she must be vigilant in her care to ensure that the patient does not fall or become very frightened of doing so. Although substitution by sight for lost kinaesthetic sense is encouraged, the use of a mirror is distasteful to some patients.

These patients must be helped to be more aware of subtle changes of position of the head than is usual and to compensate quickly if their balance and stability are threatened. Slight head movements and arm movements may correct the alignment of body segments sufficiently to maintain a sitting position or the arms may be used in a saving reaction.

A good position of the legs with the feet on the floor under the knees, a right angle at ankle, knee and hip and the legs in slight abduction gives a measure of stability to the trunk even though the patient has no control of movement and has no sensation below neck level.

Balance is practised in long sitting and in the wheelchair once the patient has gained sufficient confidence and adjustment of vasomotor function to allow this.

Self-care of the skin is taught even if the patient cannot actually do this for himself. The responsibility is his for seeing that he is lifted at frequent intervals. He must request the nursing staff or other therapists who are with him to lift him so that the circulation can return adequately to areas taking his weight.

One method of lifting a seated paralysed patient to relieve the weight on the ischial tuberosities is as follows: The patient folds his arms, the lifter stands behind with his arms, under the patient's shoulders and hands gripped over the patient's forearms (see Plate X/2). It is then possible to give a sufficiently high lift to allow the return of circulation to the buttock region. The lift must last for at least fifteen seconds. It is repeated as frequently as necessary to keep the skin in a healthy condition. Later the patient is taught to relieve pressure himself by rolling onto one buttock and then onto the other (see Plate X/3 (a), (b) and (c)).

As described previously the use of a firm base to a firm foam cushion, which is covered in sheepskin, helps to prevent pressure sores.

Training in the care of the hands is included. Gloves or special palm mittens are worn whilst wheeling the chair. Cigarette holders must be used if the patient smokes. Hot plates and mugs must not be placed in the hand or rested on the legs. Gloves must be worn in cold weather and for activities such as gardening.

The patient is responsible for requesting that the skin is inspected daily and that the urinal is not causing friction (see list of reminders at the end of this chapter).

There is a great difference in functional ability of a patient with voluntary control of elbow extension and one who has none.

A patient with control of an active triceps can support himself firmly on one or both arms, lift safely to relieve pressure on his seat and wheel his chair strongly even with no active control of the hand.

If triceps is active some use is usually possible also in the wrist extensors as these share the same segmental supply from cervical seven nerve root. With gadgets strapped to the hand, feeding, shaving, smoking, attention to personal hygiene and hair grooming are possible.

The patient, without active elbow extension, is much more disabled, he must rely on the force of gravity to extend his elbows so cannot keep them stable in any position except possibly a vertical position with the hand on a firm surface directly below the shoulder. The shoulder adductors are weak also, so the arm cannot be firmly pressed over the hand.

Activities are commenced as soon as the patient has adjusted to sitting up. Mat work is very valuable. The patient must be lifted onto the mat carefully and mat activities such as rolling, balance training in long-sitting and modified cross-sitting are taught (see Plate IX/10 and IX/11).

Some patients, particularly those with active elbow extension and radial wrist extension achieve a remarkable degree of control of activities. Some can hook their thumbs into their trouser pockets and sit up using the shoulder adductors and extensors and in the same way raise the trunk. Others get to forearm support and then to arm support.

Ball games are arranged and archery, swimming, and table tennis are possible, with adapted apparatus if needed.

Morale is aided by helping each patient to take a pride in his or her own appearance. A wig should be provided for a patient who has had to have the scalp shaved during the period on skull traction. Girls are helped to make up the face and men to shave with special electrically operated razors.

A full programme of physiotherapy, occupational therapy, bladder training, skin care, and personal hygiene is arranged. The patient must be responsible for getting himself to the correct place on time for treatment. Even those with no control of the elbow joints can have an electrically driven chair supplied so that they can be responsible for their own locomotion.

The problem of spasticity has not been discussed but it is an ever-present threat of becoming a severe complication unless sores, contractures and bladder infection can be avoided.

Standing with leg support in some form of splint such as plaster of Paris shells or a specially designed standing-frame is favoured by the medical team. The patient gains a psychological uplift from a period of standing which may not be understood by those of us who have never had to lie flat or sit immobile throughout days, weeks and years. Physiological benefits of standing include better drainage of the kidneys, some beneficial stimuli to keep the leg bones strong, a position which maintains length of hip flexors, knee flexors and calf and a means of reducing spasticity. In many cases standing improves the activity of postural muscles of the neck and upper trunk. The patients can have some apparatus supplied so that they can stand for a period daily at home when they are discharged from the spinal unit.

Occupational therapy is essential for tetraplegic patients. In the acute stage with the patient absolutely helpless in bed tape-recorded books and a suck-blow page turner for the patient's use are most valuable. These are supplied by the occupational therapist who teaches the use of the page turner. Later when the patient is sitting up simple gadgets can usually be supplied for page turning, feeding and use of an electric typewriter.

For the more disabled patients with very high lesions more complex aids may be found useful.

Art therapy is very valuable when it is available. Gadgets to hold pencils or brushes can be used by some patients or special dental devices used to paint with the mouth.

Apparatus controlled by the mouth by pneumatic control can be supplied to enable a patient to put on and off switches for lights, electric fires, radio or television sets. It can also be used to control a telephone, page turner or electric typewriter. This is known as the Patient Operated Selector Mechanism (P.O.S.M. or POSSUM).

Other apparatus designed for a tetraplegic patient include a ball-bearing feeding device, an opponens splint and flexor hinge splints. The success of these varies but details are given in books listed at the end of this chapter.

Reconstructive surgery for the hand is sometimes considered but great care is needed to ensure that no ability is lost by attempts to improve hand skill.

Motorized transport can be controlled by a tetraplegic patient who has active use of the elbows and wrists but the patient has to be lifted into and out of the car. This is facilitated by the use of a sliding board.

Resettlement presents many difficulties and the relatives must be thoroughly trained to care for the patient at home. This is done by all members of the team and should commence as soon as possible. A list of reminders to the patient and his relatives is reproduced at the end of this chapter.

Follow-up and frequent review is necessary and domiciliary visits from experienced nurses, occupational therapists, or physiotherapists are of great value.

Although the patients need a personal attendant the prognosis is more favourable for tetraplegics who return to the community than for those forced by circumstances to remain in institutional care. The future is grim for those young patients who must depend entirely on others to be fed and for all personal care and who have no family able and willing to do so.

Even those patients who can achieve some degree of self-care need adapted buildings, accommodation and some supervision, if they are to live away from home or institution.

INCOMPLETE TETRAPLEGIA

Because the cervical spine is relatively mobile and also vulnerable, injury is common and frequently produces a partial cord lesion.

As discussed previously, partial lesions present with great variation and the precise treatment needed depends on the clinical symptoms.

Treatment in the early stage

Even in *mild cases* the principles of treatment for patients with a cord lesion should be observed. If mobility at the site of injury is permitted the neurological damage may increase. Nursing care should be meticulous and an explanation is needed to gain the patient's co-operation in maintaining a good position even if he can control some movement of the trunk and limbs.

In cases with more *severe involvement* the treatment will be as described for complete lesions. Range of joints and soft tissue length must be maintained in the legs and hands and signs of sensory or motor recovery must be reported and recorded. Spinal shock will wear off rapidly in partial lesions. When muscle tone returns to the trunk and legs spasticity will be apparent and extreme care must be taken to try to avoid eliciting flexor or extensor spasms. As soon as possible an assessment is made of spared motor and sensory function but care must be taken not to raise false hope by mistaking spinal reflex activity for voluntary control of movement.

Treatment when weight-bearing is allowed through the spine

This follows the principles for all cord lesions. The individual needs of each patient must be carefully considered.

In all but the most mild cases some residual flaccid paralysis of the hands will make manipulative skills difficult or impossible. This factor with the added problem of imperfect control of the spastic trunk and lower limbs, leads to a very frustrating situation. The use of crutches or sticks may be almost impossible for a patient with weak or insensitive hands. The spasticity of the legs can be reduced by the patient's own handling if he has normal use of his arms, but this is usually impossible for incomplete tetraplegics.

As for all partial lesions, assessment of the individual abilities and difficulties of each patient is essential.

A plan of treatment must be made and co-operation is needed with occupational therapists and the medical social worker to try to help each patient to realize his potential for rehabilitation.

FEMALE PATIENTS WITH CORD LESIONS

Treatment for female patients is as described above but some added problems arise. One example is the relative shortness of arms and heavier pelvis and legs of a woman compared to that of a man. These factors make transfers difficult for all but the most slender and youthful females.

Another problem is the difficult situation of double incontinence; no really satisfactory urinal is available. Bladder training is therefore of vital importance to the female patient. Nurses are responsible for attempting to establish a regular automatic reflex-emptying of the bladder. Fluid intake is carefully regulated both in quantity and times when it is taken. The patient must understand the aim of the training and if possible learn to express the bladder manually to ensure good emptying. Menstruation brings special problems and may upset the automatic bladder function. Young patients often achieve a remarkable success in bladder training. The physiotherapist should understand the aim of training.

In spite of these physical difficulties women show great determination and courage and many paraplegics achieve complete independence.

CHILDREN WITH COMPLETE CORD LESIONS

Children with cord lesions present a challenge but no greater problems than adults, if care is taken to prevent deformity.

Because growth is retarded when normal use of a part is prevented, the lower limbs of a child with paraplegia are relatively short. This factor is an advantage as transfers and gait are facilitated if the arms are long and the lower part of the body lighter than normal.

Many children show great adaptability to physical defects and are very rewarding to train in new skills. They become almost recklessly proficient in the use of wheelchairs, take to swimming eagerly, learn swing-through gait and develop speed and expertise in this rapidly. Many children can get up from the floor unaided, gain balance in standing, place the crutches for use and walk off. Calipers are needed for these activities but do not need to be hinged at the knee for very young children.

Regular, frequent review is needed, however, to ensure that good function is preserving good joint range and length of soft tissue.

As the child grows new splints are needed and the older child needs hinged calipers to enable him to sit correctly on a stool or chair.

Bladder training is essential as it is for adults, and regular checks are made by the urologist to see that kidney function is good. Parents should be instructed in the care of skin, bladder, use of splints and shown how to give passive movements to preserve joint and soft tissue range.

If possible normal schooling should be arranged but the school authorities must be instructed in precautions against skin damage from extremes of temperature or from abrasion.

CHILDREN WITH PARTIAL CORD LESIONS

Partial cord lesion may be caused by trauma, developmental errors, infection or severe bone disease.

Treatment follows the principles of treatment for the cause and should be appropriate for the individual neurological symptoms.

Assessment should be attempted but in very young infants the examiner needs a knowledge of the normal motor behaviour and experience of handling young children with neurological defects.

Prognosis is made by the medical personnel but is aided by a concise report of examinations and observations by the physiotherapist. The habitual posture or response may be difficult to assess in a short examination session and the physiotherapist who handles the child for a longer time and more often, should be able to give a valuable account of her observations.

Methodical examination and simple, clear, well-documented, dated reports are required.

Treatment for the neurological symptoms varies according to the precise clinical defects of muscle control and sensory loss.

A careful plan of treatment is facilitated by good assessment. Methods should be selected which are appropriate to the age of the child and the exact defects, and which are found, by subsequent assessment, to be proving helpful.

The problem of deformity is increased if some muscles are active and the antagonists, flaccid or very weak. This problem arises whether the active muscles are under control of the will or are merely activated by spinal reflex activity. In the former case a difficult decision may face the medical director of the case because surgical intervention is irreversible and the possible beneficial use of innervated muscles may be permanently prevented.

Splintage must be chosen with care and its measurement, fitting and application must be meticulous to gain the maximum benefit without the risk of skin damage.

The problem of incontinence usually arises and is one of the most distressing factors for both parents and child.

Further discussion and details of treatment are given in the Chapter on Spina Bifida and associated defects, page 251 *et seq.*

CAUDA EQUINA LESIONS

A lesion of the spine below the second lumbar vertebra may cause damage to the roots of spinal nerves passing from the lower segments of the cord within the neural canal until they emerge at the corresponding intervertebral foramina.

As the nerve roots contain only nerve fibres, these may regenerate and conduction of nerve impulses along them will be restored. However, dense scar tissue sometimes prevents good recovery of function and if regeneration does occur it takes up to two years for nerve axons to grow to the most distal muscles and skin.

Treatment of the initial injury follows the principles for fractures of the spine and treatment for neurological symptoms must be appropriate for severe and extensive lower motor neurone lesions.

The latter is similar to that needed for polyneuritis and details are given in the section on polyneuritis.

If the tip of the lowest segment of the spinal cord is involved the lesion is known as a combined conus and cauda-equina lesion. In these cases some partial or complete loss of control of the external sphincters may create problems of incontinence which are permanent.

Loss of skin sensation over the buttocks may also occur and be permanent, thus appropriate training is needed in skin care.

Reminders for patients with spinal injury, and for their attendants

Care in bed

1. See there are no creases in the bottom sheet.

2. Use a firm mattress on a firm support so that the mattress does not sag.
3. Turn regularly as instructed by the nurses.
4. Do not use hot water bottles.
5. Inspect the skin each night and morning. Use a hand mirror to see posterior parts. If any redness occurs investigate and take necessary measures to prevent breakdown of skin.
6. Inspect skin of legs when calipers are removed.
7. If sheets etc. are wet these must be changed at once.

Care whilst dressing etc.
1. Do not use safety pins.
2. Do not wear tight clothing, trousers, stockings or shoes. Avoid holes in socks.
3. Keep finger and toe nails short and smooth.
4. Check temperature of bath or washing water with a thermometer to avoid scalds. Water must be below 98°F (36.5°C).
5. Check inside shoes before putting them on to ensure there are no nails or other harmful objects inside. Inspect feet when shoes have been removed.
6. Be careful not to have sharp objects in trouser pockets.

Transfers
1. Always move the legs carefully, lift them and do not drag them along, place down carefully.
2. Always lift high enough to avoid dragging buttocks over hard surfaces.
3. See the brakes are on and the wheelchair secure.
4. Do not sit on hard surfaces, use a cushion or rubber seat e.g. bath and lavatory.

Care when in the wheelchair
1. Lift every fifteen minutes for fifteen seconds.
2. High cervical lesions must be lifted every thirty minutes.
3. Do not sit too near a fire or radiator.
4. Tetraplegics wear gloves when wheeling chair.
5. Take care whilst smoking not to drop hot ash or cigarette ends etc., tetraplegics use a holder.
6. Avoid exposing the legs to extremes of temperature e.g. wrap up in a rug if outdoors in cold weather.

7. Do not expose insensitive skin to strong sunlight.
8. Do not rest hot plates or mugs on your legs. Tetraplegics use insulated mugs.

Care in motorized cars
1. Transfer with care.
2. Use a cushion.
3. Do not use a car heater.
4. Wrap up legs if weather is cold.

REFERENCES

Fulton, J. F. and McCouch, G. P. (1937). 'Spinal Shock.' Journal of Nervous & Mental Diseases (Baltimore), **86**, 125.

Kuhn, R. A. (1950). 'Alteration in Dominance of Postural and Protective Reflexes.' Brain, **73**, 1.

The Right Hon. the Baroness Masham of Ilton (1971). Report of Annual Congress. Physiotherapy, **57**, November 1971.

FURTHER READING

'*Physiotherapy*'
Guttmann, L. 'Some Problems in the Initial Management of Spinal Cord Injuries'. Physiotherapy, January 1964.

Bromley, Ida. 'The Early Stages of Physiotherapy in Paraplegia and Tetraplegia'. Physiotherapy, January 1964.

Goldsmith, Selwyn. 'Planning Homes for the Disabled'. Physiotherapy, October 1963.

Paraplegia – the official journal of the International Medical Society of Paraplegia. Livingstone, Edinburgh.

BOOKS
1. Bromley, Ida. *Tetraplegia and Paraplegia*. A Guide for Physiotherapists. Churchill Livingstone, 1976.
2. Burke, David C. and Murray, D. Duncan. *Handbook of Spinal Cord Medicine*. Macmillan Press Ltd, 1975.
3. Elson, R. *Practical Management of Spinal Injuries for Nurses*. Livingstone, 1965.
4. Fallon, Bernadette. '*so you're paralysed*', 1976. Obtainable from Spinal Injuries Association, 24 Nutford Place, London W1H 6AN.

5. Ford, Jack R. and Duckworth, Bridget. *Physical Management for the Quadraplegic Patient*. F. A. Davis and Co., Philadelphia, Pennsylvania, U.S.A., 1974.
6. Goble, R. E. A. and Nichols, P. J. R. *Rehabilitation of the Severely Disabled* – I. *Evaluation of the disabled living unit*. Butterworth, 1971.
7. Guttmann, Sir Ludwig. *Spinal Cord Injuries*. Blackwell Scientific Publications, 1973.
8. Harris, Phillip (ed.). *Spinal Injuries* – Proceedings of a Symposium, Royal College of Surgeons of Edinburgh, 1963. Morrison & Gibb, 1970.
9. Nichols, P. J. R. *Rehabilitation of the Severely Disabled* – II. *Management*. Butterworth, 1971.
10. Roaf, R. and Hodkinson, L. (Jt. eds. 1977). *The Paralysed Patient*. Blackwell Scientific Publications. Oxford.
11. Rossier, A. *Rehabilitation of Spinal Cord Patient*. Documenta Geigy Acta Clinica, Basel, 1973.
12. *Sport and Physical Recreation for the Disabled*. An Enquiry by the Disabled Living Foundation, Vincent House, Vincent Square, London, S.W.1.
13. Walsh, J. J. *Understanding Paraplegia*. Tavistock Publications, 1964.

USEFUL ADDRESSES

See list in Physiotherapy, January 1972, including

Disabled Drivers Association,
Ashwellthorpe Hall,
Ashwellthorpe,
Nr. Norwich,
NOR 89W.

Disabled Living Foundation.
346 Kensington High Street,
London, W14 8NS.

CHAPTER XI

Spina Bifida and Hydrocephalus

by OLWEN NETTLES, O.N.C., M.C.S.P.

The three major and most common neurological conditions found in the newborn are anencephaly, hydrocephalus and spina bifida cystica. The last is the most common crippling congenital condition in this country.

ANENCEPHALY

Literally this means absence of the brain and the condition is not compatible with life. It is said to be the commonest of the three conditions and it is known that it is more common in the Eastern hemisphere than in the West.

HYDROCEPHALUS

Hydrocephalus occurs when there is an increase in the cerebrospinal fluid circulating in and around the brain. Normally the fluid is formed by the choroid plexuses, circulates through the ventricular system (under increased pressure) and central canal of the spinal cord and reaches the subarachnoid space through the median and lateral foramina in the fourth ventricle. It bathes the surface of the brain and cord and is reabsorbed into the cerebral venous sinuses via the veins on the surface of the hemispheres and the granulations.

Should any blockage occur in any part of this system pressure of fluid will build up in the ventricles causing enlargement and in the neonatal stage a consequent enlargement of the skull. Occasionally hydrocephalus occurs in utero and is easily detected if the size of the head intereferes with the normal delivery of the baby. Much more often the head is normal at birth and only grows abnormally during the early months.

In 80 per cent of all cases hydrocephalus is associated with spina bifida cystica and when this condition is present the doctors will be prepared for hydrocephalus. In the remaining 20 per cent it may only be detected when the head grows abnormally and the anterior part bulges. Often the health visitor or infant welfare doctor may spot this during routine visits because they have the detailed knowledge of child development which is required to ascertain whether the circumference of the head is outside the normal limits.

Aetiology

In the 80 per cent of cases of hydrocephalus associated with spina bifida, the excess of fluid is due to malformations associated with the spina bifida. Known as the Arnold-Chiari malformation, it is a displacement of the medulla and part of the cerebellum into the foramen magnum, causing a damming up of the cerebrospinal fluid. In a few cases this blockage may be complete but in the great majority of cases it is only partial.

Hydrocephalus may occur as a result of prematurity, a precipitate birth, or toxaemia in the mother. During birth the baby's head may be damaged due to haemorrhage and this may result in an interruption in the flow of the cerebrospinal fluid. The blockage may be by a blood clot, in which case the damage may only be temporary.

Again, hydrocephalus may occur after birth if a newborn baby develops an infection causing meningitis. The inflammation of the meninges may narrow the channels through which the cerebrospinal fluid has to flow and this will produce symptoms of hydrocephalus.

When the baby is born it may be possible to recognize the hydrocephalus at once. The head may be larger than average or deformed. The brow may be bulging, the fontanelles larger than usual and bulging with a palpable pulse (see Fig. XI/1). The sutures may be wider apart than usual, especially the lambdoid sutures behind the ear. The 'setting sun' sign may be present but it is not a very reliable one. If present, the baby's eyes stare more than one would expect and the cornea is large with the sclerotic visible above but not always visible below. If there is any doubt the circumference of the head is watched closely, and a chart of this is kept. This usually gives a very accurate estimate of abnormal growth (see Fig. XI/2).

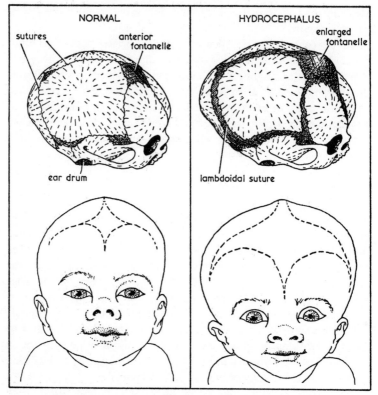

Fig. XI/1 Enlarged fontanelles and separated sutures

TREATMENT

Until 1956 no effective treatment for hydrocephalus was available, but some time before this a child whose father, John Holter, was an engineer was born in America with this complaint. This father together with a neurosurgeon, Mr. Eugene Spitz, perfected the Spitz-Holter shunt (Fig. XI/3A) which is designed to drain the excess cerebrospinal fluid from the ventricles into the circulatory system (to be disposed of in the usual way).

This shunt comprises a right-angled catheter, the 'proximal' catheter, one end of which is inserted through the skull into the ventricle of the brain while the other end is attached to a piece of clear plastic compressible tube about three-quarters of an inch long. This has at either

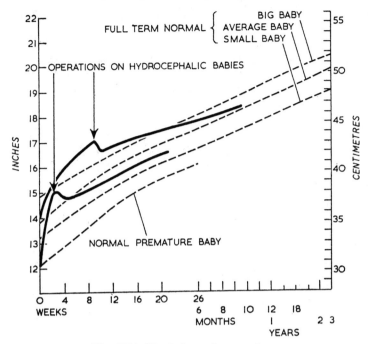

Fig. XI/2 Head circumference chart

end a non-return valve encased in metal and at the lower end is the 'distal' catheter which in turn is usually inserted into the jugular vein and thence into the right atrium of the heart. The whole shunt runs beneath the skin with the valve just behind the right ear. To a trained eye the catheter in the neck is just visible looking very much like a prominent vein, while the shunt is soon covered by the growing hair.

To insert the shunt, a half-moon incision is made behind the right ear and another one over the jugular vein. As the child grows it may become necessary to lengthen the distal catheter to ensure that drainage into the heart is maintained.

Once the shunt is in position it begins to drain away the excess cerebrospinal fluid, the bulge in the fontanelles disappears and the space between the sutures returns to normal. The valves in the shunt only work when the pressure in the ventricles is excessive, and it has been found that in many children the shunt may only be operational for short spells during the day. At the present time the shunts are not removed but remain in situ indefinitely. Other types of shunts have been used, notably the Pudenz (Fig. XI/3B).

This method of control of hydrocephalus was first used in this country by the late Mr. G. H. Macnab at the Hospital for Sick Children, Great Ormond St., London, and for some time was the standard procedure in all cases of hydrocephalus in the newborn. Nowadays the treatment is more conservative and the future quality of the life of the child is assessed before the surgeons come to a decision on surgery.

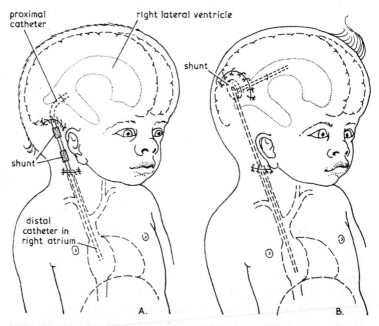

Fig. XI/3 A. Spitz-Holter shunt   B. Pudenz shunt

Spontaneous arrest of hydrocephalus does happen in a few cases. This has always been the position and it is these cases which managed to survive before the advent of the shunt.

When hydrocephalus appears without spina bifida, there is, of course, no flaccid paralysis but there may be spastic paralysis due to brain damage. Left untreated, the damage to the brain will increase especially once ossification of the skull bones has occurred. In such cases the degree of spastic paralysis will increase and mental retardation will result.

Hydrocephalus often causes a squint even when treated, but if untreated blindness may result.

PHYSIOTHERAPY
Such children are treated exactly as other children with cerebral palsy (see Chapter XII, p. 266 *et seq*).

Before a baby with a shunt is allowed home the parents are given instructions in its care. Blocking of the shunt is an ever-present danger and the ward sister makes sure that the parents know the signs to look for. The valve in the shunt can be tested by compressing the soft tube which normally empties and fills quickly. If the proximal catheter, in the brain, blocks, the valve will stay flat as no cerebrospinal fluid can pass into it when pressure is released. The onset of the symptoms may be sudden or gradual depending on the extent of the blockage.

False fontanelles

Becoming increasingly popular is the operation to create a 'false fontanelle'. Before the child's fontanelles close naturally, it is very easy to keep a check on the functioning of the shunt. If this is pumping satisfactorily the fontanelles are soft and look normal, but when there is any malfunction in the shunt the fontanelles very soon begin to bulge and this acts as a warning sign. Once they have closed naturally this method of checking is denied to the parents and medical personnel. In order to maintain this accurate indication surgeons now remove a small circle of bone, usually from behind the right ear, so that there is a more permanent aperture in the skull through which any increase in the intracranial pressure may be watched.

TYPES OF SPINA BIFIDA

There are two main types of spina bifida:
1. Spina bifida occulta
2. Spina bifida cystica (or aperta or manifesta)
   a. with meningocele
   b. with myelomeningocele

SPINA BIFIDA OCCULTA

This is a bifid or split spinal column but a perfectly normal and unaffected spinal cord (see Fig. XI/4).

In its mildest form an occult spina bifida may go undetected throughout that person's life, or may only be diagnosed if there has to be a spinal X-ray for some completely different reason, but other cases may have slight muscle imbalance, often in the muscles of the feet. This may not become apparent until the child is in his early teens when he puts on a spurt of growth during which his cord, already 'tethered', causes the nerve roots to be stretched and consequently

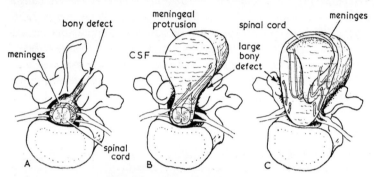

Fig. XI/4 Cross-section of spine
A. Normal vertebra (Spina bifida occulta)
B. Incomplete vertebral development (Meningocele)
C. Incomplete vertebral development with flat protruding spinal cord plate (Myelomeningocele)

damaged. The defect in spina bifida occurs in the first month of development, so the cord is 'tethered' at a much lower level in relation to the bones than the normal level in the upper lumbar vertebrae. This in turn interferes with nerve conductivity and so causes the imbalance. This usually results in a pes cavus deformity but in any unusual abnormal pattern of foot growth an occult spina bifida cannot be ruled out without an X-ray. Such cases are frequently seen in children's orthopaedic clinics.

An occult spina bifida is sometimes detected at birth by a number of outward signs. These are: a hairy patch over the vertebrae; naevi; unusual dimples; and/or a small fatty lump over part of the spine. Provided the baby exhibits all the normal reflexes and is normal in other respects, he does not require urgent surgical treatment but a careful watch is kept on his progress.

Cases of spina bifida occulta are not the ones we usually associate with the condition as they may never be diagnosed as such. Recognized cases of spina bifida cystica are those associated with either a meningocele or a myelomeningocele. In each type the baby is born with either an open wound over the area or a sac covered with skin.

SPINA BIFIDA CYSTICA

Spina bifida cystica is a neural tube defect – a defect in the structure of the bones of the spine with an incomplete closure of the vertebral canal and often associated abnormalities in the spinal cord itself, and other abnormalities in the body. It is one of the conditions that comes under the general heading of *rachischisis* (Greek: a cleft spine) an alternative name being *rachischisis posterior*. It is also known as *dysraphism*. A *raphe* is the ridge or furrow marking the line of the union of the two halves of symmetrical parts. *Dysraphism* is a failure of these two parts to join to form the raphe.

Incidence

Spina bifida occurs in about two per thousand live births in this country but its incidence varies from area to area. The Welsh and Irish have a higher incidence than the English and over the world the incidence is higher in Europe than in Asia, and, unlike anencaphaly, it is more common in the Western hemisphere than in the Eastern. It is estimated that between 2,500 and 3,000 babies with spina bifida are born annually.

The reason for the recent increase in the number of children growing up with spina bifida is the fact that before the control of hydrocephalus 90 per cent of all known cases died, leaving only about three hundred surviving annually. Some of these were only mildly affected but many were so disabled that they spent their lives in institutions and were not integrated into the community. For some years after the invention of the shunt, all affected children were operated on at birth and about 60 per cent lived beyond the age of five years and are presenting the medical, paramedical, education and employing authorities with a very big problem. With this in mind, consideration is now given to the quality of life any baby can reasonably expect before embarking on neonatal surgery.

Aetiology

The cause is unknown. Considerable research is being undertaken into hereditary factors, environment, chromosome abnormalities, etc.

There is as yet little evidence of diet, drugs, or any external factors playing any part in the development of such defects.

The defect occurs in the early weeks of pregnancy, usually the fourth week, before the mother is really sure she is pregnant. At this stage of the zygote a primitive streak develops which is later to become the brain and spinal cord. This normally becomes covered with cells which later develop into the bony casing, the skull and vertebrae, but occasionally these cells fail to fuse completely and spina bifida results. This may appear anywhere from the occipital bone in the back of the head (encephalocele) to the sacrum, but about 70 per cent are in the lower thoracic and lumbosacral region. Fig. XI/5 opposite shows the distribution of lesions and the incidence of hydrocephalus in a series of 262 cases studied by two surgeons. Spina bifida in each area has its own characteristics.

Once a child with spina bifida has been born into a family, although apparently random in the case of the first child, the chances of having a similarly affected second child is greatly increased. Whereas the initial risk of any family having a child with spina bifida is about one in five hundred, once one baby is born the risk increases to about one in twenty-five for the second and one in eight for the third.

Recently it has become possible to diagnose some cases of anencephaly and spina bifida before the child is born, by examination of the amniotic fluid surrounding the fetus. In early intra-uterine life the substance *alpha-feto-protein* (AFP) is the main circulating protein in the fetus, and some of this substance is present in the amniotic fluid. In a procedure known as *amniocentesis* a sample of this fluid is taken from the uterus, and if the fetus has a neural tube defect the amount of AFP in the sample is raised. Other tests on the same sample may show the presence of other congenital defects, notably Down's syndrome and other conditions associated with chromosome abnormalities. This test is a complicated one and is carried out during the second trimester of pregnancy, between the sixteenth and eighteenth week. If the test is positive the parents are informed and are offered an abortion. The test can only be offered to parents who are known to be at risk, e.g. those who have already had one abnormal child, or where there is a history of abnormal births in the immediate family, or where the mother is over 40 years of age (when the risk of an abnormal birth, especially Down's syndrome, is considerably greater). AFP is also present in the

DISTRIBUTION OF LESIONS			ASSOCIATED HYDROCEPHALUS PRESENT IN:—
(%)			(%)
8	ENCEPHALOCELE		70
4	CERVICAL		40
6	THORACIC		73
69	9	THORACO-LUMBAR	96
	32	LUMBAR	84
	28	LUMBO-SACRAL	82
13	SACRAL		56

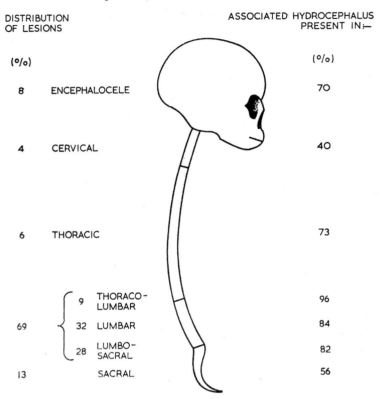

Fig. XI/5 Incidence of spina bifida

blood plasma of the mother, and the viability of screening every pregnant mother by a blood test is now under discussion. If the AFP level is raised in the plasma, the parents are offered an amniocentesis to confirm the suspicions, and if the result of this is positive an abortion will be offered, but the final decision always rests with the parents.

As has been stated, hydrocephalus occurs in 80 per cent of all cases of spina bifida and 20 per cent of affected children have hydrocephalus alone. Conversely, there are 20 per cent of spina bifida cases where hydrocephalus does not occur. These cases are usually the milder ones in any region but the majority are the ones affecting the sacral bones (see Plate XI/1).

SPINA BIFIDA WITH MENINGOCELE

This may occur at any spinal level or in the occipital bone in the back of the head. The sac or lump has a meningeal lining but no tissue of the spinal cord itself so that paralysis does not result from a meningocele. Meningoceles may be covered with a thin skin, or with an abnormally thick skin and a pad of fat, but not all lumps covered with a skin are simple meningoceles. This condition may be associated with hydrocephalus.

SPINA BIFIDA WITH MYELOMENINGOCELE

This unfortunately is much more common and in these cases the spinal cord or cauda equina protrudes into the sac or lies on the surface of an open wound. The nerve roots are malformed or damaged and this leads to a partial or complete flaccid paralysis below the site of the malformation. There may also be loss of sensation and loss of sphincter control.

Some spastic paralysis may be present in some muscles. The cord distal to the lesion may not be damaged in which case the muscle innervation is normal but the path of messages to and from the brain is interrupted (either partially or completely) by the lesion. Uncontrolled or spastic movements may occur in the limbs and in the newborn it is very difficult to decide, when movement is present, whether it is uncontrolled or volitional. This type of spina bifida may be accompanied by a bony deformity of the spine causing scoliosis, kyphosis or lordosis – either over the site or in the length of the spine. Other deformities are often present, especially foot deformities – often talipes equinovarus. The hips may be dislocated or 'at risk' with a limitation in abduction, or the child may lie with his hips fully flexed (this is usually associated with a lesion in the L.3 area) and the knees may be deformed, stiff or abducted. These deformities may be caused either by an associated skeletal defective development or by the muscle imbalance. This imbalance is due to difference in tone in opposing groups of muscles, either hypertonicity if there is uncontrolled action or hypotonicity where some muscles are flaccid. This unequal pull of the muscles will cause an abnormal bone growth and consequent deformities.

DIASTOMETAMYELIA

Diastometamyelia is spina bifida in which there is a bony spur in the spinal canal. The spinal cord splits into two, one side of which may be normal and the other damaged. This does not occur often but when it does it is recognized because one leg is virtually normal while the other is paralysed to some extent – one half of the spinal cord being affected while messages can travel normally up and down the cord in the other half. There is usually some nerve supply to the sphincters and such children are trainable. In its mild form, as in spina bifida occulta, this may only become apparent during growth.

If a mild diastometamyelia or spina bifida occulta is suspected, a myelogram may be done and this will show that the conus or tip of the spinal cord is at a lower level than normal. In spina bifida occulta the tethering is by the filium terminale – a fibrous band, whereas in diastometamyelia it may be a peg of bone or soft tissue separating the two cords.

MYELODYSPLASIA

This is a disordered development of the spinal cord associated with the bifid spine.

HEMIVERTEBRAE

Another condition associated with spina bifida in which one or more of the vertebrae are wedge-shaped or malformed in such a way that part of the vertebra is missing, causing a scoliosis.

SYRINGOCELE

This is a form of spina bifida in which herniation of the spinal cord contains a cavity.

SYRINGOMYELOCELE

A form of spina bifida in which a cavity in the protruding sac is connected with the central canal of the spinal cord and that central canal is distended.

CRANIUM BIFIDUM

A cranium bifidum is present when there is a malformation mostly of the occipital bone, but may be frontal, vertical or basal and this may produce a meningocele, but if the brain protrudes it is called an encephalocele. If the former, the prognosis may be good, although hydrocephalus is usually present. If it is accompanied by an encephalocele the outlook is poorer and the child is often mentally retarded and hydrocephalus is a complication. Expectation of life is not good.

Lesions here do not produce a flaccid paralysis as, being a brain lesion, the descending and ascending tracts may be involved with a consequent spastic paralysis. There is not usually any sensory loss or consequent circulatory sluggishness and whether or not the child can be toilet trained depends on his mental ability rather than on his muscular control. This condition may be associated with *microcephaly*, i.e. a very small brain, which also causes retardation.

From the physiotherapist's point of view, a case of encephalocele is treated as a child with cerebral palsy (see Chapter XII) and not as a child with spina bifida with the resulting paralysis.

SPINAL AREAS AFFECTED

Where a myelomeningocele has occurred the resulting damage depends on the extent of the malformation and the area in which it has occurred. Although the typical spina bifida patient is one in whom the disease is in the lumbo-sacral area, the condition is seen in all parts of the spine (Fig. XI/5).

Cervical spine

Spina bifida occurs less frequently here (about 4 per cent of all cases) than in any other area. There is often a cervical scoliosis causing a torticollis and there may be deformities of the shoulder girdle. There may also be an inability to raise the arms above the head and the fine movements in the hands are impaired, this being due to paresis and underdeveloped muscles of both arms.

Only in rare cases is the paralysis complete and lower limb paralysis, if any, is usually of a spastic nature. Control of the sphincters is unaffected and as a result there is no incontinence.

Thoracic spine

With a thoracic spina bifida there is often considerable deformity of the ribcage. This is because the ribs are attached to the thoracic vertebrae and any malformation of these will cause a scoliosis and a consequent rotation of the ribs. It is in this area, too, that hemivertebrae are most likely to appear. Occasionally a child is completely paralysed from a thoracic lesion and needs a considerable amount of splintage for walking. More often there is a paresis of the legs and sometimes a spastic paralysis; poor chest expansion and chest ailments are common and incontinence may be complete in severe cases, but many children with a thoracic lesion are trainable in this respect.

As well as the treatment given to all children with spina bifida (see pages 254–62), physiotherapists may be called on to teach breathing exercises and to train the patient to use what chest muscles are present to the full and so help to prevent frequent and debilitating chest illnesses.

Lumbar spine

This together with the last two thoracic vertebrae is the area which produces the typical spina bifida patient and 70% of all myelomeningoceles occur in this region. The flaccid paralysis may be complete or only partial and the legs may be quite flail or some groups of muscles may have slight innervation. There is also, at best, a weakness of the hip muscles, especially the extensors, resulting in unstable hip joints with hips that may be dislocated at birth or 'at risk'. The hip is a shallow joint as normally the acetabulum is not a deep socket at birth, and the joint is largely kept stable by the tone of the muscles and fascia surrounding it, so that when this tone is missing as in a flaccid paralysis, instability of the joint results.

Incontinence is common, sometimes only of urine but it may be of faeces as well. Circulation in the legs is poor due to an impairment of the sympathetic nervous system. Due to the poor circulation and lack of use, the condition of the bones is not good and they are thinner than normal. This results in frequent fractures which may go undetected as the patient cannot feel pain. The first indication that there has been a fracture may be the lump of callus formation during the healing process. These fractures are not serious as there is seldom any displacement – with the paralysed muscles there is no pull to produce this. They heal fairly quickly.

Lack of sensation is one of the more serious symptoms. The patient cannot feel hot or cold, pressure or pinpricks, and great care must be taken in the handling of such children. Parents must be taught to make the examination of the child's legs and feet an automatic part of the general hygiene of the child. Physiotherapists must be continually aware of this and avoid anything that is likely to cause continual rubbing which, in turn, causes friction burns. Hot water bottles, radiators, or anything hot are other hazards to be avoided.

Hydrocephalus is present in most cases of lesions in the lumbar regions.

Sacral spine

Spina bifida in this area causes a mild paralysis usually below the knee joint with paresis of the glutei and hip extensors. Hydrocephalus is rarely a complication and the highest survival rate is in these lesions. Conversely, incontinence is a major problem in this group, both of bladder and bowel, as innervation of the genito-urinary muscles comes largely from the sacral plexus and there is an associated sluggishness in the sympathetic nervous system. Lack of sensation is again a problem as in cases of lumbar lesions.

In all cases of spina bifida where there is some flaccid paralysis there may also be symptoms of spasticity. This is due to the fact that there may be some part of the spinal cord intact below the area of the lesion but impulses cannot travel to the brain because of the blockage caused by that lesion. Reflex action may then take place in the muscles controlled by the isolated cord and physiotherapists should be aware of this in order that they are not too optimistic when slight movement occurs. Occasionally even in fairly severe spina bifida cases some slight communication is left, although only a few fibres of the cord are intact and this (according to the nerves involved) may result in some bladder or bowel control or in some action in a few muscles.

THE COCKTAIL PARTY SYNDROME

The character of the typical child with spina bifida has been described thus – most of the children are happy, lovable extroverts with a quick wit, full of uninhibited questions and ready answers. This tends to convince their parents, and others, that they are exceptionally bright. Unfortunately only a few live up to this early prognosis and on expert assessment it is found that their retention of knowledge may not be as good as expected. In fact the intelligence of any group of children with spina bifida seems to be much the same as that found in any other group of children, i.e. 25 per cent are below the range of normal intelligence, 50 per cent within the average range and the remaining 25 per cent above normal. Physiotherapists should be aware of this and not be over-optimistic about their future scholastic prowess.

INCONTINENCE

One of the most distressing complications of spina bifida cystica is incontinence. This may be of the bladder only or of both bladder and bowel.

Incontinence of urine

This is a major problem facing the parents of a child with spina bifida. It is caused partly by lack of sensation and partly by the lack of a motor nerve supply. Those whose motor nerve supply to the sphincters may be intact may have no sensation so that they may not realize the feeling of fullness of the bladder that indicates to most of us the need to urinate. This incontinence may take three forms.

First, there may be neither control nor sensation; the bladder does not store the urine as the sphincters are always open. There is a continual trickle of urine, the patient is always wet and there is no residual urine in the bladder. These cases rarely get an infected bladder as no stasis occurs and equally they will never be trainable.

Second, no sensation at all, but there is slight involuntary control of the sphincters. The patient has no conscious control so the bladder keeps filling but as sensation is absent he cannot tell when he needs to urinate and cannot control the sphincters. The bladder continues to fill until there is an overflow or 'stress' incontinence which is followed by a dribble until pressure is eased. The bladder is never really empty, and the residue becomes stale and infected. Left untreated this infection may travel via the ureters to the kidneys and this will soon cause kidney infection with serious consequences.

Third, no sensation, but there is some muscle control. In these cases the bladder fills normally and automatically empties, but with no sensation, and the patient has no idea when the need arises. This group may be dry for long spells and are often trainable by finding out how long they can stay dry and giving them attention regularly and gradually increasing the time between this attention.

In the second type, manual expression is possible and may be advised to keep the bladder as empty as possible and perhaps keep the child dry for up to three hours. In the other two types expression has no place.

Treatment

The problem of urinary incontinence especially in girls is the social one. Changing one's own nappy when chairbound is almost impossible, there is always the danger of pressure sores (the more so when there is anaesthesia) and the risk of a smell; in fact, one is not socially acceptable when incontinent.

Boys and men can always wear a penile appliance – consisting of a plastic or rubber bag, usually strapped to one thigh to be inconspicuous, with a suitable applicator. With girls no applicator is suitable and a urinary diversion operation is now performed if the surgeons feel there is risk of infection and there is no hope of getting control. In this operation (sometimes called a uretero-ileostomy or ileal loop) a short section of the small intestine is isolated from the rest and sealed at one end – the small intestine itself being sutured together again. The ureters are then passed from the kidneys into this segment, the open end of which is passed through the body wall usually on the right hand side just below the waist. This provides a stoma (or spout) through which the urine may pass into a bag which is attached to the skin by a variety of methods (see Figs. XI/6 and XI/7).

By this means the girl becomes completely independent and is socially acceptable. This operation has proved so successful for girls that it is now being performed more and more on boys in preference to the penile appliance. It is irreversible and once done is there for life but this is preferred to the only alternative of nappies or pads. Modern diagnosis enables surgeons to decide at a very early age whether control will eventually be possible and this diversion operation may be performed while the child is still a baby so that no damage is caused to the ureters and kidneys by infection.

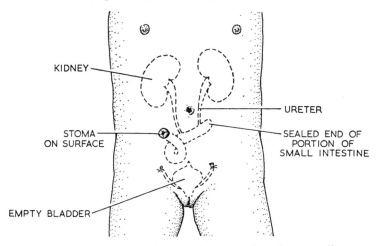

Fig. XI/6 Diagram showing stoma after operation of uretero-ileostomy or ileal loop

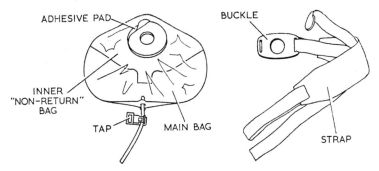

Fig. XI/7 Bag and belt for ileal loop stoma

Incontinence of faeces

Lack of bowel control occurs in a number of cases of lumbar and sacral spina bifida. It is from the same sacral roots that the pudendal and other pelvic nerves arise as are responsible for the urinary incontinence. In some cases the lumbar lesion may be complete and the sacral nerves may not be damaged so that the sphincters function but are uncontrolled by the brain as no messages can pass the lesion. There is then no idea of the need for defaecation and again the lack of sensation means that there is no feeling of fullness.

253

It is ironical that it is in children with the milder motor paralysis that the faecal incontinence is most marked, and this is the group which is sufficiently mobile to attend normal school. It is difficult for the child to do so if his bowel action is unreliable and he is not socially acceptable because of an offensive odour.

In some cases there is a continual looseness and in others a severe constipation with a large faecal mass in the rectum. This may result in an apparent diarrhoea as the spastic contraction of the sphincters does not allow the child to excrete this mass and liquid faeces are all that can pass it.

Occasionally it is necessary for a colostomy to be performed as well as a urinary diversion operation but by far the greater majority of children manage to get some control. Since the popularity of the urinary diversion operation it has been found that once such a child is dry the bowel action seems to become more controllable. Whether this is due to some sympathetic nervous reaction or whether the child, having sensed the difference in no longer being wet, makes an unconscious effort at control, or indeed whether the operation is performed at a time when the years of routine and regular training are producing results, is not known.

The use of suppositories and/or medicines may be necessary to gain regularity but this is such a highly individual problem that the answer may be different in every case.

Although physiotherapists are not directly concerned with the questions arising from incontinence, the whole subject is one of such concern to the parents that physiotherapists will inevitably be asked about it. Physiotherapists working in hospitals will be able to refer the family to the appropriate department but this knowledge is necessary for those who work in the field where specialist information may only be obtainable when the parents travel to the hospital.

TREATMENT OF SPINA BIFIDA

The active treatment of spina bifida has only become a realistic possibility since the introduction of the shunt to control the hydrocephalus. Before this the repair of the back lesion was not considered for some months as most of the babies died in the neonatal stage (i.e. within the first few weeks of life) and only when it was found that the baby survived and hydrocephalus did not develop was an operation undertaken to repair the lesion. Even then hydrocephalus sometimes developed and with no treatment to control it, the result was a grossly enlarged head with consequent brain damage and mental subnormality.

With the advent of the shunt it became the usual practice to repair the back lesion as soon after birth as possible, preferably within the first 24 hours. The theory underlying this was to prevent further damage to the exposed nerves, as nerve fibres cannot live uncovered and soon deteriorate.

Modern thinking now takes a line somewhere between these two courses of action, and before selecting any neonate for surgery many aspects of the condition are discussed. The prognosis, the probable quality of life that can be expected, the possible mental and physical abilities of the child, as well as the number of major operations likely to be needed before the child can walk, all have to be taken into account, and often surgery may be delayed for some weeks for a full assessment.

The following pages refer to the treatment of surviving babies with neural tube defects, whether they have been treated conservatively or by surgery.

Neonatal physiotherapy

As well as the paediatrician, paediatric or neuro-surgeon, orthopaedic surgeon and experienced nursing staff, the spina bifida team also includes a physiotherapist who has a very important role to play from the day the baby is born until he becomes independent.

As soon as the baby is admitted the physiotherapist is called upon to make a physical assessment of the child and this early assessment, if correctly done, can give a fairly accurate indication of the future physical ability of the child. The movement of the legs in some babies appears to improve after the back is repaired but when an assessment is made after about one year it nearly always relates very closely to the neonatal one.

This assessment – both of movement and sensation – is almost always done with the child in an incubator. It may be done by the paediatrician or it may be the responsibility of the physiotherapist. The baby may have had to travel a long distance to the hospital and has been subjected to a lot of examination and handling so it is vital for the operator to work quickly and efficiently. She needs to be very experienced and to have some knowledge of the developmental progress

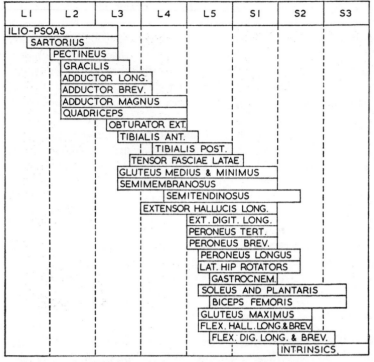

Fig. XI/8 Muscle innervation chart

of a normal newborn child for comparison in order to detect the abnormal (see Fig. XI/8). (Sheridan, 1969)

To carry out the assessment the examiner first records her general impressions – abnormal position of limbs, deformities present, movement (if any), etc. Reflexes are tested as far as possible and then groups of muscles as individual muscle testing is impossible in one so small in the time available. This is dealt with more fully elsewhere (Holgate, 1970). A sensory chart is then completed and to do this the protopathic or deeper feeling is tested with a safety-pin as testing the epicritic feeling, or light touch as with cottonwool, is unsatisfactory at this stage. The most reliable test of feeling is whether the baby cries when pricked with the pin. This obviously shows that he has felt it. If the limb moves when pricked although the movement may be an uncontrolled reflex action and if that movement is repeated when the spot is pricked again, there must be some sensation to cause it.

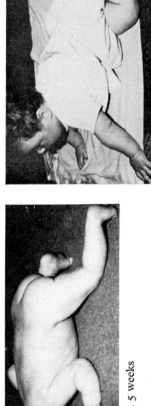

(a) Child aged 5 weeks

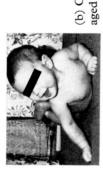

(b) Child
aged 3½ months

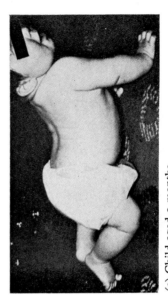

(d) Child aged 8 months

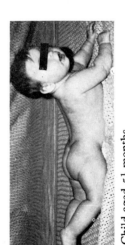

(c) Child aged 5½ months

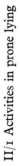

(e) Child aged 9 months

II/1 Activities in prone lying

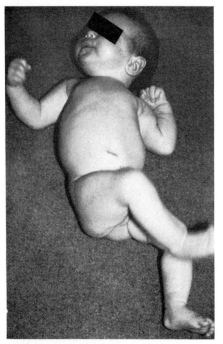

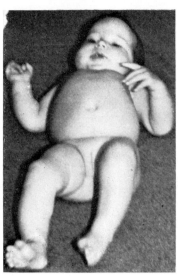

(c) Child aged 3½ months

(a) Child aged 5 weeks

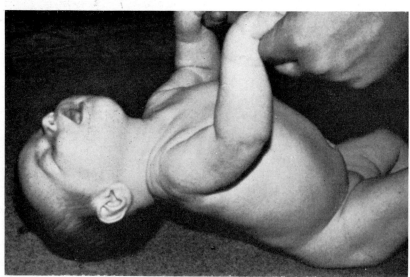

(b) Child aged 5 weeks

II/2 Activities in supine lying

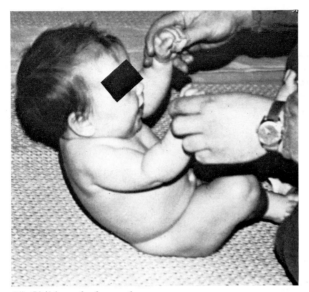

(d) Child aged $5\frac{1}{2}$ months

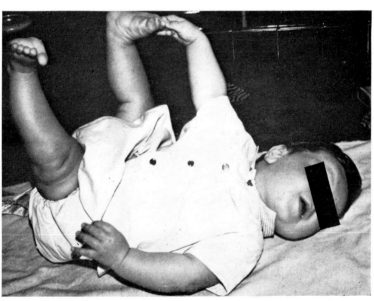

(e) Child aged $7\frac{1}{2}$ months, playing with the toes

II/2 Activities in supine lying

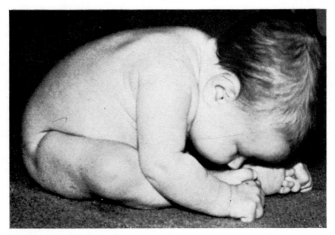

(a) Child aged 5 weeks

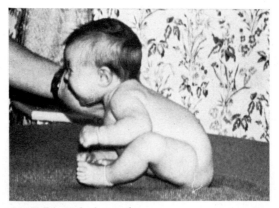

(b) Child aged 3½ months

II/3 Activities in sitting

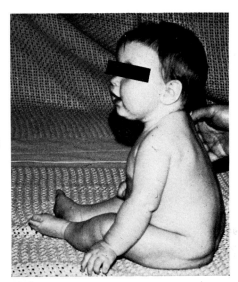

(c) Child aged 5½ months

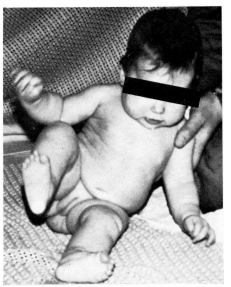

(d) Child aged 6 months

II/3 Activities in sitting

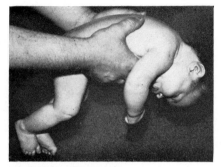

(a) Child aged 5 weeks

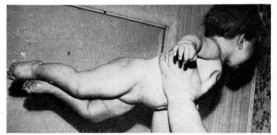

(b) Child aged $7\frac{1}{2}$ months

II/4 Ventral suspension

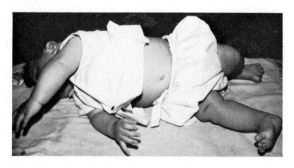

II/5 Child aged 8 months, rolling

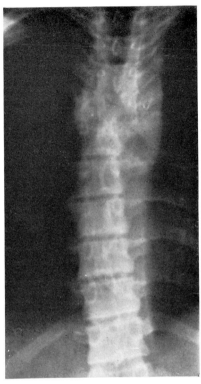

VIII/1 X-ray of spine to show
fracture dislocation

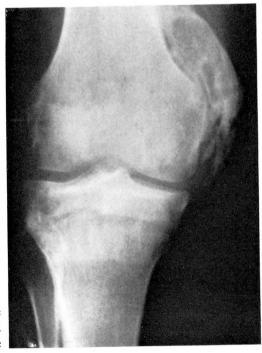

VIII/2 X-ray of knee
joint to show calcified
soft tissue

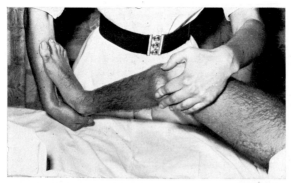

IX/1 Positioning of
contacts when handling
leg with spasticity

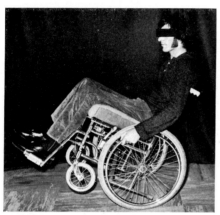

IX/2 Control of wheelchair to mount
curb, etc.

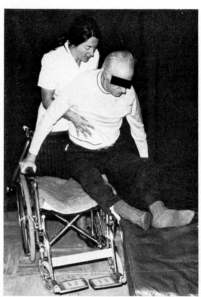

IX/3 Transfer from
chair to side of plinth

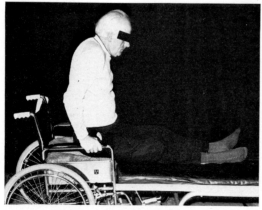

IX/4 Transfer from
chair to end of plinth

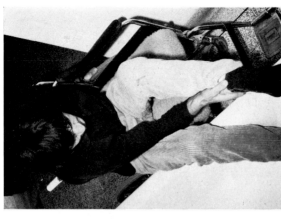

IX/7 Transfer from chair to bath from side of bath

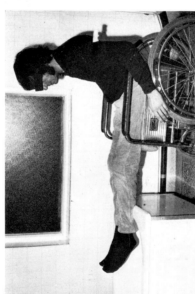

IX/6 Transfer from chair to bath from end of bath

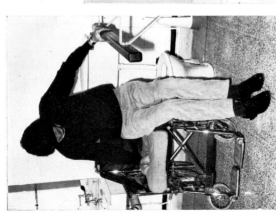

IX/5 Transfer from chair to lavatory

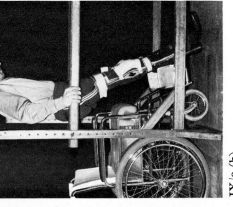

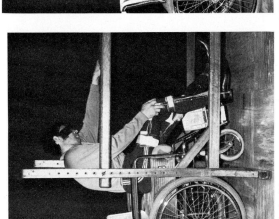

IX/9 (a)

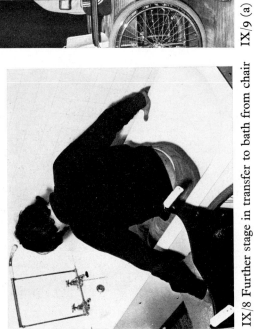

IX/8 Further stage in transfer to bath from chair at side of bath

IX/9 (b)

Stages in getting from chair to standing in parallel bars

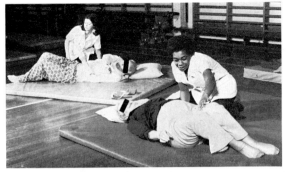

IX/10 Mat work for patients with spinal cord lesions

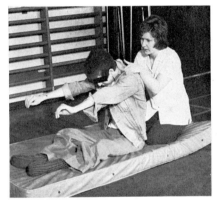

IX/11 Training in sitting balance
for a patient with a spinal cord lesion

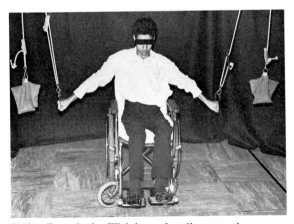

IX/12 Paraplegia. Weight and pulley exercise to
strengthen adductors of the shoulder, elbow extensors
and grip

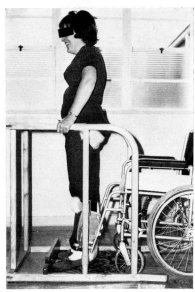

IX/13 Care is taken to see feet do not slip

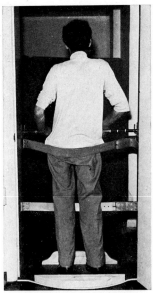

IX/14 Standing frame for home fitting and use. The patient is standing in the doorway of his home. It is a cheap, simple adaptation of the 'standing frame' idea. It can be put up in seconds once the fitments are fixed securely to the doorway

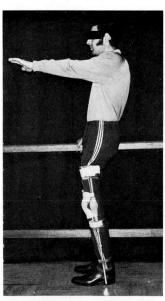

IX/15 Balance standing with one bar

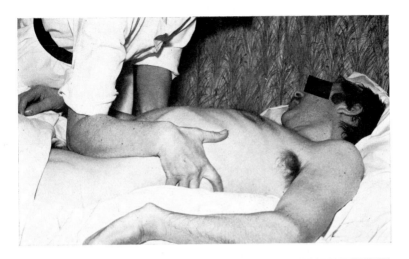

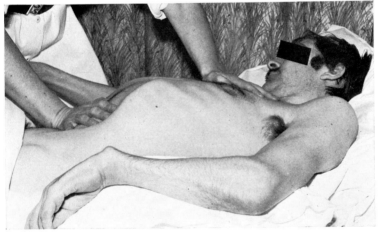

X/1 Position of hands for assisted coughing

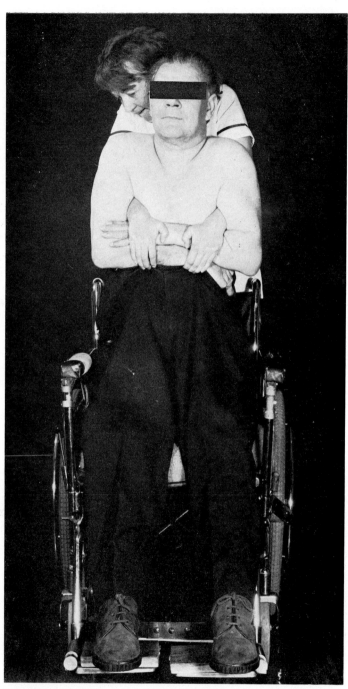

X/2 Method of lifting patient to relieve pressure

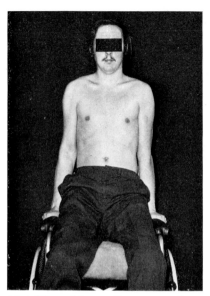

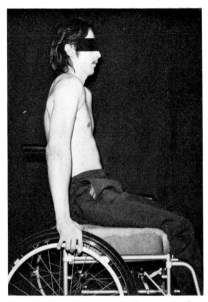

(a) A lift pushing up from arms of chair

(b) A lift pushing up from wheel of chair

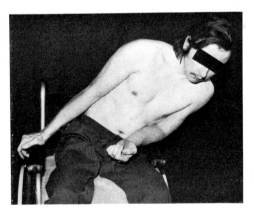

(c) To show how a low tetraplegic can roll sideways to relieve pressure

X/3 Methods of lifting to relieve pressure

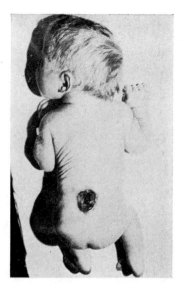

XI/1 Spina bifida

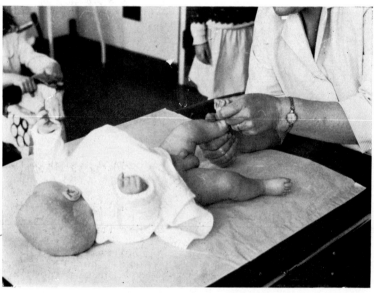

XI/2 Stretching talipes equino-varus

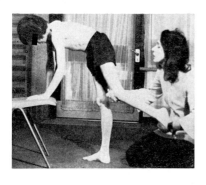

XII/1 Postural fixation: maintenance of posture of the head, trunk, pelvic and shoulder girdles

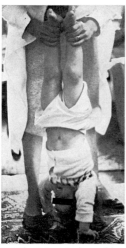

XII/2 Stimulation of saving reactions (protective extension and propping) in a spastic child

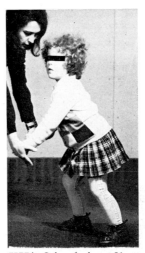

XII/3 Stimulation of locomotor reactions as the child leans forward on to the therapist's hands. The child is ataxic

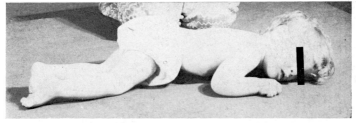

XII/4 Quadriplegic child with shoulder retraction (extension), adduction and internal rotation; elbow flexion; forearm pronation; flexed fingers and adducted thumb. Hips in flexion, adduction and tendency to internal rotation; knees semi-flexed; feet plantar flexed (extension) and equino-varus. Postural components may vary in other positions

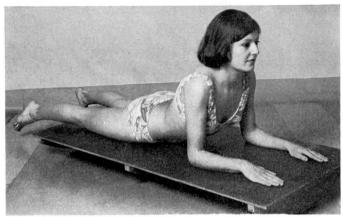

XV/1 Forearm support prone lying on balance board

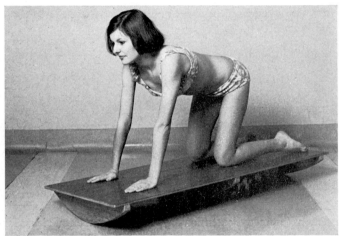

XV/2 Prone kneeling on balance board

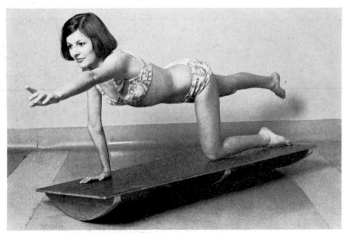

XV/3 Prone kneeling on balance board—balance reaction

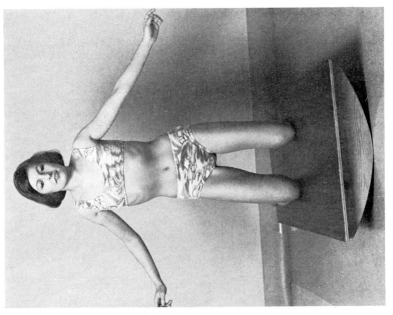

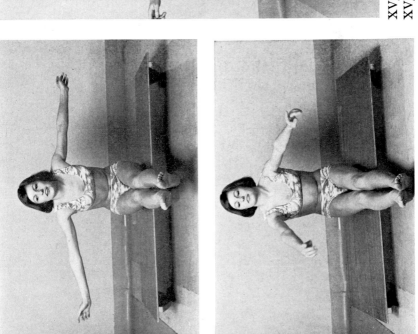

XV/4 (a) and (b) Sitting on balance board—balance reactions
XV/5 Kneeling on balance board—balance reaction

XV/4 (a)

XV/4 (b)

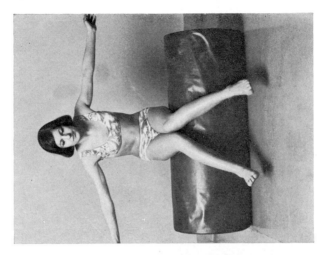
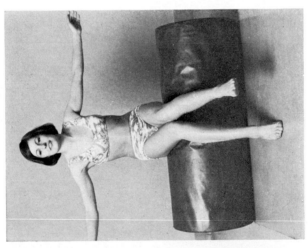
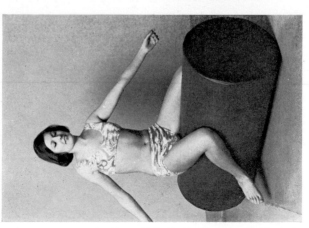

XV/6 (a) (b) (c) Sitting on roll—balance reactions

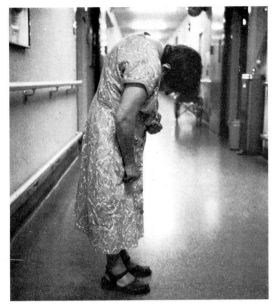

XVI/1 Typical stance of patient with parkinsonism

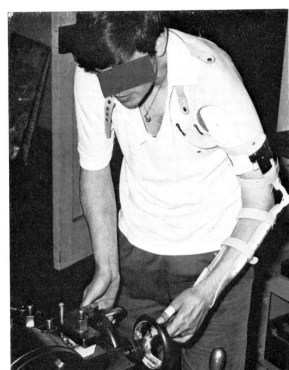

XIX/1 A C5 and 6 brachial plexus lesion wearing a splint which allows the patient to make use of the function in his hand

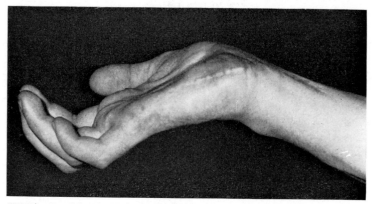

XIX/2 Combined median and ulnar nerve lesion showing flattening of the thenar eminence and clawing of the fingers

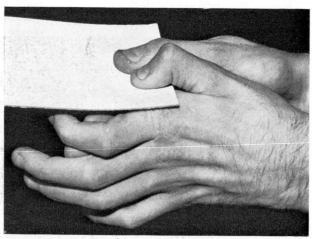

XIX/3 An ulnar nerve lesion. Note trick adduction of the thumb

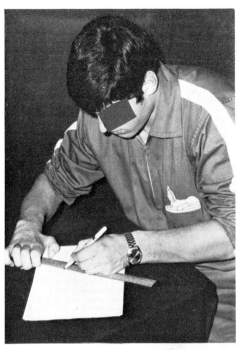

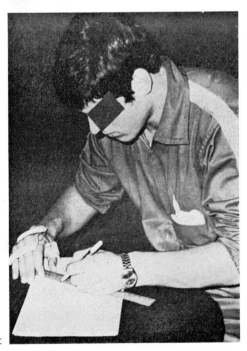

(b) wearing a lively splint

XIX/4 A patient with median and ulnar nerve lesions attempting to hold a ruler

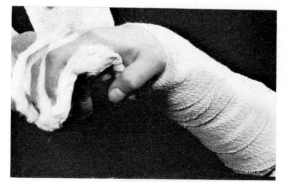

XIX/5 A median nerve lesion with adherence of the flexor tendons at the wrist having a serial stretch plaster applied

XIX/6 Sensory re-education for a recovering median nerve lesion

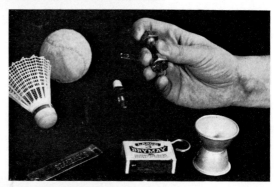

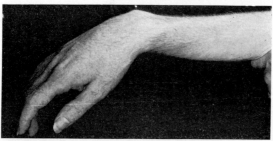

(a) showing a drop-wrist and wasting of the extensor aspect of the forearm

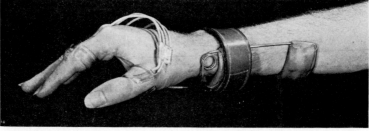

(b) splinted in a lively cock-up for the wrist and a spider splint for the fingers, allowing the interossei to extend the interphalangeal joints

XIX/7 A radial nerve palsy

While the baby is still in hospital, providing he is well enough the physiotherapist turns her attention to any deformities that may be present. Most common of these is talipes equino-varus and all will be treated according to the wishes of the consultant concerned.

Talipes equino-varus may be strapped with zinc oxide or elastic strapping, or treated by splinting. Whichever is used the physio-therapist must remember that the baby has impaired sensation, poor circulation and probably limbs that are in a poor condition generally so that she must be even more careful than usual in applying corrective measures. The limb should be coated with Tinct. Benzoin Co. (to get better adhesion and prevent sores) and a length of one inch strapping attached down the inside of the leg below the knee, around the heel to hold it in the correct position and up the lateral side of the leg to the knee but not over it. The second piece of strapping is to correct the forefront of the foot. It is attached to the dorsum of the foot at the level of the fifth metatarso-phalangeal joint, carried across the top of the foot along the line of the joints, under the sole and again up the lateral side of the leg. This is under tension so that the deformity is corrected as far as possible. Some prefer this length of strapping to be started on the plantar side of the fifth metatarso-phalangeal joint before being carried across the dorsum, but by using this method there is more danger of constricting the circulation. Short lengths of strapping are then passed around the leg (not under tension) to keep the first two in position. One length around the calf may be enough but a second piece near the ankle may also be necessary. A continuous piece of strapping used as a bandage is not advised in cases of spina bifida because of the poor skin condition and danger to the circulation. Once in position the feet must be watched for any interference in the circulation.

Different consultants like different methods of strapping for talipes equino-varus but the principle is the same – to strap the foot into eversion and dorsiflexion to correct the varus and equinus (i.e. inversion and plantarflexion) of the feet. Occasionally the feet may lie in a calcaneo-valgus position (in eversion and dorsiflexion) when strapping or splinting, if used, is into plantarflexion and inversion. In either case the physiotherapist will be called upon to stretch the feet (Plate XI/2).

The hips may be dislocated or 'at risk' from birth and the physio-therapist will be instructed accordingly. She will know the preferences of the consultant in charge and will only treat according to his wishes.

The baby may be nursed in a splint to keep his legs in abduction and lateral rotation and again the same precautions must be taken to prevent pressure and sores especially as there is the danger of wetting and soiling from the nappy.

Some splints used to maintain the abduction and lateral rotation are the Barlow, Von Rosen and Denis Browne (Fig. XI/9). The Barlow and Von Rosen are made of light malleable metal suitably padded to prevent undue pressure. The Barlow is in the form of the letter X, the upper arms of which are bent over the shoulders while the lower ones are put round the legs in the correct position. The Von Rosen is very similar but is H-shaped. The Denis Browne is just a straight bar with two cuffs into which the abducted and laterally rotated legs are placed; there is an oval pad in the central back to avoid pressure on the lesion and sometimes a harness to keep the splint in position. The choice of splint is the consultant's but in every case the damaged area of the back must be avoided and this may be the deciding factor. All the precautions against any pressure must be rigorously observed. Other deformities are individual to each baby and are treated accordingly.

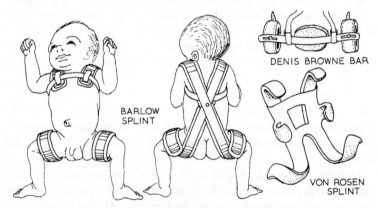

Fig. XI/9 Congenital dislocation of hip appliances

Subsequent treatment

When the baby is sent home a new but equally important team of workers look after the child and his family. This will include the family doctor and probably an infant welfare doctor, the health visitor, district nurse, social services department and a physiotherapist. Later this team will be extended to include a teacher at the child's school. (See also Chapter XXI.)

The physiotherapist is an essential part of this team – she may be the one to act as liaison between the team and the hospital concerned and her work will include far more than pure physiotherapy. It will be 'healing by physical means' in the truest sense by becoming an adviser in the physical management of the child.

Most spina bifida children are treated in paediatric hospitals with a large catchment area and frequent visits to the out-patient department may be impossible; the physiotherapist becomes a vital link here as she sees the child and parents regularly for treatment. With tact and understanding she can help the family to accept the baby as he is – a normal child born with a disability.

Acceptance by the family from the beginning and their future attitude to the child are very often dependent on the attitudes of the professional people who advise them. If the physiotherapist, while not showing undue optimism, can accentuate what the child *can* do and do her best to improve what is difficult and minimize what is impossible, then not only the family but also the child himself is likely to have a practical outlook for the future.

Physiotherapy

Physiotherapy already started while the child was in hospital is continued at home for many reasons – to treat any deformities present and to prevent others developing; to encourage what movement there may be in the limbs and to strengthen the muscles producing it; to exercise limbs that the child cannot exercise himself and by so doing improve the circulation; to encourage the child to keep up with his peers in his milestones i.e. rolling over, crawling, sitting up etc., and in later stages to teach him to walk in whatever calipers are necessary.

The experienced physiotherapist will be aware of any particular treatment advocated by the hospital concerned and a frequent exchange of ideas and information is helpful but the principles are the same in all cases.

Treatment of any deformities started in hospital will be continued and all joints will be exercised in their full range to prevent contractures. In general the flexor muscles are stronger than the extensors and this especially applies to the hips, even though the difference may be only slight. Hip flexion is often present and with the consent of the ortho-paedic surgeon, hip extension stretching should be routine as well as teaching the mother to place the baby in a prone position during play-time, preferably on the floor. It is hip flexion that causes the marked lordosis that is characteristic of older children with spina bifida.

Any movement present must be noted and encouraged and if there is any sensation in the legs this can be used to stimulate movement by tickling or touching. There may be little or no sensation present and until the baby can respond to toys most of the movement will be passive. These passive movements must be given in as full a range as possible to all joints starting with the toes, then the tarsal joints, ankles, knees and hips. This not only helps to keep them supple but it gives the circulation the pumping action that normal babies provide by their kicking. Mothers must be taught how to carry out these movements and advised to do them each time they change the baby's nappy.

Arm movements can be started as soon as the baby responds and exercises to strengthen the shoulder girdle gradually introduced. This is necessary because most patients with spina bifida will need to rely on sticks or crutches to help them to walk and a strong shoulder girdle is very necessary.

A knowledge of the developmental progress and milestones of a normal child is necessary to be able to assess when a disabled child is ready to be encouraged to attempt another skill such as rolling over, sitting up and even his own brand of crawling (see also Chapter II). The physiotherapist must be alert to his development and start instruct-ing him in the next step just before he is ready for it. The mother is encouraged to prop him up as soon as he shows an interest in his sur-roundings. In the past children have become more disabled simply because having been told that their child is disabled, the parents have not realized and have not been told that their child needs all the challenges and stimuli he can get to develop his potential to the full in the same way as any other baby.

Play therapy forms a very important part of the general physiotherapy. As soon as the baby begins to respond, brightly-coloured toys and those that make a noise are excellent to encourage any movement – squeaky toys to press on, coloured balls to push away, miniature cars to make a bridge for (a useful exercise for gluteal contractions, see Fig. XI/10) all have their place. As the child gets older, bigger toys can be introduced

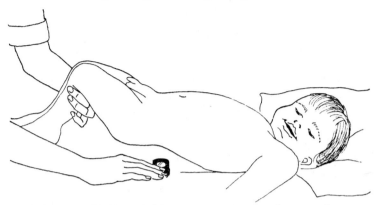

Fig. XI/10 Making a bridge to encourage gluteal contractions

– nursery slides to pull *up* rather than slide down, to strengthen the shoulders, and small trampolines to teach the child to sit on an unsteady surface and later to stand on it.

The ingenuity of the physiotherapist will be taxed to the full to make the treatment interesting and so get the child's full co-operation because routine exercises are boring to small children and they rarely respond.

Proprioceptive neuromuscular facilitation (P.N.F.) has very little use in the early treatment of spina bifida partly because of the lack of sensation and partly because physiotherapy is of most use when the child is too young to respond to the kind of instructions necessary. Resisted exercises can however be devised to encourage action in muscles which are innervated, i.e. putting baby's feet with knees and hips flexed on one's chest and saying 'push me away' is useful in some sacral lesions where hip and knee action is present, but weak.

If spasticity is present, treatment is given on the usual lines for cerebral palsy (see Chapter XII, p. 266).

Ambulation

Early ambulation is now regarded as necessary for the normal development of a spina bifida child. All babies – except some retarded ones – walk some time between their first and second birthdays, a few a little before and some slightly later. This is the psychological time for walking and most spina bifida children despite their slow start, are no exception. If they can be fitted with suitable appliances to help them to walk, then the physiotherapist has nature and the innate desire of the children to help her and her task is lighter. Once this stage has passed and the children realise they are different the barrier of 'conditioned inability' creeps in. The longer walking is delayed the deeper this conviction becomes and the greater will be the work of the physiotherapist to overcome this barrier.

Whether early ambulation will overcome the tendency of children to give up walking and become wheelchair-bound at adolescence it is too early to tell since treated children are only just reaching this stage, but in any case wheelchairs should not be encouraged any more than can be helped as wheelchair addiction is only too easy to acquire.

In order to enable children with spina bifida to walk some sort of calipers will be necessary in all but a few cases. In general the higher in the back the lesion is the greater will be the splintage needed. Those with a dorsal lesion often need calipers with both pelvic and chest bands, while dorso-lumbar lesions usually need calipers with a pelvic band and sacral lesions manage with only below-knee irons.

In general the physiotherapist should aim at having the child walking independently (albeit with sticks, crutches, or some other aid) by the time he is due to go to school. The physiotherapist will still be necessary as adviser in management in the school as well as to prevent any deterioration in walking and for post-operative physiotherapy when the child comes home but the greater part of the education in walking and independence should be finished by then.

Surgery

The attitude of the general public towards disabled children has improved markedly in recent years and this, coupled with enlightened medical treatment, means that children born with a disability can look forward to finding their rightful place in the community. This especially applies to those with normal intelligence and the physical ability to obtain a good degree of independence. Many cases of spina bifida are in this category, but to do this, education and training are essential to enable the children to develop to their full potential. Doctors therefore try to arrange that all major surgery is, if possible, carried out during the pre-school years so that the child's education is interrupted as little as is practicable.

This means that before he is five the child may have been in and out of hospital many times. Occasionally the shunt may block and replacement prove necessary. As the child grows the distal catheter may need to be replaced with a longer one. Orthopaedic surgery may be necessary to correct deformities, so enabling the child to wear calipers and become mobile. Lastly, the 'ileal loop' or urinary diversion operation as described earlier may be carried out any time in the first five years.

Education

The problem of schooling has probably worried the parents from the beginning and a good physiotherapist needs to know what facilities are available in her district. She will be asked by the team to give her judgement on what type of school the child is physically best suited for. Educational suitability will be assessed by the educational psychologist but the authorities often depend on the opinion of the physiotherapist as to whether the child can cope with a normal school or whether a school for the physically handicapped would suit his disability best. Once the child starts in a normal primary school the teachers welcome the advice of the physiotherapist in his management; whereas if he goes to a school for the physically disabled there are usually physiotherapists on the staff.

Training

More and more avenues are opening for disabled adolescents and given the ability and desire (and a certain amount of adjustment by all concerned including the adolescent and his family) many trades and professions welcome disabled members.

During adolescence the full impact of his disability may hit the victim and this is the time when the early training in acceptance will help, but there is often a period of depression and withdrawal when he realizes that he will never be normal. Such a teenager should be encouraged to join as much as he can in the social life of the community. There are many activities at which the spina bifida youngster can excel – horseriding, archery, table-tennis are but a few where he can compete with normal people.

There are a few training colleges specially designed to cater for the training of disabled people in many skills, but most universities, teachers' training colleges and colleges of further education are only too willing to accept disabled young adults if it is at all possible.

Marriage

The question of marriage and reproduction is another one that has occupied the thoughts of parents and is often discussed by them during physiotherapy sessions. As the treated spina bifida cases are only now reaching adolescence, there are not many statistics to quote and the only experience we have is in those untreated survivors who managed to grow up without the modern treatment. In general it may be said that spina bifida girls can marry and have children, some of whom may be quite normal, but in men the sex act depends largely on sensation and where that is absent the man will probably be impotent, but this is a very complicated matter and other factors are involved.

Spina bifida cystica is now the biggest single cause of congenital physical handicap. The invention of the shunt has had very far reaching results, the impact of which is only just being realized. It is presenting the medical profession in general and physiotherapists in particular with a challenging problem. Physiotherapists should accept this challenge by widening their horizons and becoming an integral part of the various teams who work together to give such children as normal a life as their disability will allow.

FURTHER READING

Cook, Richard C. M. 'Spina Bifida and Hydrocephalus'. Brit. Med. J. (1971), **4**, 796-799.

Eckstein, H. B. 'The Child with Myelomeningocele'. Midwife & Health Visitor (November 1967), Vol. **3**.

Field, Allen. *The Challenge of Spina Bifida.* William Heinemann Medical Books, 1970.

Holgate, Leonie. 'Physiotherapy for Spina Bifida'. Published by Queen Mary's Hospital, Carshalton.

Lorber, John. 'Your Child with Spina Bifida' and 'Your Child with Hydrocephalus'. Published by the Association for Spina Bifida and Hydrocephalus.

Nettles, O. R. 'The Spina Bifida Baby'. Published by the Scottish Spina Bifida Association.

Nettles, O. R. 'Growing up with Spina Bifida'. Published by the Scottish Spina Bifida Association.

Physiotherapy. August 1969, April 1970, February 1971, April 1971, etc.

Sheridan, Mary. 'The Developmental Progress of Infants and Young Children'. HMSO, 1968.

Swinyard, Chester. 'The Child with Spina Bifida'. Published by the Association for the Aid of Crippled Children, New York.

Watkins, Arthur G. 'Spina Bifida Cystica'. Nursing Times, 8 March 1968.

Webster, Barbara. 'Clothing for the Spina Bifida Child'. Published by the Association for Spina Bifida and Hydrocephalus.

'Equipment and Aids to Mobility'. Published by the Association for Spina Bifida and Hydrocephalus.

CHAPTER XII

Cerebral Palsy

by SOPHIE LEVITT, B.SC.(PHYSIOTHERAPY, RAND)

CEREBRAL PALSY, MENTAL HANDICAP AND DEVELOPMENTAL DELAY

The physiotherapy in cerebral palsy is intimately involved with child development. Most of the techniques, therefore, are used in the field of mental subnormality and any other developmental delay in children besides that associated with cerebral palsy.

Definition

Cerebral palsy, or more accurately, the cerebral palsies are a group of motor disorders caused by damage or maldevelopment of the brain that occurs prenatally, peri-natally or postnatally. Although the lesion is non-progressive, since the brain and nervous system develop in the presence of the lesion, the clinical picture of disordered movement and posture will change as the child gets older. Despite its name the cerebral palsies present not only 'palsies', or motor problems, but many other problems in these children. They often have multiple handicaps.

Incidence

In various countries this varies between 0·6 and 5·9 per 1,000 births. In Britain the incidence is given as 1·7 per 1,000 (Asher & Schonell), 1·9 per 1,000 (Woods) and 1·99 per 1,000 (Ingram).

Multiple Handicaps

.Damage or malfunction of the brain of the infant and young child may disrupt not only motor function but also other functions of the brain. The lesion is often diffuse. There may be speech and communication problems, hearing or visual disorders, epilepsy, perceptual disturbance, apraxias, mental defect and general behaviour problems. Fortunately not all of these may be present in the same child!

The non-motor handicaps may be due to the original organic lesion or they may be secondary to the motor handicap. Secondary handicap occurs because the child is unable to acquire normal learning experience because he cannot move normally and explore his environment. He cannot creep, crawl or walk, nor use his hands to discover the meaning of space and direction, of textures, of shape or temperature. He may not be able to look at, reach or touch different parts of his face and body in order to learn his body image and its spatial relationships. This paucity of normal everyday experiences disrupts normal perceptual and conceptual development. This and his poor motor development affect speech and language development. If, say, he cannot even control his head, he cannot observe what makes a specific sound and he cannot easily communicate with eye to eye contact with another person. Without head control he also misses perceptual information; he cannot observe perceptual aspects such as the relationships of objects to himself and to each other which give meaning to words. He has not experienced the meaning of such words as 'far, near, up, down, in, out, beside'.

Socially and emotionally the child is handicapped as he cannot run up to join his friends at play, cannot fling his arms around his mother's neck or even push an annoying child away.

In addition, the stress on the family having a handicapped child creates emotional problems, some of which may handicap the cerebral palsied child as well. The family's attitudes and their socio-economic problems are important influences on the cerebral palsied child's function.

With all these problems to face, it is, therefore, not surprising that an intelligent cerebral palsied child may appear mentally subnormal or, if he is mentally low, may appear even more subnormal than he is. The contribution of the physiotherapist to the cerebral palsied child's motor development, therefore, has far-reaching effects on the child's total development.

Aetiology

There are many causes in pregnancy, labour and delivery which may result in cerebral palsy. The most common causes are associated with abnormal labour and delivery, including forceps delivery, asphyxia of the newborn, neonatal jaundice and especially prematurity. Postnatal causes may be trauma, meningitis, encephalitis, high fever, a vascular accident or tumours. The cause may not be clear and a number of possible causes may be present or there may even be a history of normal pregnancy, labour and birth. Genetic factors may exist. Brain damage may also be associated with hydrocephalus and spina bifida and similar problems encountered as in cerebral palsy.

Clinical Features

The causes of mental subnormality or the 'clumsy child' or minimal brain dysfunction are often the same as the causes of cerebral palsy. The severity varies from severe mentally and physically handicapped children to the clumsy child who is intelligent but who has specific learning problems.

Classification

Cerebral palsied children are classified differently in different clinics. The most commonly accepted classifications are the Diagnostic Types given as follows.

Diagnostic Types

1. Spastics.
2. Athetoids or Dyskinesias.
3. Ataxics.
4. Rigid and Dystonics (sometimes classified under the Dyskinesias).
5. Mixed types.

Atonic type usually changes to become one of the above. It is more common to have some mixture in these types of cerebral palsy.

There is also:

Classification of Distribution

1. Hemiplegia. One side of the body affected.
2. Bilateral hemiplegia or quadriplegia. All limbs are affected (mainly the upper limbs).
3. Diplegia. All limbs are affected (mainly the lower limbs).
4. Triplegia. Lower limbs and one arm affected.
5. Paraplegia. Lower limbs affected.
6. Monoplegia. One limb affected (very rare).

Topographical classification should *not* be so dogmatic as to prevent the physiotherapist from checking the function of the other parts of the body.

Classification of Severity

This varies greatly from clinic to clinic. In general:

1. Mild. Where the child is independent and even so mild that he only appears to be clumsy. The non-motor handicaps may be the greater problem in these children.
2. Moderate. Where the child can achieve partial independence and requires aids for most activities.
3. Severe. When the child is totally or almost totally helpless and a wheelchair is inevitable. The accuracy of this classification is poor as it is too general for the physiotherapist.

Any classification or diagnosis is only *a beginning* and the physiotherapist must make a detailed assessment, especially of the motor skills or functions in each child at his levels of development.

SIGNS AND SYMPTOMS

Slow Acquisition of Motor Skills

Cerebral palsied babies and children have not acquired the motor skills seen in normal children of their own age.

Abnormal Performance of any Motor Skills

The few motor skills that are acquired by the child are frequently carried out in an abnormal way. The abnormal performance may simulate the pattern of posture and movements seen in infants or children younger than the cerebral palsied child. In addition there are postures and movements which are not seen at earlier levels in any normal children but are pathological. These pathological postures and movements result from spasticity, rigidity, involuntary movements of various kinds and from ataxia.

Abnormal Reflexes or Reactions

These are of three kinds. (*i*) The abnormal reflexes of the upper motor neurone lesion such as the brisk tendon jerks. These reflexes do not affect the physiotherapist directly and are diagnostic. (*ii*) The reflexes or neurological reactions present in the newborn which do not disappear as in normal development. Techniques to counter these in older children may be needed. (*iii*) The neurological reactions which appear in the maturing nervous system. Techniques to stimulate these reactions are frequently needed. (*iv*) Pathological reflexes seen in upper motor neurone lesions, e.g. associated reactions and withdrawal reflexes, extensor thrusts, symmetrical tonic neck reflex, asymmetrical tonic neck reflex and tonic labyrinthine reflex (see also Chapter I).

The physiotherapist must know what all these reflexes look like and whether they are present in her patients. For example, in the author's experience the tonic neck and labyrinthine reflexes are rarely present as such in cerebral palsied children. However, what is even more important is to recognize only those reflexes or reactions which disrupt function or cause deformity. There are many reactions which are diagnostic and of no direct interest for physiotherapy.

The most important reactions which should appear with maturation or motor development and which require physiotherapy are the following.

(The presentation is taken from Purdon-Martin who studied these postural reactions in adults.)

POSTURAL FIXATION
Maintenanee of posture of the head, trunk, pelvic and shoulder girdles (see Plate XII/1).

COUNTERPOISING
Maintenance of posture whilst counterpoising the movement of part of the body such as an arm or leg (see Plate XII/1).

TILTING REACTIONS
If the child is tilted off the horizontal he adjusts his balance using his neck and trunk muscles.

SAVING OR PROTECTIVE REACTIONS
If the tilt of the child is so great that his tilt reactions cannot save him from falling, he will fling his arms and legs out to save himself (see Plate XII/2).

RISING OR RIGHTING REACTIONS
These are used to rise from the floor to sitting, hands and knees, or to standing and other positions. Change of posture is dependent on these reactions.

LOCOMOTION REACTIONS
To initiate a step, continue walking and to stop walking (see Plate XII/3).

SPECIFIC SIGNS AND SYMPTOMS

The Spastic Type

The clinical description of spasticity differs in different systems of treatment. In general the observations are:

RESISTANCE TO SUDDEN PASSIVE STRETCH IN SPASTIC MUSCLE GROUPS
Sudden passive stretch results in a resistance given by an increase of muscle tension. This occurs at a threshold in the passive range of movement. Such spasticity is of the 'clasp-knife' variety, also called hyperactive stretch reflex. Spasticity occurs mainly in the shoulder flexors, retractors, adductors, internal rotators, elbow flexors and pronators, wrist flexors, flexors of fingers and thumb, hip flexors, internal rotators, adductors, knee flexors, plantar flexors, evertors, invertors of the feet.

ABNORMAL POSTURES OF A GREAT VARIETY
The spastic muscle groups above usually shorten and have a tight pull on the joints contributing to their abnormal positions. There is apparent

weakness of their antagonists which do not counteract these abnormal joint positions. The abnormal postures must be studied in the whole child, that is, his limbs, trunk and head, as they are almost never localized to one joint. The abnormal postures are deformities, which at first are unfixed but become fixed deformities or contractures if not treated adequately.

ABNORMAL VOLUNTARY MOVEMENT

Spasticity is not paralysis; the movements are present but often laboured, weak and look abnormal.

(*i*) *The synergies or patterns* of movements are similar to the postures and vary in each child and at different developmental levels. The following synergies are common examples. *Arm*: Shoulder protraction, adduction, internal rotation. Elbow flexion, pronation or extension-pronation. Wrist and hand flexion and ulnar deviation. *Leg*: Hip semi-flexion, adduction, internal rotation. Knee flexion. Foot plantar flexion or eversion or inversion.

Total extensor or total flexor synergies may be seen occasionally. More commonly the abnormalities are the abnormal combinations of flexion at some joints with extension at others together with abnormal abduction, adduction, internal or external rotation (see Plate XII/4).

(*ii*) *Weakness is present* in the antagonists to the spastic synergies. The spastic muscle groups themselves are often weak and do not act throughout their full range of motion.

(*iii*) *Isolated movements* of one joint are difficult or impossible, thus the discrete movements of finer co-ordination of say, the hands, are difficult.

(*iv*) *Associated reactions.* Movement of one part of the child's body may have an associated increase in spasticity in other parts of the child's body.

The spastics may have squints, a variety of intelligence levels and perceptual problems. Poor posture-balance mechanism is present (see above). Involuntary movements occasionally occur in distal joints.

The Athetoid Type

INVOLUNTARY MOVEMENTS OR ATHETOSIS

These are purposeless slow or fast movements which may be unpatterned or patterned. They may be writhing, jerky, tremor, swiping or rotary patterns which may be present at rest, or only aroused on effort to move or speak, on excitement or even deep thinking. Some athetoids have involuntary movement at rest and on activity. Involuntary movements may be uncontrollable or the child can learn to control them. Fatigue, drowsiness, fever, prone-lying or holding the child's full attention decrease the involuntary movements. Athetosis may be present in all parts of the body including the facial grimacing and tongue musculature.

VOLUNTARY MOVEMENTS
These are usually possible but may be disrupted by the involuntary movements or hypertonia, if present. Poor fine movements and weakness are common.

HYPERTONIA OR HYPOTONIA
Hypertonia or hypotonia or fluctuations of tone are possible. The hypertonia may be rigidity or dystonia which resists passive stretch throughout the range of movement, i.e. the 'lead pipe' variety (see also Chapter III). There may also be spasticity in athetoids and sudden spasms of flexion or extension.

Athetoids often have high intelligence which may be masked by the severe grimacing and involuntary movement, instability and muscle tension. Eye movements, especially upwards, may be absent. There is often a high frequency hearing loss in the athetoids due to severe neonatal jaundice (kernicterus). Poor posture-balance mechanism (see above).

SUB-CLASSIFICATION
There are many different kinds of athetoids so that one should never discuss the 'treatment of athetoids', but describe the problems. Sub-classification of these patterns varies from clinic to clinic. The tremor type of cerebral palsy is usually treated similarly to the athetoids.

The Ataxic

DISTURBANCE OF POSTURE-BALANCE MECHANISM
The absence or abnormality in the postural reactions presented above (according to Purdon-Martin) is the most significant symptom. How-

ever, this also occurs in spastics and athetoids so that a pure ataxia is rare.

VOLUNTARY MOVEMENTS

Voluntary movements are present, clumsy and unco-ordinated. The child overshoots or undershoots the mark he aims for. This is also known as 'dysmetria'. An intention tremor may accompany movements.

HYPOTONIA

Hypotonia is usual.

NYSTAGMUS, LOW INTELLIGENCE, SLURRED SPEECH

These are often present.

Evolution of Signs and Symptoms

The specific signs and symptoms of the spastic, athetoid, ataxic, rigid and any other types of cerebral palsy are rarely seen in infants and babies. They may be rigid and become floppy or more often floppy and become spastic, athetoid or ataxic after a few years. Athetosis may appear as late as three years of age.

The babies are delayed in development with abnormal neurological reactions. They often have feeding problems and may be irritable. However, some *normal* babies start life this way and so it is difficult to know when to treat and when to 'wait and see'. On the whole physiotherapists prefer early treatment as it prevents deformity and stimulates the best possible motor performance in cerebral palsy children. In addition parents are shown how to handle their baby so that they can play, feed, dress, wash and later toilet train him. In carrying these activities out correctly there is stimulation of the best patterns of posture and movement in each child's damaged nervous system. Until medical prognosis is possible it is better to give 'developmental stimulation' to babies and correct any abnormal positioning until the diagnosis can be made.

TREATMENT

There are many systems of treatment in cerebral palsy and some of the most well-known approaches will be reviewed.

Muscle Education and Bracing

Dr. W. M. Phelps, an orthopaedic surgeon in Baltimore, U.S.A., encouraged physiotherapists, occupational therapists and speech therapists to form themselves into teams to treat cerebral palsy children. The main points of this treatment programme were as follows:

1. A specific diagnostic classification of the cerebral palsied child was the basis for specific treatment techniques. This included five types of cerebral palsy and many sub-classifications.

2. A list of fifteen 'modalities' or methods were taught to the therapists. These consisted of massage, passive motion, active assisted motion, active motion, resisted motion, rest, conditioned motion, confused motion, combined motion, balance, reach and grasp, skills, relaxation, movement from relaxation and reciprocation.

3. Braces or calipers were specially designed and developed by Phelps. He prescribed braces to correct deformity and braces to control athetosis.

4. Equipment for daily living. Many aids for dressing, washing and feeding, and for sitting and locomotion were developed.

5. Muscle education for spastics and training in joint control for athetoids was the emphasis of the largely orthopaedic view of cerebral palsy. Motor development was seldom discussed as a foundation for therapy.

Muscle education for spastics was also developed in specific ways by a number of other cerebral palsy authorities such as Pohl in America, Plum in Denmark and many orthopaedic therapists and doctors in Britain.

Although many people today dismiss Phelps' approach, there is much of interest which we can still use for our patients. Braces (calipers) are needed by some children although they need not be as extensive or used for as many years as Phelps recommended. Muscle education is necessary before and after orthopaedic surgery. Many of the aids devised at Phelps' clinic form the basis of occupational therapy today.

In Tardieu's work in Paris, there is not only neurological assessment but also detailed 'factorial analysis' of muscles in spastics to explain the abnormal movements and deformities. He recommends bracing, some muscle education, alchohol injections into the motor point of a particular spastic muscle, orthopaedic surgery and developmental training.

Progressive Pattern Movements

The main points of this approach devised by Temple Fay are:

1. The recommendation that the cerebral palsied be taught motion according to its development in evolution. Fay regards motor development as evolving from reptilian squirming to amphibian movements, through mammalian reciprocal motion 'on all fours' to the advanced skill of walking. He argues that as early movements of progression are carried out by lower animals with a simple nervous system, they can similarly be carried out in the human in the absence of a normal cerebral cortex. The primitive patterns of movement and reflexes can be stimulated in the handicapped parts of the body, through the spine, medulla, pons and midbrain. Fay's 'pattern movements' are based on these ideas.

The author has found the pattern movements useful for co-ordination, reciprocal motion, concentration and rhythm.

2. The movement patterns begin with prone lying, head and trunk rotation or primitive squirming followed by a primitive creeping with a homolateral pattern of the arm and leg on the same side, then a contralateral pattern of arm and leg on the opposite sides. After creeping the child is trained to crawl on hands and knees and then 'elephant walk' on hands and feet and finally the walking pattern of man.

3. A strict sequence of this phylogenetic development is stressed.

4. The creeping movements are taught with passive motion or 'patterning' by adults. The child is much later encouraged to carry this out alone.

5. No braces and no aids are used.

6. Reflex movements or 'unlocking' reflexes are used to relax spasticity, e.g. reflex withdrawal of hip and knee into flexion abduction to 'unlock' adductor extensor spasticity.

Proprioceptive Neuromuscular Facilitation

Kabat disagrees with the training of isolated muscles or isolated joint motion which he says are almost never used as such in voluntary activities.

The main points in this approach, which have been developed by Margaret Knott, Dorothy Voss and others are:

1. Movement patterns rather than muscle education of individual muscle groups are recommended. However, the movement patterns taught should be those used by man in such functions as rolling over, getting up, locomotion and various daily skills using the upper limb.

2. The diagonal and rotary aspects of movement patterns were observed by Kabat. Every movement pattern used in the therapeutic techniques has a diagonal direction. Internal-external rotation and flexion-extension and abduction-adduction are the elements of the patterns.

3. Sensory (afferent) stimuli were shown to stimulate motion. Proprioception is emphasized although the techniques include touch, auditory and visual stimuli as well as the stimuli from stretch, pressure and muscle contraction.

4. Resistance is used to facilitate stronger muscle action within the synergic patterns of movement. Various methods are used to adjust the degree of resistance. It is also important to know where to apply resistance to get a local effect or an effect in another part of the body associated with the movement pattern.

5. Ice treatments are used to relax or inhibit hypertonus. Relaxation techniques of a special kind are also included for selected cases.

These methods are useful in many cerebral palsied children, are particularly good for weakness in any condition, and can be used to train motor skills. Although not mentioned by most authorities writing about proprioceptive neuromuscular facilitation, the author has found that modifications should be made when treating the various types of cerebral palsy (see References).

Neuromotor Development

Eirene Colles was a British pioneer of cerebral palsy treatment. She stressed neuromotor development as a basis for treatment. Her developmental milestones were dogmatically presented. She also considered it important to plan the whole day of the child and not rely solely on short physiotherapy sessions. Colles suggested that there should be 'cerebral palsy therapists' rather than separate professions of physiotherapists, occupational therapists and speech therapists. She thought this would help the child to have a more successful total therapeutic day, and also counteract the isolation of the different professional disciplines.

Neurodevelopmental Treatment with Reflex Inhibition and Facilitation

Dr. Karl Bobath, a neuropsychiatrist, and Mrs. Berta Bobath, a physiotherapist, base assessment and treatment on the premise that the fundamental difficulty of cerebral palsy is lack of inhibition of reflex patterns of posture and movement. The Bobaths associate these abnormal patterns with abnormal tone due to overaction of tonic reflex activity. These tonic reflexes and asymmetrical tonic neck reflexes have to be inhibited. Once the abnormal tone and reflex patterns have been inhibited, there should be facilitation of more mature postural reflexes. All this is carried out in a developmental context. The main features of their work are:

1. '*Reflex inhibitory patterns*' specifically selected to inhibit abnormal tone associated with abnormal movement patterns and abnormal posture.

2. *Sensory motor experience*. The reversal or 'breakdown' of these abnormalities gives the child the sensation of more normal tone and movements. This sensory experience is believed to 'feed back' and guide more normal motion. Sensory stimuli are also used for inhibition and facilitation and voluntary movement.

3. *Facilitation* techniques for mature postural reflexes.

4. '*Key points of control*'. The inhibition of abnormal postures and movements in reflex inhibiting patterns, and the facilitation of more desirable patterns are carried out by correct manual handling of the child by skilful use of 'key points of control' and by various sensory stimuli.

5. *Developmental sequence* is followed and adapted to each child.

6. *All-day management* should supplement treatment sessions. Parents and others are advised on daily management and trained to treat the children. Nancie Finnie has written a book for parents on the subject of handling a child in the home (see References).

A rather simplified example of the features of this approach may be applied to a spastic child who is excessively extended in supine. This extensor spasticity is considered to be due to the tonic labyrinthine reflex (see page 34). In order to inhibit the spasticity one of the *reflex inhibitory patterns* might be to flex the child's head and shoulders and hips and knees manually, or in a hammock, for everyday management. The flexion may be carried out actively. The *keypoints of control* might be that if the head is held flexed, the legs may be able to flex actively or if the hips are held in flexion, as a keypoint of control, then the child may be able actively to flex his head to look at his knees. Flexion of his head, off the couch, is also part of the more *mature postural reaction* of head righting in supine. This head righting is *facilitated* whilst there is a reflex inhibitory pattern to inhibit the extensor spasticity. The *developmental sequence* is involved in that a reflex inhibitory pattern may be sitting with hip and knee flexion rather than the earlier level of supine lying with hip and knee flexion. In facilitating the head righting in supine, this would be possible if the child is approximately at about the 6 months normal developmental level when this postural reaction is expected. Once again in the all-day management, the child may be carried correctly in a flexed position, placed in chairs which are designed to flex his hips and knees and have his shoulders flexed forward instead of retracted into extension. Play activities are given to motivate flexion at the child's developmental level.

Every child is individual and the above example does not apply to every child with extensor spasticity, but is only an example to clarify some of the features of this approach.

Sensory Stimulation for Activation and Inhibition

Margaret Rood, a physiotherapist and occupational therapist, bases her approach on many neurophysiological theories and the literature. The main features of her approach are:

1. *Afferent stimuli.* The various nerves and sensory receptors are described and classified into types, location, effect, response, distribution and indication. Techniques of stimulation, such as – stroking, pressure, brushing (tactile) – icing, heating (temperature) – bone pounding – slow and quick muscle stretch – joint retraction and approximation, muscle contractions, muscle pressure (proprioception) are used to activate, facilitate or inhibit motor response.

2. *Muscles* are classified according to various physiological data, including whether they are for 'light work muscle action' or 'heavy work muscle action'. The appropriate stimuli for their actions are suggested.

3. *Reflexes* other than the above are used in therapy, e.g. tonic labyrinthine reflexes, tonic neck, vestibular reflexes, withdrawal patterns.

4. *Ontogenetic development sequence* is outlined and strictly followed in the application of stimuli.

(*i*) Total flexion or withdrawal pattern (in supine).

(*ii*) Roll over (flexion of arm and leg on the same side and roll over).

(*iii*) Pivot prone (prone with extension of head, trunk and legs).

(*iv*) Co-contraction neck (prone, head over edge for co-contraction of vertebral muscles).

(*v*) On elbows (prone and push backwards).

(*vi*) All fours (static, weight shift and crawl).

(*vii*) Standing upright (static, weight shifts).

(*viii*) Walking (stance, push off, pick up, heel strike).

5. *Vital functions.* A developmental sequence of respiration, sucking, swallowing, phonation, chewing and speech is followed. Techniques of brushing, icing and pressure are used.

Reflex Creeping and Other Reflex Reactions

Dr. Vaslav Vojta, a neurologist working in Czechoslovakia, developed an approach based on the work of Temple Fay, Kabat and his own ideas. The main features are:

1. *Reflex creeping.* The creeping patterns involving head, trunk and limbs are facilitated at various 'trigger' points or 'reflex zones'. The creeping is an active response to the appropriate 'triggering' from the zones with sensory stimuli. The muscle work used in the normal creeping patterns or 'creeping complex' have been carefully analysed. The therapist must be skilful in the facilitation of these normal patterns and not provoke 'pathological patterns'.

2. *Sensory stimulation.* Touch, pressure, stretch and muscle action against resistance are used in many of the triggering mechanisms, or in the facilitation of creeping.

3. *Resistance* is recommended for action of muscles. Various specific techniques are used to apply the resistance so that either a tonic or phasic muscle action is provoked. The phasic action may be provoked on a movement of a limb creeping up or downwards. The tonic action, or stabilising action is obtained if a phasic movement is fully resisted. Therefore the static muscle action of stability occurs if resistance is applied so that it prevents any movement through the range.

Conductive Education

Professor Andras Peto in Budapest, Hungary, originated Conductive Education. Since Professor Peto's death, his work has been continued by Dr. M. Hari. The main features are the integration of therapy and education by:

1. *A conductor* acting as mother, nurse, teacher and therapist. She is specially trained in the habilitation of motor disabled children in a four-year course. She may have one or two assistants.

2. *The group* of children, about fifteen to twenty, work together. Groups are fundamental in this training system.

3. *An all-day programme.* A timetable is planned to include getting out of bed in the morning, dressing, feeding, toileting, movement training, speech, reading, writing and other school work.

4. *The movements.* There are sessions of movements, mainly taking place on and beside slatted plinths (table/beds) and with ladder-backed chairs. The movements are devised in such a way that they form the elements of a task or motor skill. The tasks are carefully analysed for each group of children. The tasks are the activities of daily living, hand skills including hand function, balance and loco-motion. The purpose of each movement is explained to the children. The movements are repeated, not only in the movement session of, say, the 'hand class' or 'plinth work', but also in various contexts throughout the day. The children are shown in practice how their 'exercises' contribute to daily activities.

5. *Rhythmic intention.* The technique used for training the elements or movements is 'rhythmic intention'. The conductor and the children state the intended motion, 'I touch my mouth with my hands'. This motion is then attempted together with their slow, rhythmic counts of one to five. Motion is also carried out to an operative word such as 'up, up, up' repeated in a rhythm slow enough for their active movement. Speech and active motion reinforce each other.

6. *Individual sessions* may be used for some children to help them to participate more adequately in the work of the group.

7. *Learning principles* are basic to the programme. Conditioning techniques and group dynamics are among the mechanisms of training discussed. 'Cortical' or conscious participation is stressed, as opposed to involuntary and automatic, unconscious reflex therapy.

The Eclectic Viewpoint

It is difficult to prove which treatment approach is superior to the other. All claim good results and to date no approach can be scientifically proved superior by a controlled study. There are many variables such as intelligence, home background, personality of the child and of the therapist as well as different associated handicaps, which could affect the result of physiotherapy. Untreated controls are difficult to obtain, and it is also difficult to match the treated children in a study.

Theoretical considerations are controversial and none of the approaches have the complete answer to the understanding of the cerebral palsies. The lack of a complete 'answer' is not surprising as neither what is happening in the brain of the cerebral palsied nor the effect of therapy on the neurological and psychological mechanisms is fully understood as yet. From practical experience many physiotherapists find that each child is so individual in his clinical picture and needs, that it is difficult to confine all the children to any one set of techniques or approach. The facilities for treatment will also affect what techniques can be used.

In order to draw on various schools of thought and treatment systems it may be helpful to use the following general principles. These are the common factors the author has found after a study of many different systems of treatment.

MOTOR DEVELOPMENT
Follow the normal motor developmental sequences (gross and fine motor) and *modify them* according to each child. A detailed developmental assessment of each child is essential for treatment. The motor skills at each developmental level, such as head control, rolling, creeping, crawling, sitting, standing, walking and hand function should be facilitated with techniques from any treatment system. A physiotherapist may invent her own methods to obtain these motor activities and she must work particularly closely with the occupational therapists.

AFFERENT STIMULI
Various techniques are used with afferent stimuli to obtain desirable activity and decrease hypertonus.

PREVENTION OF DEFORMITY
Any methods to stimulate a variety of corrective movements should be

used. Splintage, bracing, correct furniture, footwear and frequent changes of posture are important in the prevention of deformity. Orthopaedic procedures, using plaster of Paris or surgery, may be indicated in selected cases.

INHIBITION AND FACILITATION

Inhibition of hypertonus can be obtained as a result of facilitation of active corrective movements and postures. These activities are best carried out within the function or context of the motor skills of child development. Correct training of, say, hand function, head control, rolling over, creeping, crawling, sitting, standing and walking will, at the same time, inhibit hypertonus and involuntary movement.

However, special techniques of inhibition of hypertonus may also be needed in some children. Both facilitation and inhibition techniques are available from many different approaches.

MOTIVATION TECHNIQUES

Motivation techniques with songs, toys, adventure playgrounds, play equipment, group games, group exercises, playgroups, music and horse riding can be subtly arranged to obtain active corrective movements, posture and equilibrium.

MOVEMENT PATTERNS AND MUSCLE WORK

Most modern systems train movement patterns rather than muscle education. However, specific muscle groups may be particularly weak or spastic or both and need concentrated therapy. They may be treated in isolation or 'in pattern', depending on the child.

TEAMWORK AND ALL-DAY CARE

It is not enough to see the treatment of the child as only a half-hour session in a day. The physiotherapist should check that her aims of treatment are not hampered by incorrect management throughout the day. She must check the furniture used by the child, his toys, the way he is carried, his feeding, washing, toileting and any other activities involving posture and movement. She will have to advise parents, teachers, other therapists, housemothers, and anyone handling the child as to what postures and movements to avoid and what to encourage.

In order to understand the child as a whole, and to treat him in a total habilitation programme, it is obvious that the therapist must function as part of a team of cerebral palsy workers. It is easier if the personnel handling the child are all working in the same building so that contact can be maintained. Staff conferences are useful, but informal discussions in the staff room are as important for team work.

It is essential to explore the different ways in which various professions overlap for the sake of total habilitation of the child. It is unrealistic for each professional person of a cerebral palsy team to isolate herself in her own department. The overlapping of therapies and education does not mean that there is still not a need for the benefits of the specialized knowledge and training. Clearly the parents must be part of this team work. Where cerebral palsy teams do not exist, parent participation is the only way a child can be treated.

INCREASE GENERAL SENSORY-MOTOR EXPERIENCE

The physiotherapist should make sure that in giving the child postures and movements and added independence, he uses these achievements to explore space, textures, shapes, temperatures and other everyday experiences. If he is learning to crawl or walk he should try not only on the floor of the physiotherapy room, but on grass, rough ground, in sand, on inclines and so on. He should get into boxes, cupboards, under tables, go into different rooms in his house and so on. Any visits to shops, the country and the zoo must be encouraged.

EARLY TREATMENT

The advantages of early treatment are that not only is motion stimulated but it is stimulated in the best possible patterns. An intelligent baby can be motivated to move by an enterprising mother. However, he will move in the way which comes easiest to him. In other words, the abnormal patterns of movement will be used. If there is a potential for more normal patterns in the baby's nervous system, correct early physiotherapy can facilitate this, and prevent the abnormal patterns from being established as habitual. If abnormal patterns are used, this can lead to deformities and later contractures.

LEARNING PROCESSES

Physiotherapy systems are preoccupied with orthopaedic and neurophysiological techniques. However, this is not the only way a child learns to move. Whilst working within multidisciplinary teams, physiotherapists should obtain information and be guided by educationalists and psychologists. The physiotherapist should also study principles of learning movement from the field of education, human movement studies, child development and psychology.

Techniques of Treatment

It is not possible to describe these in a chapter. The physiotherapist must attend courses, gain clinical experience, study the literature and carry out study visits in order to learn how to treat cerebral palsy. She must collect a repertoire of methods and understand the purpose of each method she decides to use. The methods must be relevant to each child's problems.

In selecting techniques for each child, the physiotherapist naturally selects the technique which she can carry out skilfully. Some techniques require more supervision and training than others.

In selecting techniques it is important to focus on the stimulation of motor function in daily life and the correction of the way in which they are performed. Techniques are, therefore, on three related aspects:

(*i*) Techniques only used by specially trained paediatric physiotherapists.

(*ii*) Techniques which can be shown to parents, nurses, playgroup workers, teachers and others stimulating movement or caring for cerebral palsied children.

(*iii*) Selection of equipment to reinforce techniques, or to be used with techniques of movement training.

REFERENCES

BOOKS

Blencowe, S. M. (ed., 1969). *Cerebral Palsy and the Young Child.* Churchill-Livingstone.

Bobath, B. (1971). *Abnormal Postural Reflex Activity caused by Brain Lesions.* Heinemann Medical Books.

Bobath, B. and Bobath, K. (1975). *Motor Development in the Different Types of Cerebral Palsy.* Heinemann Medical Books.

Bobath, K. (1966). *The Motor Deficit in Patients with Cerebral Palsy.* Heinemann Medical Books.

Decker, Ruby (1962). *Motor Integration.* Charles C. Thomas, U.S.A.

Egel, P. F. (1948). *Technique of Treatment for the Cerebral Palsied Child.* C. V. Mosby, St. Louis. (Phelps approach).

Finnie, Nancie (1974). *Handling the Young Cerebral Palsied Child at Home*. Heinemann Medical Books.

Foley, J. (1964–74). Personal communication. Lectures at the Cheyne Walk Centre for Spastic Children, Chelsea, London.

Foley, J. (1965). 'The Treatment of Cerebral Palsy' in *Physical Medicine in Paediatrics*, ed. B. Kiernander, Butterworth.

Gillette, Harriet E. (1969). *Systems of Therapy in Cerebral Palsy*. Charles C. Thomas, U.S.A.

Holt, K. S. (1965). *Assessment of Cerebral Palsy – Motor Function*. Lloyd-Luke.

Ingram, T. T. S. (1964). *Paediatric Aspects of Cerebral Palsy*. Churchill-Livingstone.

Knott, M. and Voss, D. E. (1969). *Proprioceptive Neuromuscular Facilitation Techniques*. Harper & Row, New York.

Levitt, Sophie (1962). *Physiotherapy in Cerebral Palsy*. Charles C. Thomas, U.S.A.

Purdon-Martin, J. (1967). *The Basal Ganglia and Posture*. Pitman Medical, London.

Woods, Grace (1975). *The Handicapped Child*. Blackwell Scientific Publications, Oxford.

PAPERS

American Journal of Physical Medicine, **26**(1), February 1967. 'An Exploratory and Analytical Survey of Therapeutic Exercise'.

Bobath, B. and Bobath, K. (1963). 'Treatment, Principles and Planning, in Cerebral Palsy'. Physiotherapy, April 1963. Also many other reprints, available from The Western Cerebral Palsy Centre, 20 Wellington Road, London, N.W.9.

Cotton, Ester (1970). 'Integration of Treatment and Education in Cerebral Palsy'. Physiotherapy, April 1970.

Cotton, Ester (1974). *The Basic Motor Pattern*. The Spastics Society, London.

Fay, Temple (1954). 'The Use of Pathological and Unlocking Reflexes in the Rehabilitation of Spastics'. Amer. J. Phys. Med., **33**, 347–52.

Levitt, Sophie (1966). 'Proprioceptive Neuromuscular Techniques in Cerebral Palsy'. Physiotherapy, **52**, 46.

Levitt, Sophie (1970). 'P.N.F. in Cerebral Palsy' in *Proceedings of the World Congress in Physical Therapy*, Amsterdam, Holland.

Levitt, Sophie (1974). 'Common Factors in Various Treatment Systems in Cerebral Palsy'. Cahiers (English edition), Paris.

Levitt, Sophie (1975). 'Stimulation of Movement: A Review of Therapeutic Techniques' in *Movement and Child Development*. Spastics International Medical Publications, Heinemann.

Levitt, Sophie (1976). 'Survey of Physiotherapy Approaches' in *Motor Learning in Children, Normal and Abnormal*. Workshop at the Institute of Child Health in association with Anstey College of Physical Education.

FURTHER READING

Bobath, K. and Bobath, B. (1964). 'The Facilitation of Normal Postural Reactions and Movements in the Treatment of Cerebral Palsy'. Physiotherapy, 50(8), 246.

Crothers, B. and Paine, R. S. (1959). *The Natural History of Cerebral Palsy*. Oxford University Press.

Gesell, A. (1966). *The First Five Years of Life*. Methuen.

Holt, K. S. (1965). *Assessment of Cerebral Palsy*. Lloyd-Luke.

Illingworth, R. S. (1966). *The Development of the Infant and the Young Child, Normal and Abnormal*. Third edition, Churchill-Livingstone.

Sheridan, M. (1968). *The Developmental Progress of Infants and Young Children*. H.M.S.O.

'Training the Multiply Handicapped Child', Physiotherapy, September 1971.

Note: This chapter on Cerebral Palsy was based on materials used by the author in a book *The Treatment of Cerebral Palsy and Motor Delay* to be published by Blackwell Scientific Publications, Oxford.

CHAPTER XIII

Hemiplegia – I

by JENNIFER M. BRYCE, M.C.S.P.
revised by JENNIFER M. TODD, M.C.S.P.
and PATRICIA M. DAVIES, M.C.S.P., DIP.PHYS.ED.
(*based on the work of* DR. and MRS. K. BOBATH)

Lesions which result in hemiplegia occur in the brain or upper segments of the spinal cord and can affect any age-group. The characteristic feature of hemiplegia is the loss of voluntary movement with alteration of muscle tone and sensation throughout one side of the body.

Causes

Hemiplegia in infants is caused by birth injury, congenital malformations, specific fevers, or space-occupying lesions. The above lesions affect an immature brain, and the additional management and handling required come under the umbrella of cerebral palsy (see Chapter XII).

In young adults hemiplegia may be brought about by trauma, vascular causes (e.g. thrombosis, haemorrhage or embolism), or space-occupying lesions (e.g. tumour or abscess).

In the middle-aged or elderly hemiplegia is caused by cerebral thrombosis, cerebral haemorrhage, or space-occupying lesions. Cerebrovascular accidents resulting in hemiplegia occur most frequently in later life because of degenerative changes in blood vessels and raised blood pressure.

ANATOMY AND PATHOLOGY

The two internal carotid and the two vertebral arteries carry the blood

288

supply to the brain. A linkage between these arteries at the base of the brain is called the circle of Willis. The main vessels arising from the circle are the anterior, middle and posterior cerebral arteries, each responsible for supplying important regions in the cortex, basal ganglia and upper brain stem.

Collateral circulation may be sufficient to compensate for a slowly-forming occlusion of any one of the main vessels supplying the brain, but a sudden, complete occlusion or lesion of one of the terminal branches of the circle of Willis usually produces clinical signs.

Hemiplegia due to vascular lesions commonly has its origin in a thrombotic or embolic process originating in the internal carotid arteries in the neck. A similar clinical picture may arise from occlusion of any of the major branches of the circle of Willis. Branches of the middle cerebral artery supply not only a major part of the main motor and sensory areas, including the speech area, but also the internal capsule. The internal capsule, closely related to the basal ganglia, has a concentration of fibres coming from many parts of the cortex, and occlusion of even a small vessel supplying this section can cause considerable damage. The anterior cerebral artery supplies the more medial parts of the anterior hemisphere, and near its origin has an important role in areas concerned with the maintenance of consciousness as well as higher intellectual functions.

Where haemorrhage causes localized destruction of brain tissue, there is additional damage to surrounding areas as a result of pressure from reactionary swelling. *Both thrombosis and embolism* obstruct the blood supply and cause infarction of brain tissue as a result of anoxia. Once brain cells or fibres are damaged they are gradually removed by neuroglial phagocytic cells, leaving either a cystic space or a fibrous scar.

The normal postural reflex mechanism

To assess and treat the problems of the hemiplegic patient the factors underlying normal movement must be understood. The normal postural reflex mechanism which provides a background for movement has two types of automatic reaction: righting reactions and equilibrium reactions.

Righting reactions allow the normal position of the head in space and in relation to the body, and normal alignment of trunk and limbs.

289

They give the rotation within the body axis which is necessary for most activities (see also page 35).

Equilibrium reactions maintain and regain balance. More complex than the righting reactions, they may be either visible movements or invisible changes of tone against gravity. Basic patterns of movement evolve from the righting reactions of early childhood, which later become integrated with the equilibrium reactions (see also page 36).

The brain is continuously receiving sensory impulses from the periphery, informing it of the body's activities. All movement is in response to these sensory stimuli and is monitored by proprioceptors (in muscles and joints), extroceptors (in skin and subcutaneous tissue) and telereceptors (the eyes and ears). Without sensation human beings do not know how to move or how to react to various situations, but in the conscious state intention may govern these reactions (see page 32).

Normal function of the body depends on the efficiency of the central nervous system as an organ of integration. Every skilled movement depends on:

1. NORMAL POSTURAL TONE
Postural tone, which is variable, provides the background on which movement is based, and is controlled at a subcortical level. It must be high enough to resist gravity yet still permit movement. Hypertonicity is loss of dynamic tone, giving stability without mobility. Hypotonicity precludes the stable posture necessary for movement. With each movement posture changes, and cannot be separated from it.

2. NORMAL RECIPROCAL INNERVATION
Reciprocal innervation allows graded action between agonists and antagonists. Proximally the interaction results in a degree of co-contraction which provides fixation and stability. Distally, skilled movements are made possible by a greater degree of reciprocal inhibition.

3. NORMAL PATTERNS OF MOVEMENT
Movement takes place in patterns that are common to all but there are slight variations in the way different people perform the same activity. The brain is not aware of individual muscles, only of patterns of movement produced by the interaction of groups of muscles.

DIFFICULTIES ASSOCIATED WITH HEMIPLEGIA

When treating the hemiplegic patient it must be remembered that the problem is loss not only of motor power but also of normal movement patterns, with abnormal tone, abnormal sensation and the presence of stereotyped associated reactions.

I. WEAKNESS

The inability to initiate movement is due to disturbed tone and reciprocal innervation and not to actual muscle weakness.

2. ALTERATION IN TONE

After the onset of hemiplegia the abnormal quality of postural tone appears initially as hypotonus, but at a very early stage increased tone may become apparent in certain groups, e.g. finger flexors or retractors of the scapula, so that a mixture of flaccidity and spasticity is present. Tone usually changes and increases as the patient becomes more active. The basic tone may change gradually for 18 months or longer. When hypotonicity is present the tone is too low to initiate movement. There is a lack of resistance to passive movement and the patient is unable to hold a limb in any position. When hypertonicity develops there is resistance to passive movement and active movement is difficult or impossible. The increase in tone is usually more marked in certain patterns involving the anti-gravity groups of muscles, i.e. the flexor groups in the arm and the extensor groups in the leg.

Alterations in posture may also affect the distribution of tone, e.g. there may be resistance to extension of the arm when it is held by the side but resistance to flexion if held above the head. If marked co-contraction is present, resistance to all passive movement may be felt (see also Chapter VI).

3. SENSORY DISTURBANCE

Loss of sensation impairs the patient's ability to move and balance normally. In many cases, the deficit can be attributed to inattention toward the affected side rather than actual loss of feeling. Sensory deprivation can be improved with treatment, and there would seem to be many exceptions to the traditional belief that sensory deficit precludes functional recovery and that the loss is greater in the arm than the leg (see also Chapter V).

4. LOSS OF ISOLATED MOVEMENT

Although many patients with hemiplegia appear able to move all parts of their bodies, they may be unable to move one part in isolation without other muscles acting simultaneously in a stereotyped pattern of movement, e.g. they may only be able to grip while the elbow flexes and the shoulder adducts, or stand up with the hip and knee extended and the foot plantarflexed. Similarly dorsiflexion of the foot may only be possible when the hip and knee flex.

5. LOSS OF BALANCE REACTIONS

With every movement, posture must be adjusted to maintain balance, but with altered tone present the required reactions are impaired or absent.

6. ASSOCIATED REACTIONS

Associated movements occur in the normal person during strenuous activity, but with hypertonicity they appear as associated reactions in abnormal stereotyped patterns which inhibit function.

7. SPEECH

Speech may or may not be affected, but speech difficulty is usually associated with right-sided hemiplegia. It is sometimes purely a sensory-motor problem, where correct articulation is hampered by loss of voluntary control, or in other cases there is difficulty in interpreting the written or spoken word, and in expressing ideas. Often there is a combination of varying degrees of affliction. Everyone who is in contact with the patient must be aware of and understand his individual difficulties.

APPROACH TO TREATMENT

The unilateral approach

It is generally accepted today that patients who have suffered a stroke need not spend the rest of their lives in bed, but most traditional methods of treatment are directed towards gaining independence by strengthening and training the sound side to compensate for the affected side. Many disadvantages are inherent in such methods:

1. The resultant one-sidedness accentuates the lack of sensation and awareness.

2. Relying on a tetrapod or stick for balance not only increases spasticity and abnormal associated reactions, but prevents use of the unaffected hand for functional tasks (the hand being solely involved in maintaining the patient in an upright position).

3. One-sidedness requires increased effort to perform any function, making movement tiring and difficult. Consequently, spasticity increases and movement becomes more abnormal.

4. Progressive spasticity in the lower limb demands increasingly complex appliances which are difficult, if not impossible, for the patient to apply himself, and which may ultimately fail to control the position of the foot.

5. Increased tone in the upper limb leads to a distressingly obvious deformity which hinders mobility and everyday activities including washing and dressing.

The bilateral or symmetrical approach

Preferable methods stress the need to re-educate movement throughout the body, realizing that as the quality of movement improves function will automatically improve. They aim to normalize tone and to facilitate normal movement, thus providing the sensorimotor experience on which all learning is based. If the patient learns to move with abnormal muscle tone and in an abnormal manner, such movement will be all he knows and correction afterwards will be more difficult. Everyone, regardless of age, should be treated in a way which gives the opportunity to develop maximum potential. Even if dramatic motor recovery is not achieved they will be better able to function and live more normally. Time and social circumstances will determine whether they will live at home or in an institution.

All treatment should be directed toward obtaining symmetry with normal balance reactions throughout the body. The affected side should be bombarded with every form of stimulation possible to make the patient aware of himself as a whole person again. Re-education of bilateral righting and equilibrium reactions in the head and trunk are vital if independent balance is to be regained.

From the beginning, the patient must be discouraged from using the good arm to assist every movement as this could prevent return of control in the affected side.

The patient should never struggle to perform an activity which is

293

too advanced for him. Any movement he is unable to manage himself should be assisted to make the action smooth and easy without being passive. Excess effort induces abnormal tone and unwanted associated reactions. Assistance should be gradually lessened until he performs the movement unaided. Repetition re-establishes a memory of the feeling of normal movement.

When and if movement returns to the limbs it will be in abnormal patterns. These stereotyped patterns must be corrected at once to prevent them becoming established habits.

If everyone in contact with the patient reinforces the approach from the start, hours of physiotherapy time will be saved and the final result far more satisfactory. Because it is an overall management of the patient, he is never 'too ill to treat'.

INSTRUCTION FOR NURSES AND RELATIVES

Careful instruction and involvement of nurses and relatives is of paramount importance and will eliminate or minimize many of the complications associated with hemiplegia.

For the nurses

POSITION OF THE BED IN THE WARD
The patient benefits if the position of his bed in the ward or room makes him look *across* his affected side at general activity or items of

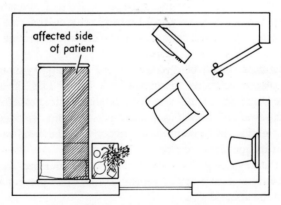

Fig. XIII/1 Position of bed in ward

interest (e.g. television) (see Fig. XIII/1). Similarly, with the locker on his affected side, he has to reach across the mid-line for a glass of water, tissues, etc.

NURSING PROCEDURES

Great therapeutic value can be incorporated in routine procedures by encouraging the patient's participation. While bathing him in bed, the nurse can focus his attention on each part of the body by naming it, and asking for his help to facilitate washing, e.g. rolling onto his side with her aid, and holding up the affected arm with the sound hand; or rolling actively as she is making the bed. When bed-pans, medicines or food are brought to the patient, the approach should be from his affected side, thereby increasing his awareness of it (see Fig. XIII/2).

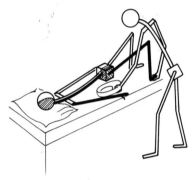

Fig. XIII/2 Presentation of bed-pan by nurse (The right side of the patient is affected and is shown in black)

POSITIONING THE PATIENT IN BED

The bed must have a firm mattress on a solid base and the height should be adjustable. It will need to be lowered to enable easy and correct transfer of the patient into a chair. Five or six pillows will be required to maintain the correct alignment of the head, trunk and limbs. The patient's position should be changed frequently to avoid chest complications, pressure sores and discomfort. Two to three-hourly turning is advisable in the early stages while the patient is confined to bed. Even when he is out of bed during the day and more active, correct positioning at night must continue.

POSITION LYING ON THE AFFECTED SIDE
(See Fig. XIII/3)

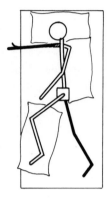

Fig. XIII/3 Position of patient lying on the affected side

1. The head is forward with the trunk straight and in line.
2. The underneath shoulder is protracted with the forearm supinated.
3. The underneath leg is extended at the hip and slightly flexed at the knee.
4. The upper leg is in front on one pillow.
5. Nothing should be placed in the hand or under the sole of the foot because this stimulates undesirable reflex activity, i.e. flexion in the hand and extensor thrust in the leg.

POSITION LYING ON THE SOUND SIDE
(See Fig. XIII/4)

1. Patient is in full side lying, not just a quarter turn.
2. The head is forward with the trunk straight and in line. If necessary a pillow under the waist will elongate the affected side further.
3. The affected shoulder should be protracted with the arm forward on a pillow.
4. The upper leg is in front on one pillow. (The foot must be fully supported by the pillow and not hang over the end in inversion.)
5. A pillow is behind the back.

6. Nothing should be placed in the hand or under the sole of the foot.

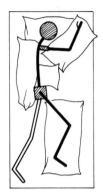

Fig. XIII/4 Position of patient lying on sound side

POSITION IN SUPINE
(See Figs. XIII/5(a) and (b))

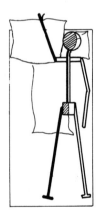 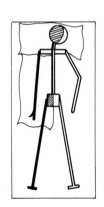

Fig. XIII/5

(a) Position in supine with arm elevated
(b) Position in supine with arm at side on pillow

1. The head is rotated to the affected side and flexed to the good side.

2. The trunk is elongated on the affected side.

3. The affected shoulder is protracted on a pillow with the arm elevated or straight by the side.

4. A pillow is placed under the hip to prevent retraction of the pelvis and lateral rotation of the leg.

5. Nothing should be placed in the hand or under the sole of the foot.

In the supine position there will be the greatest increase in abnormal tone because of the influence of reflex activity, and this position should be avoided whenever possible.

SITTING IN BED
(See Fig. XIII/6(a) and (b)

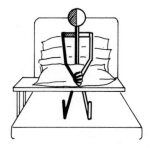 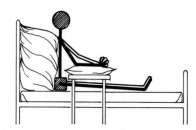

Fig. XIII/6
(a) Sitting in bed – from front
(b) Sitting in bed – from side

Sitting in bed for meals is not desirable, but may be necessary to fit in with staffing and ward routine. The half-lying position should never be used, as there is increased flexion of the trunk with extension in the legs and greater risk of pressure sores.

1. The patient should be as upright as possible with the head and trunk in line and his weight evenly distributed on both buttocks.

2. The affected arm is protracted at the shoulder, both hands are clasped together and placed forward on a bed-table.

3. The legs are straight and not laterally rotated.

TRANSFERRING FROM BED TO CHAIR
(See Fig. XIII/7)

Much damage can be done to the patient's shoulder as well as to the

298

nurse's or therapist's back during this manoeuvre if it is performed incorrectly. It can also be a very frightening time for the patient if he is suddenly transferred without any explanation or chance to move himself. The following is an easy, safe, therapeutic way of transferring a patient from bed to chair.

The chair is placed in position on the affected side and the patient is rolled or assisted onto his affected side. The helper places one hand under the patient's affected shoulder, swings his legs over the edge of the bed with her other hand, and brings the patient to the sitting position. During this phase elongation of the trunk occurs, and if a pause is needed to rearrange clothes, etc., the patient can be propped on the affected elbow and take weight through it (see Fig. XIII/7(a)).

The patient is moved to the edge of the bed by rocking or wriggling from side to side. The assistant's arms are placed under the patient's shoulders with her hands over the scapulae while her legs wedge the patient's feet and knees (see Figs. XIII/7(b) and XIII/7(c)). The patient's arms are placed round the helper's waist or on her shoulders, but he must not grip his hands together. If he does he will pull on the assistant's neck so that she takes his weight instead of him bearing weight through his legs. His trunk is then pulled well forward and he is brought to standing by pressure forward and down on the shoulders, so that his weight goes equally through both legs. No attempt is made to lift him up at all. The assistant's weight counter-balances the patient's, and with shoulders and knees fixed he is pivoted round to sit on the chair (see Fig. XIII/7c and d).

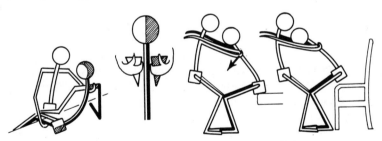

Fig. XIII/7 Transferring from bed to chair

(a) Bringing the patient from lying to sitting over the side of the bed
(b) Starting position for transfer, from behind patient
(c) Starting position for transfer from side
(d) Pivot round to chair – seat well back in chair

Transferring in such a way emphasizes the hemiplegic side and encourages weight-bearing and weight transference to that side.

SITTING IN A CHAIR

A better sitting posture can be obtained in an upright chair.

1. The chair should be of sufficient height to allow the patient's hips, knees and ankles to be at approximately right angles when he sits well back in the chair (see Fig. XIII/8).

2. His head and trunk are in line with the body-weight evenly distributed over both buttocks. His hands are clasped and placed well forward on a table in front of him.

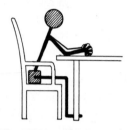

Fig. XIII/8 Sitting in chair

For the relatives

Within the first few days the physiotherapist should meet the patient's relatives and explain his difficulties and how they can help to overcome them. They enjoy being involved, and having something concrete to do while visiting, and often have more time to spend with the patient than either nurses or therapists.

When visiting the hemiplegic patient, relatives tend to sit on his unaffected side as his head is usually looking that way, and it is easier to gain his attention. They should sit on his affected side and be shown how to turn his head toward them by placing a hand over his cheek and applying a firm prolonged pressure until the head stays round. They should then strive to attract his attention by encouraging him to look at them and talk to them, etc. Their conversation and presence will stimulate him and help to restore his state of awareness. Holding his affected hand will give sensory stimulation and bring awareness of the limb. Interested relatives can encourage the patient to do his self-assisted arm exercises (see page 304).

CHAPTER XIV

Hemiplegia – II

by JENNIFER M. TODD, m.c.s.p.
and PATRICIA M. DAVIES, m.c.s.p., dip.phys.ed.
(*based on the work of* DR. AND MRS. K. BOBATH)

Treatment must commence immediately after the onset of hemiplegia. Progress will be more rapid if the patient is treated two or three times a day in the early stages, even if only for ten minutes at a time.

The patient's ability and tolerance are directly related to the site and severity of the lesion and his physical condition prior to the illness rather than to the length of time since the incident. Treatment must progress accordingly.

Most patients will sit out of bed within a few days and it is important for them to move from the ward or bedroom so that they are stimulated by the change of surroundings. Shaving, wearing make-up, dressing in everyday clothes all help to overcome the feeling of being an invalid.

Rehabilitation in a hospital department has the advantage of invaluable contact with other people and patients with similar problems as well as the stimulation of leaving home and dealing independently with new situations. Many stroke patients never attend hospital and are treated in their homes. The physiotherapist in attendance must use all her ingenuity to provide a complete rehabilitation without special apparatus and to overcome the limitations of space and over-protective relatives.

The following outline of physiotherapy is not a fixed regime or programme for all patients but suggestions for activities which will be of benefit to many. Careful and continuous assessment must be made as the problems arising from hemiplegia will be different for each individual and may alter from day to day. Treatment must be carefully selected and progressed.

For simplicity the activities have been divided into sections but the therapist must be aware that one part of the body cannot be treated in isolation, e.g. working on the leg in sitting or standing may adversely affect the trunk and arm if they are flexing and retracting with effort. Similarly attention must always be given to the trunk before normal movement of the limbs can be achieved.

ACTIVITIES IN LYING

Mobilizing the arm

Although most hemiplegics with severe paralysis will never regain functional use of the affected arm, it is important that it should remain fully mobile. A stiff painful arm impedes balance and movement of the whole body, limits treatment and interferes with daily living. If full passive elevation of the arm is performed every day the complication need never arise.

ELONGATION OF THE TRUNK (Fig. XIV/1)

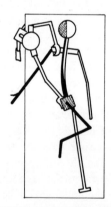

Fig. XIV/1 Elongation of the trunk

The patient lies in half crook lying with his affected leg flexed and adducted. Place one hand on his pelvis, the other hand over his shoulder and elongate his trunk until his hip remains forward off the bed.

302

MOVEMENT OF THE SCAPULA (Fig. XIV/2)

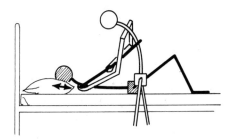

Fig. XIV/2 Mobilization of scapula

Place one hand over his scapula, the other supporting his arm. Protract his shoulder and slowly elevate and depress his scapula until spasticity releases and it moves freely. Ease his arm into lateral rotation while moving the scapula.

ELEVATION OF THE ARM (Figs. XIV/(3a), (b))

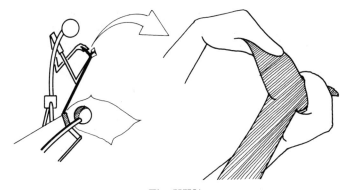

Fig. XIV/3
(a) Elevation of the arm
(b) Close-up of hand grip

Maintaining lateral rotation at the shoulder, extend his elbow and lift his arm into elevation. Continue until full elevation is obtained with supination of the forearm, extension of the wrist and fingers and wide abduction of the thumb. Move his arm until it will stay in elevation without pulling down into flexion.

303

ABDUCTION OF THE ARM (Fig. XIV/4)

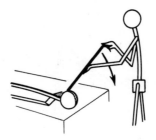

Fig. XIV/4 Arm out to abduction

From full elevation take his arm out to the side in abduction and up again maintaining the extension at the elbow, fingers and wrist with supination of the forearm.

SELF-ASSISTED ARM MOVEMENTS (Fig. XIV/5)

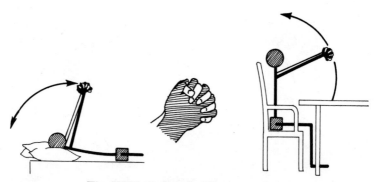

Fig. XIV/5 Self-assisted arm movement

Teach the patient at an early stage to clasp his hands together, inter-lacing the fingers, and to lift them up into full elevation. The movement should begin with protraction of the shoulders and extension of the elbow. The patient must be encouraged to perform this activity frequently throughout the day and to continue this when he is sitting in a chair.

Moving the leg

To prevent associated reactions his hands can be clasped in elevation or forwards with the shoulders protracted and the elbows extended.

HIP AND KNEE FLEXION OVER THE SIDE OF THE BED
(Fig. XIV/6)

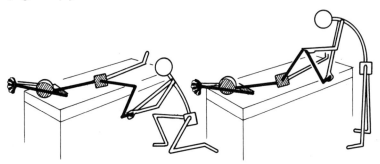

Fig. XIV/6 Hip and knee flexion over side of bed

Place his leg over the side of the bed with his hip extended and hold his knee in flexion and his foot in full dorsiflexion until there is no resistance. Maintain the position of the foot and knee and guide the leg up onto the bed while he actively assists. Repeat the movement preventing any abnormal pattern occurring, e.g. extension of the knee or lateral rotation of the hip.

If the exercise is perfected the patient will be able to bring his leg

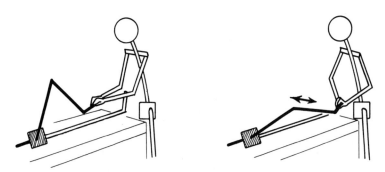

Fig. XIV/7 Control of knee extension through range

through when walking and climb stairs in a normal manner, one foot after the other.

KNEE EXTENSION WITH DORSIFLEXION (Fig. XIV/7)
Hold his foot in dorsiflexion, and move his leg from full flexion into extension without his toes pushing down and without rotation at the hip. The patient takes the weight of his limb, making it feel light throughout.

HIP CONTROL WITH THE FOOT ON THE BED (Fig. XIV/8)

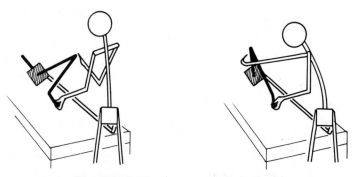

Fig. XIV/8 Hip control with foot on bed

In crook lying, the patient moves alternate knees smoothly into medial and lateral rotation without his other leg moving and without tilting his pelvis.

HIP CONTROL WITH THE HIP IN EXTENSION (Fig. XIV/9)

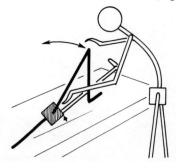

Fig. XIV/9 Hip control with hip in extension

In half crook lying with his affected leg flexed and adducted the patient lifts his affected hip forward off the bed and, maintaining hip extension, moves his knee out and in.

ISOLATED KNEE EXTENSION (Fig. XIV/10)

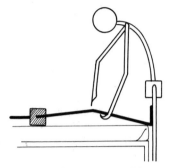

Fig. XIV/10 Isolated knee extension

Place the patient's foot against your thigh to maintain dorsiflexion and ask him to straighten his knee without pushing down with his foot.

Bridging

BRIDGING WITH ROTATION OF THE PELVIS (Fig. XIV/11)

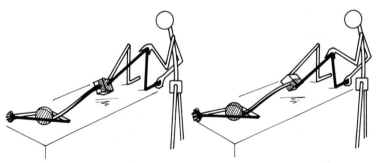

Fig. XIV/11 Bridging with rotation of pelvis

Maintaining good extension at the hips the patient rotates his pelvis equally to either side while preventing any associated movement in his affected leg.

307

BRIDGING ON THE AFFECTED LEG (Fig. XIV/12)

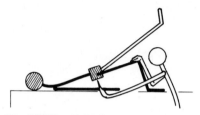

Fig. XIV/12 Bridging on affected leg

The patient bridges on both legs and lifts his sound foot off the bed while maintaining the same position of the pelvis and affected leg.

Progress to raising and lowering his hips several times.

Rolling

Correct rolling brings awareness of the affected side, release of spasticity by rotation between the shoulder girdle and pelvis and facilitates active movement in the limbs.

TO THE AFFECTED SIDE (Fig. XIV/13)

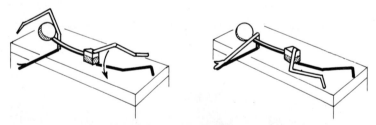

Fig. XIV/13 Rolling to affected side

Place his affected arm in abduction and ask him to lift his head and bring his sound arm across to touch his other hand. Instruct him to lift his sound leg across his affected leg without pushing off.

TO THE SOUND SIDE (Fig. XIV/14)

Guide the patient's affected leg over his other leg giving less and less assistance until he can perform the action himself. He can clasp both

308

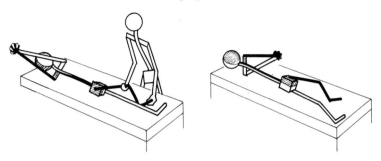

Fig. XIV/14 Rolling to sound side

hands together and rotate his upper trunk by moving both arms to the sound side.

ACTIVITIES IN SITTING

The patient should be moved into sitting as soon as possible even if he is not fully conscious, to stimulate balance reactions.

WEIGHT TRANSFERENCE FROM SIDE TO SIDE
(Figs. XIV/15 and XIV/16)

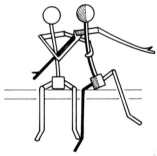

Fig. XIV/15 Weight transference in sitting to affected side

Sit on the patient's affected side and draw his body towards you so that his body weight passes through one buttock only. Elongate his trunk on that side and inhibit any flexion in his arm. His good leg is then free to be raised in the air.

Shift his body weight over his sound side and place his head in

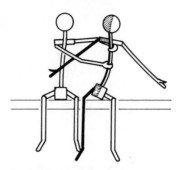

Fig. XIV/16 Weight transference in sitting to sound side

position if it does not right automatically. Facilitate side flexion of his trunk on the affected side by giving pressure at his waist with your hand and encourage him to lift his buttock clear of the bed.

Repeat the movement in a rhythmic manner until automatic head and trunk righting occurs to both sides.

MOVING IN SITTING (Fig. XIV/17)

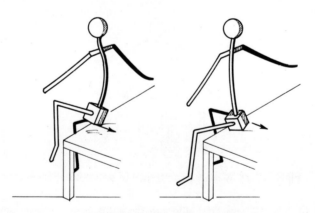

Fig. XIV/17 Moving in sitting

The patient must move in sitting without using his hand. Teach him to shuffle or walk on his buttocks forwards and backwards and later sideways. Help him by placing one hand under each hip or thigh and then rock and move him from side to side.

WEIGHT TRANSFERENCE THROUGH THE ARMS BEHIND

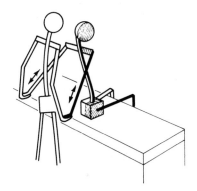

Fig. XIV/18 Weight transference through the arms behind

Take both arms carefully behind the patient with his hands supported on yours. Facilitate extension by using a sharp push-pull action up through his arms until they support his weight. Progress by shifting his weight from one side to the other without his elbow bending.

WEIGHT TRANSFERENCE THROUGH THE ARM SIDEWAYS
(Fig. XIV/19)

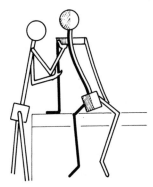

Fig. XIV/19 Weight transference through the arm sideways

Practise a similar activity with his affected arm at the side. Place his hand flat on the bed or plinth and with one hand under his axilla and the other supporting his elbow, draw the patient towards you elongating his trunk at the same time.

INDEPENDENT MOVEMENT OF THE LEGS (Fig. XIV/20)

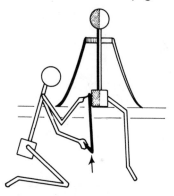

Fig. XIV/20 Lifting one leg at a time in sitting

To prepare for walking teach the patient to move his legs without moving his trunk. Lift one leg at a time asking him to make it feel light by taking the weight himself. He must maintain control while his leg is lowered onto the bed. Ask him to keep his trunk still and not to lean back throughout the activity.

INHIBITION OF EXTENSOR THRUST (Fig. XIV/21)

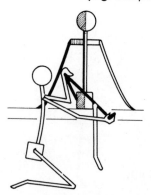

Fig. XIV/21 Sitting with affected leg crossed inhibiting extensor thrust

Cross the patient's affected leg over the sound one and hold it in full flexion and lateral rotation with the foot and toes in full dorsiflexion until it will stay in position on its own. Maintain inhibition at his foot and ask the patient to uncross his leg and lower it, making it feel light and to raise it once more across his other leg.

RAISING THE HIP IN SITTING WITH THE LEGS CROSSED
(Fig. XIV/22)

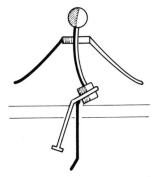

Fig. XIV/22 Sitting with crossed legs raising alternate hip
off bed

While one leg remains crossed make the patient transfer his weight onto the hip of his underneath leg and lift his other buttock off the bed. Facilitate flexion of his trunk with pressure at his waist.

Repeat the same activity to both sides.

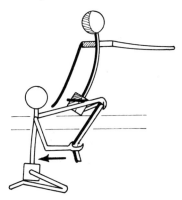

Fig. XIV/23 Lift both legs together and rotate them

313

BALANCE REACTIONS OF THE UPPER TRUNK AND HEAD
(Fig. XIV/23)
Facilitate increased balance reactions of his head, trunk and upper
limbs by lifting both legs together and rotating them to either side.
Alter the speed and position to obtain the required reaction in the
rest of his body.

STANDING FROM A HIGH BED OR PLINTH TO THE GROUND
(Fig. XIV/24)

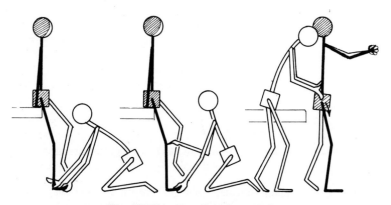

Fig. XIV/24 Standing from sitting
(a) Affected leg on ground with foot dorsiflexed
(b) Isolated knee extension
(c) Coming off onto affected leg

The patient wriggles to the edge of the bed and puts his affected leg
to the floor without his foot pushing down. If necessary mobilize his
foot by pressing down over the front of his ankle to ensure that his
heel is on the ground and dorsiflexion possible.

When his affected foot is on the floor practise isolated knee extension before bringing his hip forward to take full weight through the
leg. The plinth will prevent his hip pushing back in a pattern of total
extension.

Do not allow his affected knee to snap into extension as his sound
leg is taken off the bed. Take the same precautions when lifting his
sound buttock up first to return to the sitting position.

STANDING FROM A CHAIR (Fig. XIV/25)

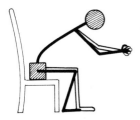

Fig. XIV/25 Standing from a chair

Place the patient's feet together with his affected foot slightly behind the the sound one to ensure good weight bearing as he comes to standing. Make him lean forward until his head is vertically in front of his feet and to stand without pushing up with his hand. If his trunk and arm retract too much at first the patient can assist standing by pushing his arms out in front of him with hands clasped together. When returning to sitting his affected foot remains behind and his head is kept well forward while his bottom is placed far back in the chair. He must not put a hand down on the chair as this spoils the symmetry and alters the weight bearing. Instead he should look behind and back up until he is correctly aligned with the chair.

MOVING IN SITTING WITH THE FEET ON THE FLOOR
(Fig. XIV/26)

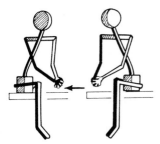

Fig. XIV/26 Moving bottom from side to side in sitting

Practise a similar action when the patient moves in sitting. With his feet on the ground he can place his bottom forward or back and from one side to the other.

315

TRUNK CONTROL (Figs. XIV/27 and XIV/28)

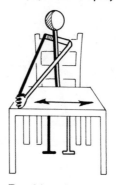

Fig. XIV/27 Reaching sideways and forwards

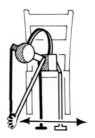

Fig. XIV/28 Reaching down to feet

With his hands clasped in front of him, and elbows extended, he can practise reaching out to either side, well forwards and down to his feet.

ACTIVITIES IN STANDING

It is of no benefit to practise walking with a patient who is unable either to take weight on his affected leg or bring it forward in a reasonably normal manner. The same applies to a patient who walks with a poor gait pattern. The difficulties should be assessed and relevant activities practised. Preparation for walking can be carried out adequately in an area of one square yard.

Weight-bearing on the affected leg
(Preparation for the stance phase of gait)

i. Standing on the patient's affected side draw his weight toward you, giving as much support as he requires. Ask him to take steps forward with his sound leg. Prevent his knee from snapping back into extension by keeping his hip well forward.

ii. In the same position ask the patient to place his sound foot lightly on and off a step in front of him (Fig. XIV/29).

iii. Repeat the activity with the step placed well out to the side.

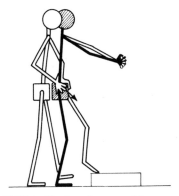

Fig. XIV/29 Placing the sound leg on a step

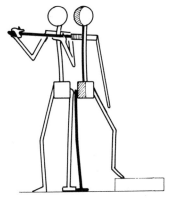

Fig. XIV/30 Stepping out to side with sound leg

Encourage the patient to keep his affected hip against your hip (Fig. XIV/30).

iv. Still preventing his knee from locking back ask the patient to draw large letters on the floor with his sound foot, ensuring weight-bearing on a mobile leg (Fig. XIV/31).

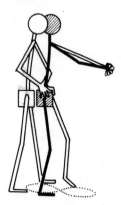

Fig. XIV/31 Making figure of eight with sound leg

v. Make the patient stand on his affected leg and lightly place his sound foot at right angles in front or behind the other foot, without transferring his weight onto it (Fig. XIV/32).

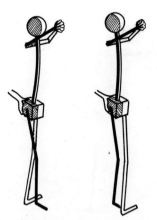

Fig. XIV/32 Putting sound foot at right angles to hemiplegic foot

318

If the activity is performed accurately it help him to gain control of the hip abductors and extensors.

vi. Place the patient's affected leg on a 6 inch step in front of him. With your hand pushing down on his knee and keeping his weight well forward, he steps up onto the step (Fig. XIV/33).

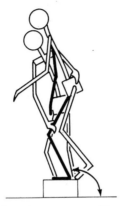

Fig. XIV/33 Stepping up onto step with affected leg on step

vii. Practise stepping down with his sound leg placing it further and further back, and tapping it on the floor behind keeping the weight forward on his affected leg (Fig. XIV/34).

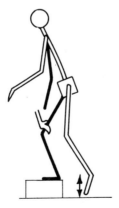

Fig. XIV/34 Putting sound leg behind further and further back (Eros)

319

viii. Put his affected leg on the step and help the patient to push up and step right over and back again (Fig. XIV/35).

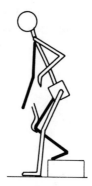

Fig. XIV/35 With affected leg on step, step up and over

Releasing the knee and moving the hemiplegic leg
(Preparation for the swing phase of gait)

i. The patient stands with his feet close together. Guide his pelvis forward and down to release his knee on the affected side. Instruct him to straighten it again without pushing his whole side back. His heel must remain in contact with the floor, only possible if his pelvis drops forward (Fig. XIV/36).

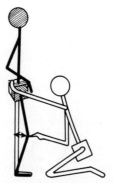

Fig. XIV/36 Releasing hemiplegic leg in standing

320

ii. Practise the same activity in step standing with his affected leg behind, and the weight forward over his extended sound leg (Fig. XIV/37).

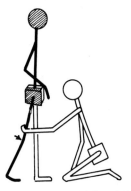

Fig. XIV/37 Releasing knee with hemiplegic leg behind

iii. The patient stands with the weight on his sound leg. Facilitate small steps backward with the other foot by holding his toes dorsiflexed and instructing him not to push down. Do not allow him to hitch his hip back (Fig. XIV/38).

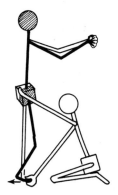

Fig. XIV/38 Taking small steps backward with affected leg

iv. Make the patient walk sideways along a line crossing one foot in front of the other. When his sound leg takes a step, keep his affected hip well forward so that his knee does not snap back into extension (Fig. XIV/39).

321

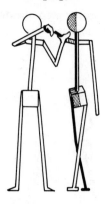

Fig. XIV/39 Walking sideways behind a line

Stairs

Practise climbing stairs at an early stage, even before independent gait is achieved, as it is both therapeutic and functional. Teach him to perform the activity in a normal manner, i.e. one foot on each step and without the support of the hand-rail.

ASCENDING
In the early stages it may be necessary for you to lift his affected leg onto the step rather than allow him to struggle. Support his affected

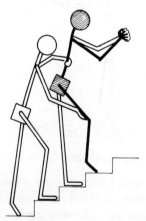

Fig. XIV/40 Climbing stairs assisting affected leg up

knee as he steps up with his sound leg and keep his weight well forward (Figs. XIV/40 and 41).

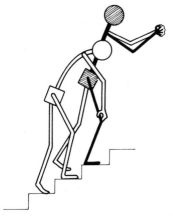

Fig. XIV/41 Climbing stairs supporting affected knee to step up

DESCENDING

Guide the pelvis well forward on his affected side as he puts the foot down, preventing the leg pulling into adduction. Your hand on his knee will give support as he steps down with his sound leg (Fig. XIV/42).

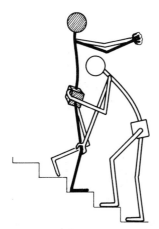

Fig. XIV/42 Descending stairs – hand supporting affected knee

Activities on the tilt board

The tilt board is not essential for treatment but is most helpful when re-educating correct transference of weight.

i. Stand on the floor behind the patient and help him to step onto the tilt board with one foot on either side. His feet should be parallel to one another throughout the exercise. Tilt the board slowly from side to side, pausing at each extreme to correct the patient's position and

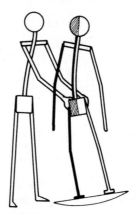

Fig. XIV/43 Stride standing on tilt board – side lengthening as weight comes over affected side

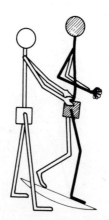

Fig. XIV/44 Step standing on tilt board – hemiplegic leg in front – weight over front leg

make sure that his hip comes right over his foot, that his side lengthens and that his pelvis does not rotate (Fig. XIV/43).

ii. The patient turns on the board so that he is in step standing across it with his affected leg in front. Tilt the board slowly forward and back, stopping at the extreme of movement to check his position. Make sure that his weight is taken well forward over the front foot without the pelvis rotating. His feet must remain parallel (Fig. XIV/44).

iii. The same activity is performed with his affected leg behind.

Facilitation of gait

Once the patient has sufficient tone and movement in his leg, walking can be assisted. Hold his pelvis on either side from behind and facilitate the action, making it as smooth and rhythmic as possible. Keep the affected hip well forward during the stance phase on that side so that the knee does not snap back into extension. Press down on the pelvis during the swing phase to help him release his knee instead of hitching his hip to bring the leg forward.

As walking improves facilitate a normal reciprocal arm swing by lightly rotating his pelvis or shoulders with your hands.

Activities on the mat

To assist the patient getting down onto the mat stand behind him and ask him to step forward with the sound leg and kneel down on his affected leg. Support the affected hip with your knee to prevent him from collapsing as he brings the other knee down (Fig. XIV/45).

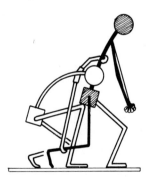

Fig. XIV/45 Assisting patient to kneel down on the mat

i. In kneel standing support him from behind, with your arms over the front of his shoulders and your hands behind each side of his pelvis. Move his weight sideways over his affected leg, with his trunk lengthening on that side and his hip kept well forward. Repeat the movement to the sound side. The patient should practise holding the position with the weight fully over each side, with less and less assistance (Fig. XIV/46).

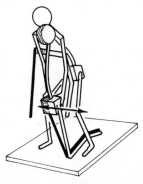

Fig. XIV/46 Kneel standing – transfer weight over affected leg – hip forward

ii. Also in kneel standing make the patient take steps forward and back with his sound knee, while keeping his affected hip stable (Fig. XIV/47).

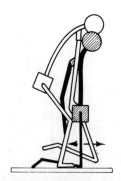

Fig. XIV/47 Stepping forward with sound knee – affected hip stable

iii. Assist the patient as he sits down to either side, and learns to balance in side sitting without using his hands to support him (Fig. XIV/48).

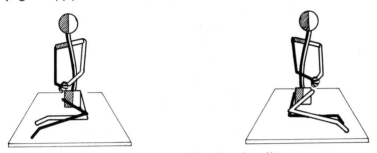

Fig XIV/48 Side sitting from kneeling

iv. Instruct the patient to step forward with his sound foot and practise activities balancing in half kneel standing. Make him tap lightly on the floor with his foot (Fig. XIV/49).

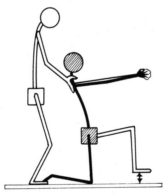

Fig. XIV/49 Half kneel standing – tapping with sound foot

v. The patient can get up from the floor by kneeling up on both knees, stepping forward with his sound foot, and standing up. Assist him at first from behind, putting your hands under his shoulders to guide him well forward as he pushes up to standing (Fig. XIV/50).

It is worth mastering these activities as they will enable the patient to get in and out of the bath without any aids.

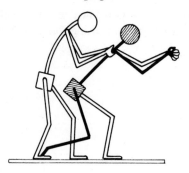

Fig. XIV/50 Assisting the patient to stand from kneeling

ACTIVITIES FOR THE RECOVERING ARM

When the hemiplegic arm shows signs of recovery every effort must be made to encourage movement and restore function as much as possible.

There is usually difficulty in isolating movement to one part of the limb, and in stabilizing proximal joints while the hand performs more skilled actions. Total patterns of movement tend to dominate.

In lying

i. After inhibiting the arm fully in elevation ask the patient to let it stay there, and then move it slightly in all directions with the elbow

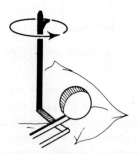

Fig. XIV/51 Small circles in air with elbow extended

328

extended. Gradually increase the range until he can lower it slowly to his side and lift it again, and take it out sideways to full abduction and up to vertical again (Fig. XIV/51).

ii. Ask the patient to touch his head (and lift his hand up again) without his elbow pulling down to his side. He can also place his hand on the opposite shoulder and lift it again. You can assist by maintaining extension of his fingers and thumb as he does so and by reminding him that his elbow must remain in the same position (Fig. XIV/52).

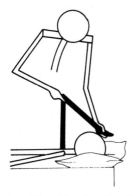

Fig. XIV/52 Touching head and up again

iii. While you hold his hand in extension and his forearm supinated, ask him to extend and flex his elbow; small movements without the shoulder participating (Fig. XIV/53).

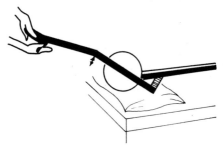

Fig. XIV/53 Flexion and extension of elbow with hand in dorsiflexion

iv. a) Holding a pole with both his hands let him lower it and raise it slowly while maintaining elbow extension (Fig. XIV/54).

329

b) Practise walking his hands along the pole, while it is held in elevation.

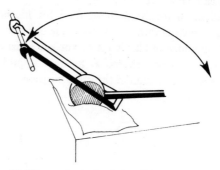

Fig. XIV/54 Holding pole in both hands, lowering and raising it.

In sitting

i. Practise protective extension sideways with his hand on your hand, giving small quick pushing movements up through the extended arm, until the arm can remain straight even when you let it go and the outstretched hand lands on the plinth (Fig. XIV/55).

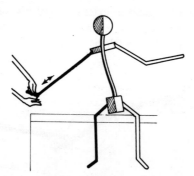

Fig. XIV/55 Protective extension sideways – hand outstretched

ii. The patient holds a towel in his affected hand and allows you to swing it round freely without him letting go, or pulling into total flexion to maintain his grip (Fig. XIV/56).

330

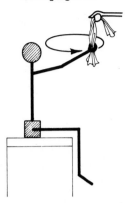

Fig. XIV/56 Holding towel in affected hand

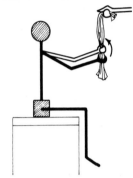

Fig. XIV/57 Holding rolled towel vertically – walk hand upwards

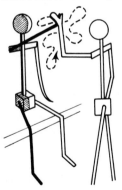

Fig. XIV/58 Place hand flat against therapist's hand and move without resistance

iii. Hold the rolled towel vertically in front of him and ask him to grip and release it, while walking his hand upwards. He must maintain elbow extension and shoulder protraction (Fig. XIV/57).

iv. Place his hand flat against yours and ask him to follow your hand whenever it moves without resistance (Fig. XIV/58).

In standing

i. Lift the patient's arm into elevation and ask him to leave it there when it feels light. The movement will be easier if his weight is on his affected leg.

ii. The patient places both his hands flat on a table in front of him. Assist him to extend his elbows and maintain the elbow extension by keeping his shoulders forward. He then walks his feet away from the table and back again without changing the position of his arms (Fig. XIV/59).

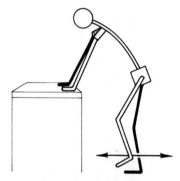

Fig. XIV/59 Weight-bearing through extended arms

Ask him to turn his feet until he is sideways on to the table and reach out with his sound arm while his affected arm remains in position (Fig. XIV/60).

iii. The same activities can be practised with his arms outstretched and hands flat on a wall or mirror in front of him. He can also bend and straighten his elbows slightly without his hands sliding down (Fig. XIV/61).

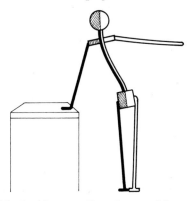

Fig. XIV/60 Weight-bearing on affected arm while rotating trunk away

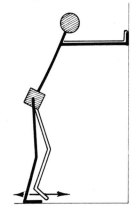

Fig. XIV/61 Hands flat on wall – lift sound arm

METHOD OF STIMULATION

Stimulation improves sensation and facilitates movement. Spasticity must be inhibited before any stimulation is given, and stimulation must be carefully graded as hypertonicity as overstimulation will cause undesirable abnormal movement.

Weight-bearing is usually the most effective way of bringing awareness and activity to the affected limbs.

THE VOICE AND USE OF WORDS
The way in which you use your voice and choose words can help the

333

patient to move correctly without excessive effort. The volume, inflection and speed of your instructions can increase or decrease tone. Choose words which give the patient the feeling of the movement required, and change the words until you find the one which evokes the required response from the individual.

ICE

a. Plunging his hand into a bucket of melting ice brings intense awareness of the part and often improves movement. For the best results, crushed or shaved ice should be mixed with just sufficient water to allow his hand to be easily submerged.

b. Stroking or teasing his hand or foot with a piece of ice will often evoke movement by sensory stimulation.

PRESSURE TAPPING

With your fingers pressed together tap firmly over the dorsum and lateral aspect of the patient's foot to encourage dorsiflexion. Elbow and hip extension can also be facilitated by tapping.

HEEL BANGING

The patient sits in a chair or stool and you hold his foot in full dorsiflexion with toes extended. With one hand on his knee bang his heel on the floor to facilitate active dorsiflexion. In the same position rub his heel firmly backwards and forwards on the floor to make him aware of the heel.

TICKLE OR FLICK HIS TOES UPWARDS to gain isolated dorsiflexion and extension of the toes. A bottle-brush can be used in the same way to excite movement.

CONCLUSION

If the methods of treatment described are carefully followed many complications and failures will be avoided.

THE PAINFUL SHOULDER

Careful mobilization of the shoulder after full release of spasticity around the scapula and in the trunk will soon free the shoulder and relieve pain.

A sling should never be worn as it reinforces the pattern of spasticity and enforces immobility – both of which contribute to the condition in the first place. Once the patient has learned to move his arm with the assistance of his other arm the problem ceases to exist.

THE SWOLLEN HAND

When the patient's hand suddenly becomes swollen for some reason, the therapist must take immediate steps to relieve the situation. If the swelling persists the hand will become contracted and even if movement returns may never become fully functional.

A small cock-up splint made of plaster of Paris and firmly bandaged with a crèpe bandage should be worn continuously till the swelling subsides. The hand should be placed in the ice bucket twice daily, the arm positioned in elevation at all times and the patient encouraged to do his self-assisted arm movements. If correctly treated the swelling should subside within a few days.

USE OF A STICK

Avoid the use of a tetrapod at all costs as it is clumsy, unsightly and prevents the patient from using his sound hand for more skilled tasks. If balance is properly trained the patient should not need to lean on a stick.

CALIPERS

It is far better to retrain dorsiflexion and correct weight-bearing than to resort to the early use of a caliper. Only use a caliper when all other methods of re-education and training have failed.

REFERENCES

Bobath, B. (1970). *Adult Hemiplegia: Evaluation and Treatment.* Heinemann Medical Books.
Bobath, B. (1971). *Abnormal Postural Reflex Activity caused by Brain Lesions.* Heinemann Medical Books.

FURTHER READING

Brunnstrom, S. (1970). *Movement Therapy in Hemiplegia.* Harper & Row.
Consumers' Association, 14 Buckingham Street, London, W.C.2. *Coping with Disablement.*

Jay, P. E. (1966). *Help Yourselves.* Butterworth.

Kingdom Ward, W. *Helping the Stroke Patient to Speak.* J. & A. Churchill.

Luria, A. R. *The Working Brain.* Penguin Edition 1973. *Restoration of Function after Brain Inuury.* Pergamon Press, 1963.

Facilitation of Movement Dec./Jan. 72/73. Adult Hemiplegia Nov./Dec. 1974. Reprints from *Physiotherapy.*

Taylor, M. *Understanding Aphasia.* Institute of Physical Medicine and Rehabilitation. New York.

CHAPTER XV

Multiple Sclerosis and Friedreich's Ataxia

by SHEILA KELLY, M.C.S.P., DIP.T.P.

MULTIPLE SCLEROSIS
(DISSEMINATED SCLEROSIS)

Multiple sclerosis is a chronic disease affecting the white matter of the
brain and spinal cord and sometimes spreading into the grey matter
of the cerebral cortex and cranial and spinal nerve roots. The course
of the disease is most often characterized by remissions and relapses,
eventually resulting in the patient becoming seriously disabled.

Changes

Small patches develop in which the myelin of the nerve fibres is
destroyed and the axons become thinner than normal or disappear.
There is proliferation of the neuroglia and the final state is a patch,
irregular in shape, sclerotic, and greyish and shrunken in appearance.
The effect is either to destroy the nerve fibres or to interfere seriously
with their conductivity. If there are only small isolated patches the
symptoms arising from these focal lesions may gradually disappear as
the patch shrinks and other nerve fibres may take over the work of
those affected. If, however, the disease progresses and more and more
plaques develop and tend to coalesce, symptoms become permanent
and are added to as more 'attacks' occur.

Etiology

Many theories have been advanced as to the cause of the disease but
none has yet been proved. At one time it was thought that the initial

337

lesion was caused by destruction of the oligodendroglia (the neuroglial cells responsible for the formation and maintenance of myelin). This would cause the characteristic loss of myelin. More recently the theory of infection has been reconsidered but as yet no proof of this has been obtained. Some favour the theory that an auto-immune process in the nervous system is responsible, while others believe that there is a disturbance in the circulation causing transient or permanent ischaemia of the areas involved.

Certain factors appear to precipitate the onset and relapses but how they achieve this effect is not known. Trauma, influenza, sepsis, surgery, infections all appear to be responsible.

Multiple sclerosis usually attacks young adults, the greatest number of cases occurring in the age group 20-40. Its onset is rare before 10 or after 60 years of age. In England it is found more commonly in women than in men though it has been stated (Brain and Walton, 1969) that in most published data elsewhere the reverse is the case. The disease is rare in the tropics and most prevalent in Northern Europe and Switzerland.

Mode of onset and course

The disease usually begins with one or more isolated lesions giving rise to local symptoms. In a series of 100 cases (Brain and Walton, 1969) one-third started with a sudden weakness of one or both lower limbs, one-third with visual symptoms and the remainder with miscellaneous symptoms of which numbness and paraesthesia were most usual.

Usually these symptoms disappear over a few days or weeks and a long remission period of months or even years follows. Eventually further attacks occur, more plaques develop, more nerve fibres are destroyed, patches coalesce and stable symptoms, depending on the areas involved, arise. Further symptoms are superimposed as subsequent attacks occur until in many cases the patient becomes seriously disabled.

Occasionally the onset is acute, the disease beginning with headache, giddiness, vomiting and widespread involvement of the white matter. There may then be mental symptoms, bladder disturbances, hemiplegia, ocular palsies, and ataxia. Death can occur in a few months though sometimes there is a remission and the disease then follows the chronic course.

Symptoms

The optic nerve and optic chiasma are often involved early in the course of the disease and blurring of vision, soon reduced to near blindness, may be the first symptom. Tenderness of the eyeballs on pressure and pain on movement will lead to a diagnosis of retro-bulbar neuritis – a diagnosis which in young people is very often a guide to the recognition of early multiple sclerosis. Paresis of ocular muscles due to lesions in the mid-brain or pons may lead to diplopia, ptosis or strabismus, though these are less common early symptoms. These eye symptoms may last for only a few days and then pass off, and no further symptoms may appear for some months or even years. The next attack may affect the same area or other areas and fresh signs such as slight frequency in micturition, paraesthesia, a feeling of heaviness in one leg which tends to drag a little, exaggerated deep reflexes in upper and lower limbs and loss of the superficial abdominal reflexes, may appear.

Many patients will now show mental changes, and euphoria is the most striking. In nearly all patients the lower limbs become most affected, the nerve fibres to the legs presenting a longer course to be attacked.

When the condition is more advanced and symptoms more stable, the outstanding characteristics will depend upon the region suffering from most sclerotic patches. Should the lesions predominate in the cerebellar system, hypotonus and ataxia will be the main problems. If the plaques are in the pyramidal pathways, spasticity and exaggerated reflexes are most marked. If the posterior columns of the spinal cord are most involved there will be sensory ataxia, diminished appreciation of vibration and postural sense and sometimes impairment of cutaneous sensibility.

In each patient, however, other symptoms will almost certainly be present. Thus, for example, the patient showing spasticity will probably have some ataxia. A very common form of disease is a mixture of symptoms – most probably weakness and spastic type of hypertonicity and a cerebellar type of hypotonia, affecting the head, neck, arms and trunk. This presents as jerky spastic patterns of movement in the legs and as nystagmus, intention tremor, weakness and inco-ordination of arm movements, and lack of postural stability of the trunk and proximal limb joints.

339

LESIONS PREDOMINATING IN THE CEREBELLAR SYSTEM

Hypotonia, especially of deep postural muscles, causes instability and defective postural reactions. There is a lack of resistance to passive movements of joints. The muscles feel flabby and the limb sways if an attempt is made by the patient to hold it in one position. Balance is impaired because the patient is unable to make the necessary postural adjustments before and during the performance of voluntary activities.

The hypotonia in postural muscles of the trunk and proximal limb joints gives a lack of stability so that on attempting voluntary movement the part sways and the distal end cannot be placed precisely (intention tremor). This overshooting of the mark is also exaggerated because all muscles are hypotonic and consequently the antagonists of the muscles producing the movement do not pay out slowly enough to slow the movement down or check it at the precise moment.

Ataxia arises because it is the function of the cerebellum to regulate voluntary movement. The loss of fixation of one segment for movement of another makes voluntary movement difficult. Thus walking may be impossible because the pelvis is not stable and eating may be impaired because of the instability of the head, trunk and shoulder girdle.

Because the various muscle groups necessary for movement are not co-ordinated, movement becomes jerky, and rapidly alternating movements are impossible. Inco-ordination is particularly noticeable in the fine movements of the fingers. Nystagmus arises from inco-ordination of the ocular muscles and dysarthria from inability to co-ordinate the lips, larynx and tongue – this may be manifest in the form of slurring, jerky, explosive speech or in the words being broken up into syllables – the 'scanning' form of speech.

The combination of hypotonia and inco-ordination produces a staggering gait rather resembling that of a drunken man. This is only noticed at first when walking round objects, turning, going up and down stairs, but gradually the gait worsens until the patient cannot walk without aid.

LESIONS PREDOMINATING IN THE PYRAMIDAL SYSTEM

Here **hypertonus** and **exaggerated reflexes** are the characteristic features. The symptoms usually begin with slight spasticity in the calf muscles, and weak dorsiflexion so that the foot is slightly dragged. The legs feel heavy and tire easily. There is an extensor plantar response and exaggeration of knee and ankle jerks. Gradually spasticity spreads until the total spastic pattern of extension, adduction and medial rotation has developed. Knee and ankle clonus are then present and the superficial abdominal reflexes lost. In addition there may be numbness and diminished vibration sense and exaggerated tendon jerks in the upper extremities.

Later as more patches develop flexor spasms begin to appear. At first these may be only occasional and slight, but they gradually increase until little stimulus is required to produce them. Eventually the total spastic pattern may change to flexion, abduction and lateral rotation. Adapive shortening of tendons, fascia and ligaments occurs and irritation resulting from this increases spasticity. At this stage bladder problems usually arise and in addition there may be some ataxia. The trunk may well be involved and unsupported sitting may be difficult. If the legs become fixed in flexion pressure sores can easily develop.

LESIONS PREDOMINATING IN THE POSTERIOR COLUMNS

In this case kinaesthetic sense is impaired. The patient, unaware, unless he watches, of the position of the joints, is unable to perform co-ordinated movement. Walking becomes ataxic and if cutaneous sensation in the soles of the feet is impaired the gait will closely resemble that of the tabetic patient.

Treatment

There is no cure for multiple sclerosis but the patient can be helped by advice on leading a sensible regulated life. It is valuable to continue the normal occupation provided overwork and fatigue can be avoided. If the condition worsens part-time work can sometimes be substituted for full-time. Where possible, infections should be avoided.

There is no known drug which has a certain effect on the course of the illness. During an acute exacerbation corticotrophin is often helpful, bringing about a rapid remission and sometimes apparently slowing deterioration, but it has little permanent effect. When spasticity is present anti-spasmodic drugs such as diazepam are valuable and intrathecal phenol injections relieve flexor spasms. When spasm has resulted in contractures tenotomy may prove useful.

If the patient eventually becomes bed-ridden nursing care is most important to prevent pressure sores, deal with incontinence and prevent respiratory complications.

Physiotherapy

As the signs and symptoms which these patients present vary greatly, careful and continual assessment must be made of each patient, so that treatment is relevant to the individual. Treatment and management of patients will differ considerably according to the progress of the disease. The stages will therefore be considered separately. It must be remembered, however, that the stages merge into each other, and are not clearly defined, and many patients will never reach the stage of gross disablement. The stages are based on the grouping advised by McAlpine and Compston (1952). They are:

Grade I. Unrestricted: without restriction of activity for normal employment and domestic life, but not necessarily symptom-free.

Grade II. Restricted: able to walk unaided for up to half a mile, and able to use public transport.

Grade III. Markedly restricted: capable of moving out of doors with difficulty for up to a quarter of a mile, usually with the aid of sticks, often unable to use public transport.

Grade IV. Mobile at home: able to move with difficulty about the house with support from furniture, unable to climb stairs.

Grade V. Immobile at home: confined to a chair or wheelchair.

Grade VI. Bedridden: requires assistance for nearly all activities.

Early stages (Grade I merging to Grade II)

The patient may complain of a feeling of heaviness in the legs, dragging of one leg, paraesthesia and numbness in the feet, or eye symptoms, e.g. diplopia.

If the neurologist refers the patient for physiotherapy, assessment should include careful observation of the patient's movement patterns and any deviations from normal should be noted. Observation should be done with the patient in various starting positions, e.g. lying, prone lying, side-lying, sitting and standing. These positions will show if there are variations in muscle tone, lack of postural fixation of proximal joints, or lack of precision of movement. Many patients in the early stages show minimal signs in the test positions, but if asked to run, hop, jump or skip, the problem of inco-ordinated movement becomes more apparent, e.g. spasticity in the lower limbs becomes obvious due to lack of reciprocal relaxation of the hypertonic groups when they are antagonistic to the movement.

Sensory testing should include investigation of joint and muscle sense, deep and light touch, vibration and stereognosis.

During assessment, any problems which the patient is having at home, at work or in leisure activities should be discussed and borne in mind when planning the treatment programme.

TREATMENT

At this stage, the patient is usually on a regime of active exercises. The Rest Exercise Programme (R.E.P.) prescribed by Ritchie Russell has proved useful. The patient is advised to take short rest periods of ten to twenty minutes two or three times a day, preceded by stressful mat exercises. These exercises are based on the hypothesis that the lesions are due to circulatory insufficiency in the white matter of the spinal cord, and that these areas of ischaemia would be less likely to occur if the circulation were maintained in a good state. The exercises are usually performed by the upper limbs to encourage a hyperaemic response in the circulation to the upper spinal cord and brainstem. Exercises may include press-ups, weight-lifting exercises while lying supine, or the use of springs to exact maximal effort in a short time. The exercises should be carried out until the patient is dyspnoeic, and the heart rate increased.

The patient should be carefully instructed in his Rest Exercise Programme. It is helpful if he can be admitted to hospital for a week of instruction. Treatment at this stage can be illustrated by the following case of a young woman who had experienced dragging of her left foot periodically over the previous six months. She complained of catching her toe under mats, on the edges of steps when going upstairs, and of wearing out the toe of her left shoe. On assessment, she was found to have minimal hypertonus of her left calf muscles and an extensor plantar response on that leg. She was working full-time as a teacher, and living with her husband in a second-floor flat.

After resting in bed for 24 hours, she was instructed in her Rest Exercise Programme over the following four days. She came to the physiotherapy department three times daily, and performed the following regime:

1. Press-ups . . . in number.
2. Lying on back with 7lb weight between hands, lift weight from above shoulder to opposite hip . . . times.
3. Lift weight above head and down to waist . . . times.

343

4. Lift weight towards ceiling and back to chest . . . times.

The number of times each exercise was performed was gradually built up, so that the maximum was reached by the fourth day. Each exercise programme was followed by 15 minutes rest, lying flat on the floor (no pillow if possible).

The programme was discussed carefully with the patient and a card with the exercises and number of times they were to be performed given to the patient. A time for doing the exercises was worked out with the patient. She felt that fitting them into a busy day might prove difficult, as she always felt very tired after returning home from work. However, on returning home, she persevered with them, helped by her husband doing some extra household chores. Prior to her leaving hospital, her husband had come to the physiotherapy department and discussed the programme with his wife and the physiotherapist.

As well as doing the exercise programme, the patient should be encouraged to do other exercises. Skipping is a useful exercise as it is enjoyable and easy to perform. Again, the patient should be carefully instructed and her movement observed. Any abnormal patterns must be corrected or the exercise adapted; if continued, they will reinforce the abnormal at the expense of the normal. Video-tape or ciné-filming can be of use in keeping an objective record of the patient's progress.

Participation in sport should be encouraged and the patient advised to participate in swimming, badminton, tennis or keep-fit classes at the local evening school. Walking is especially valuable. The amount of exercise additional to the Rest Exercise Programme that the patient is able to do will vary with the patient's occupation and other commitments.

Patients during this early stage may find it helpful to attend follow-up sessions every two or three months, so that their exercise programme can be adjusted, and any other problems discussed. Regular out-patient physiotherapy should not be necessary, nor encouraged.

Middle stage (Grades III–IV)

As the disease progresses, the signs and symptoms become more obvious and the patient may show considerable fluctuation in disability during periods of exacerbation and remission. Reassessment is necessary, and should be continual, and the effects of treatment should be constantly observed.

Before a detailed assessment is carried out the therapist should discuss with the patient the problems he is having at home or at work. Possible problems might include: can he get on and off the bus ? does his present occupation involve walking long distances ? is he having trouble with incontinence ? or, in the latter part of this stage, can he perform the normal activities of daily living, e.g. dressing, washing, cooking, etc. ?

Discussions with relatives are often helpful, as patients tend to be rather unrealistic and over-optimistic about their abilities. The physiotherapist works as a member of a team, and should be ready to ask for help for the patient from other colleagues, e.g. social workers, nursing staff, occupational and speech therapists, and dieticians.

Detailed assessment of the patient should be carried out as described in Chapter IV. After the detailed assessment, a suitable treatment programme should be planned. The patient may be treated as an in-patient in hospital, as an out-patient attending two or three times weekly, or in his own home. The last mentioned has the advantage of allowing the physiotherapist to observe the patient in his own surroundings.

TREATMENT

Treatment at this stage can be illustrated by a young man who was employed by an engineering firm, doing work which required a high degree of precision. He lived with his parents, and travelled to and from work in his own car. Over the past two years he had become increasingly disabled and was now unable to drive his car or to do the precise work his job entailed. He was admitted to hospital for investigations and intensive physiotherapy. Assessment showed that he had hypertonicity in both lower limbs, of the spastic type. There was increased tone in the extensors, adductors, and medial rotators of both hips, in the extensors of the knee, and in the plantar flexors and invertors of the feet. His lower limbs were held in a typical spastic extensor synergy. His trunk muscles showed hypotonus and his balance and equilibrium reactions were poor. Head control was still fairly good. His arms showed lack of proximal fixation at the shoulder-girdle, and intention tremor.

Because of these problems, his gait was stiff and jerky. He found some difficulty in turning over in bed, and in getting from lying to sitting. Getting from sitting to standing and from standing to sitting also proved difficult, due to increased tone in his legs and the weakness of his trunk muscles. All movements of his arms tended to be clumsy: his writing had become very poor, eating was becoming a problem, and also doing up zips and buttons. He was, however, able to look after himself, and moved around the house, holding on to the furniture. The stairs were becoming a daily hazard.

A programme of treatment was planned for the patient, who attended the physiotherapy department twice daily, with a rest period after both sessions. The main object of the treatment was to help the patient remain as independent as possible, while continuing to live at home with his parents. In order to achieve this, treatment was given to inhibit abnormal neuromuscular activity, to facilitate normal movement patterns, to improve balance and equilibrium reactions, and to gain better control of his arm movements. Functional activities were constantly practised as better movement was obtained. His scheme of treatment included the application of ice-packs to the hypertonic muscle groups in his lower limbs. These were applied in prone lying to avoid supine lying, which increased the extensor hypertonia in his legs. When the cold had reduced the spasticity, more normal movement was possible.

The patient was treated on mats on the floor, starting in side-lying with both legs slightly flexed (see Fig. XV/1a). Rhythmical passive trunk rotation was given to reduce spasticity. When this was achieved, active trunk rotation was practised to facilitate rolling and turning in bed. Passive movements were given to the lower limbs, working from the proximal to the distal joints. Shaking was used, to ease out any extra muscle tightness. Spastic muscles must never be forcibly stretched, they should be carefully and gradually eased out to their full length.

From side-lying, the patient rolled into forearm support prone lying, with the legs slightly flexed on pillows or a wedge (see Fig. XV/1b). In this position, rhythmical stabilizations can be given to the muscles of the shoulder-girdle. Pressure can also be given through the long axis of the humerus to facilitate co-contraction of the muscles around the shoulder and elbow joints. The patient then practised reaching forward to touch objects placed in front of him (Fig. XV/1c). This encouraged controlled, co-ordinated movement, after facilitating the proximal fixation.

The patient then moved to side-sitting to the right and left (Fig XV/1d). Rhythmical stabilizations were given to the trunk muscles. The free arm was encouraged to move in natural diagonal patterns

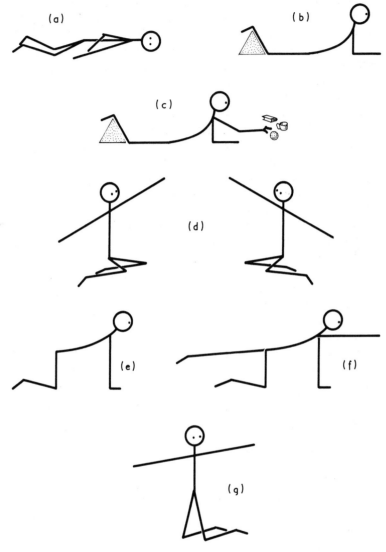

Fig. XV/1 Exercise sequence used in Stage II (Grades III to IV)

(a) Side lying, (b) (c) Forearm support, prone lying and reaching for objects. (d) Side sitting. (e) (f) Prone kneeling and balance reactions. (g) Kneeling

347

using the slow reversal technique. Head and neck movement may be combined with these. In prone kneeling, rhythmical stabilizations were given to the shoulder and pelvic regions, and also to the limbs as they were moved in the natural diagonal patterns (Fig. XV/1e, f). Counting or music may be used to obtain greater precision of movement.

The patient then practised balance and equilibrium reactions on a roll and balance board. He sat astride the roll with the physiotherapist facing him (see Plate XV/6). The physiotherapist could then gently rock the roll from side to side, so stimulating the patient's natural balance reactions. The patient could lie, sit or kneel on the balance board (see Plates XV/1 to 5).

During treatment, the patient was carefully observed. Any exercise which caused abnormal movement was avoided. Abnormal movement will facilitate abnormal movement.

Gait training was then given. This involved training the patient in transference of weight over the weight-bearing limb, while moving forwards, backwards and sideways. Natural patterns of hip and knee flexion and heel-toe gait were encouraged. Rhythmical stabilizations were given to the shoulder and pelvis, care being taken not to increase the hypertonus in the legs. After a week's intensive training, the patient was able to walk with one stick, which he only used to steady himself when necessary.

As the patient's movements improved, functional tasks were continually added. Getting from sitting to standing, going up steps, slopes and stairs, walking out of doors on rough ground, and getting in and out of the passenger seat of a car, were practised. Newly attained normal patterns of movement must be used functionally, to be of value to the patient. Towards the end of the patient's stay in hospital, the physiotherapist and occupational therapist went home with the patient to see if he could manage, and if any suggestions could be made to help the patient and his family.

The scheme of treatment outlined above does not include all techniques available, but was decided upon after assessment of the particular patient concerned. See also Chapter VI.

Advanced stage (Grades V–VI)

Most patients take years to reach this stage, and many may never reach it at all. A few may reach it very quickly.

Assessment is again important. There should be discussions with the patient about his increasing problems as and when they occur, at home, in a unit for the chronically sick, or in hospital. Emphasis should shift from treatment to the management of the patient's problems. Can the patient get on and off the lavatory? in and out of bed? can he feed himself? and manage his toilet? Close liaison is needed between all members of the health care team, doctors, nurses, social workers, occupational therapists, physiotherapists, general practitioners, and the patient's relatives and friends.

MANAGEMENT

Management of the patient in the advanced stage can be illustrated by a middle-aged woman living at home with her husband and teenage daughter. The patient was referred by her general practitioner as she was having increasing difficulty in transferring from bed to her wheelchair, and from her wheelchair to the lavatory. Her husband was out at work all day, and her daughter attending secretarial college. The patient was admitted to hospital for a period of assessment.

The physiotherapist, occupational therapist and nurses discussed the problems of the patient. She showed hypertonus in both lower limbs, which were tending to go into a position of flexor withdrawal. There was gross weakness of the trunk, and inco-ordination of both arms. Because of these problems, she found difficulty in turning in bed, and in getting from lying to sitting, and in moving around in bed. Transfer from the bed to chair proved very difficult for the patient to manage on her own.

During discussion with the patient and her husband and daughter, suggestions were made to help them manage at home. They were shown how to turn the patient with minimal effort, and how to give passive movements to her legs to prevent flexion contractures, and how to give longitudinal pressure through her straightened legs to try and stimulate an extensor response, and so prevent the patient going into further primitive flexion. The use of sheepskins to prevent pressure sores was discussed, and the need for regular turning stressed.

Transfers proved a problem, and a hoist was suggested. This was tried out, and the Oxford Hoist was found satisfactory. The patient's husband and daughter were also shown the 'Australian lift', which can be of value where it is not possible to use a hoist. The patient's wheelchair was discussed, and a deeper cushion with a space for a receiver was suggested. This would save the patient having to transfer on to the lavatory while her husband and daughter were not at home.

Every patient must be assessed individually, and their many problems considered. This necessitates a visit to the patient's home, as patients' requirements vary considerably according to the situation in which they live, and the help that is available.

The physiotherapist must be realistic in her approach and be ready to help the patient with problems as they arise. If necessary, help should be sought from special centres, e.g. Mary Marlborough Lodge, Oxford, and St. Mary's Hospital, Roehampton, where doctors and therapists are experts in the field of severe disablement. Patient and therapist may visit these centres, or the patient may be admitted for a period so that various different aids may be tried out and those most suitable for the individual patient supplied. Aids must be practical, and the patient and his helpers shown how to use them correctly, preferably in the patient's normal environment. Hoists can prove a problem in a small house with little space in bedroom and bathroom. No aid should be supplied without careful instruction in its use.

Group discussions for patients and their families can prove very useful; common difficulties and new ideas can be exchanged. The Multiple Sclerosis Society has many local branches, which are very helpful in this way.

CONCLUSION

It has been seen that the various stages of multiple sclerosis merge into each other, and methods of treatment are not confined to one phase.

The Rest Exercise Programme carried out by patients in the early stages can still be used by those who have deteriorated further, and is particularly useful in helping to maintain the strength of the upper limbs. The treatment techniques used in the middle stages can be adapted and used for patients in the advanced stage. Treatment, however, must always be appropriate to the need of the individual patient.

At all stages, the physiotherapist should be involved in helping the patient to live to his fullest capacity within the community, and not simply in treatment programmes. These are a means to an end, the quality of life of the patient. (See also Chapter XXI.)

FRIEDREICH'S ATAXIA

This is one of the commonest forms of hereditary ataxia. It is a familial and hereditary condition characterized by primary degeneration of nerve fibres involving demyelination, destruction of axons and reactionary gliosis. The posterior columns are most affected but cortico-spinal and posterior spinocerebellar tracts are also involved. Degeneration also occurs in the posterior nerve roots. Fatty degeneration and fibrosis of the heart muscle is another feature of this disease. The heart becomes enlarged as a result of these changes.

The disease affects both sexes equally and the first symptoms usually appear between the ages of 5 and 15.

Symptoms

The first symptom is usually unsteadiness of gait due to the loss of position sensibility. As the disease progresses this unsteadiness increases, the patient walks with a broad base and cannot stand without support. Usually he is worse if his eyes are shut or if he is in the dark. Weakness appears in the legs. Tone of the muscles varies. If diminished sensation from joints and muscles is most marked, tone is decreased, but if the cortico-spinal tracts are more affected there will be spasticity. Gradually the afferent side of the reflex arc degenerates and deep reflexes disappear. The plantar response becomes extensor and the superficial abdominal reflexes are lost.

Intention tremor appears in the arms and eventually will make co-ordinated movements difficult. Nystagmus and staccato speech are present and there are often fine movements of the head.

There is impairment of light touch and postural and vibration sensitivity in the lower extremities.

The mental condition is usually normal until the later stages when there may be some impairment of intelligence.

Nearly all these patients suffer from pes cavus and spinal deformities.

Prognosis

The disease usually progresses slowly, the patient eventually being unable to stand or walk. Occasionally it becomes arrested but more usually the patient succumbs from infection or heart failure within about 20 years of the onset of symptoms.

Treatment

No treatment arrests the course of the disease but symptomatic treatment is valuable. Physiotherapy will be directed towards the ataxia, weakness and deformities and is carried out on the lines indicated for patients suffering from multiple sclerosis.

For references and further reading see end of Chapter XVIII.

CHAPTER XVI

Parkinsonism

by JOAN CASH, B.A., F.C.S.P., DIP.T.P.
revised by HELEN W. ATKINSON, M.C.S.P., DIP.T.P.

The parkinsonian syndrome comprises a set of signs and symptoms which together form a definite clinical picture. The outstanding features are tremor, rigidity, slowing and poverty of movement and defective or lost postural reflexes resulting in disturbances of posture and balance.

Degeneration and loss of cells takes place in the basal ganglia but in spite of years of research the exact site of degeneration in each form of parkinsonism is still not clear.

In idiopathic parkinsonism the main changes appear to occur in the substantia nigra. There is a loss of melanin from the pigment cells, a decrease in the number of neurones and an increase in neuroglia. Similar changes are found in the reticular formation, dorsal nucleus of the vagus and hypoglossal nucleus, and in the brain stem. Less severe degeneration occurs in the globus pallidus and putamen.

With loss of cells there is a depletion of the chemical transmitter dopamine normally present in considerable quantities in the cells and nerve terminals of the substantia nigra. This upsets the delicate balance between the various chemical transmitters, especially between the inhibitory effects of dopamine and the excitatory effects of acetylcholine.

SIGNS AND SYMPTOMS

TREMOR

This appears at some stage in the disease in all patients suffering from parkinsonism. It consists of a rhythmically alternating contraction of opposing muscle groups in the area involved. Usually the tremor begins in the fingers of one hand spreading to the foot of the same side and then to the opposite side. The jaw, head and trunk may also be involved. At first the fingers flex and extend at the metacarpophalangeal joints. When the thumb joins in, a pill-rolling movement results. The head has a rotatory movement, the jaw opens and closes, the tongue is protruded and withdrawn.

The tremor occurs at the rate of about 5 to 6 times per second. It is present at rest, absent in sleep and in active movement, but is increased by emotion, excitement or fatigue and if the patient feels he is being watched.

Extensive research has been undertaken into the subject of tremor in this condition, and though no certain explanation has been established Calne (1970) states that it is suggested that damage to inhibitory nigro-striatal pathways causes excessive excitatory output from the striatum resulting in facilitation of oscillatory bursts of activity in thalamic neurones which then drive localized areas of the cerebral cortex.

RIGIDITY (see also Chapter III)
This is a uniform increase in tone in all muscle groups of the areas involved. It is felt as a resistance throughout the whole range of passive movement and may be one of two types. It may be a smooth rigidity – the 'lead-pipe' type, or the muscles may seem to yield in a series of jerks – the 'cog-wheel' type. The rigidity can be decreased if the part is supported and the patient taught to relax. It is increased by mental concentration and active movements of the other parts of the body. The hypertonus is often most marked in the neck and forearm muscles. Martin (1967) suggests that it is an exaggerated form of postural fixation and is a release phenomenon. It may be partly, at least, the cause of the unnatural immobility of these patients, the absence of the usual 'fidgety' movements, and the lack of both expression and arm swinging.

Rigidity is reduced by surgical incision in the globus pallidus and by the administration of L-dopa.

SLOWNESS AND POVERTY OF MOVEMENT (bradykinesia, hypokinesia)
Certain disturbances of motor function are characteristic of diseases of the basal ganglia. Voluntary and automatic movements are slow and reduced in amplitude and range – this can be seen in the writing

of patients, which is usually very small, and in the loss of the swing of the arms in walking. There is often delay in the initiation of voluntary movement. A considerable latent period between the stimulus and response occurs, so, for example, there is a pause between the desire to get up from a chair and the actual performance. Fine movements are particularly difficult, giving rise to problems in such activities as dressing, toilet and eating.

The patient often finds difficulty in modifying the range and speed of movement once it is initiated, creating problems, for example, in walking. There is usually inability to maintain repetitive movements or to perform rapidly alternating movements. The rotation element in movement is especially lacking. This leads to difficulties, for example, is a patient approaches a door obliquely he may fail to turn to negotiate the doorway and consequently he may bump into the doorpost. When walking towards a chair he may not turn sufficiently as he sits down so that he 'sits' to the side of the chair and falls to the ground.

Thoracic expansion is reduced and there is danger therefore of respiratory complications. In general, motor activity is greatly reduced and the patient tends to sit still. There is little movement of the facial or ocular muscles with consequent mask-like appearance and, since blinking is rare, the patient appears to stare. Both mastication and swallowing may be affected, at least partly due to rigidity. Constipation is often a problem. This may be partly due to slowness and difficulty in chewing and swallowing which will lead to a restricted diet, and partly because of rigidity of abdominal muscles and lack of trunk movements. Speech is often affected, due partly to rigidity of the muscles of the larynx and partly to slowness and limited movement of the tongue. In advanced cases the patient may speak rarely and only in whispers, or he may mumble or his speech be slurred and monotonous.

DEFECTIVE POSTURAL REFLEXES
With the exception of the anti-gravity mechanisms, the postural reflexes – postural fixation, protective reactions, righting reflexes, tilting reactions and locomotive reactions – may all be disordered.

The head tends to sink forward in sitting, standing and when on all fours, although the patient can lift it voluntarily. When sitting the trunk may sink forward or backward and in standing the patient has difficulty in keeping the knees straight and the trunk erect, so that a typical flexed position of the whole body is often a feature of parkinsonism (see Plate XVI/1). If the patient is put into, or takes up, a position he tends to 'stick' in this position but, should the position be disturbed, he finds it difficult to bring the centre of gravity back over the base (due to defective equilibrium reactions) and consequently he can easily fall or be pushed over – he is 'at risk'. These defects are increased if the patient cannot see what he is doing.

Since righting reflexes are often defective the patient has difficulty in obtaining the erect position from lying. There seems to be a reversion to primitive movement patterns in one plane only and rotation in movement seems to be particularly lacking. Thus turning over is sometimes impossible. The eyes and head may turn but the shoulders fail to follow and instead of using the free arm to assist rotation the patient tends to press the free hand against the ground. If the neck muscles are rigid failure to turn the head means the response to the labyrinthine righting reflexes cannot be elicited. Rigidity of trunk muscles interferes with the impetus they give to rolling over. If the patient can roll over and get on to all fours he may not be able to get to the erect position because he is unable to get his centre of gravity over his feet.

Locomotion is much impaired. Some patients are unable to get the lateral movement or the upper trunk sway which enables the centre of gravity to be taken over the supporting foot and the other foot to be freed from the ground for stepping. In severe cases walking can then only occur from the knees in the form of a shuffle. A gentle push to the right when the right foot reaches the ground and *vice versa* will greatly assist walking.

To gain propulsion in normal walking the trunk is tilted forward and this forces the walker to take a step. Some patients, possibly owing to rigidity as well as loss of postural reflexes, cannot tilt the trunk forward and consequently stepping is not stimulated. Other sufferers cannot control the forward tilt and therefore either fall or take rapid short steps forward (the festinant gait), continuing until they are stopped by any object which gets in the way. If the walking patient is pushed backwards or forwards he tends to run back or forward (retropulsion and propulsion). Initiation and actual walking are often improved if transverse broad lines are drawn on the floor in a contrasting colour or if a series of 2 to 3 inch blocks are placed for the patient to step over. This appears to give visual reinforcement and may be the explanation of why patients find climbing stairs easier than walking.

Martin (1967) quotes the case of a man who always carried newspaper balls in his pocket to drop in front of him when he wanted to start walking.

SENSORY SYMPTOMS
Sensation is normal in these patients but on the other hand they often suffer from pain and aching. This is probably partly due to muscular rigidity, partly to faulty posture and so strain on ligaments, and partly to inability to move easily and adjust the position.

STRETCH REFLEXES
These are often difficult to elicit and reduced in amplitude. The plantar reflexes are usually flexor.

AUTONOMIC SYMPTOMS
Excessive salivation, flushing of the skin and uncomfortable sensations of heat often give rise to considerable discomfort. The patient tolerates cold better than heat and elderly patients may therefore suffer from hypothermia.

MENTAL STATE
Most patients remain mentally normal but if the condition is due to encephalitis or cerebral arteriosclerosis other areas of the brain will be affected and the patient may then show mental deterioration, extreme depression and suicidal tendencies.

VARIETIES OF PARKINSONISM

Various factors may cause changes in the basal ganglia and produce the parkinsonian syndrome. The degeneration may be idiopathic, may be due to encephalitis, poisoning, cerebral arterio-sclerosis or trauma. Because of these varieties of causation, differences arise both in the age of onset and the incidence of the signs and symptoms.

Idiopathic parkinsonism

This implies parkinsonism of spontaneous and unknown cause. This form is seen rather more often in men than in women, its onset usually occurring between the ages of 50 and 60. Tremor is most often the first symptom though slowness of movement and difficulty in the fine movements of the hands are often early features. The disease is progressive, but progress may be slow. The patient may eventually become completely immobilized and helpless. Death is usually the result of pressure sores or pneumonia.

Postencephalitic parkinsonism

This type followed the epidemics of encephalitis lethargica which occurred between the years 1917 to 1926. The disease is rare today, but parkinsonism from this cause is still seen among older people. The neurological symptoms tended to develop insidiously several years after the acute illness. The changes in the brain are more widespread than in idiopathic parkinsonism, affecting in addition to the substantia nigra, the putamen, thalamus, hypothalamus and sometimes the oculomotor nuclei (Lewis 1971). Rigidity was usually an earlier and more pronounced feature together with slowness and weakness of movement. Disturbances of behaviour and dementia are much more common than in idiopathic parkinsonism and oculogyric crises tend to occur.

Arterio-sclerotic parkinsonism

This is found as part of a generalized cerebral arterio-sclerosis usually appearing in late middle or old age. Areas of softening occur in the basal ganglia. Slowness and weakness of movement are usually more pronounced than tremor and the disease tends to progress rapidly. Other symptoms of cerebral disease are usually present and eventually the condition progresses to dementia.

Toxic parkinsonism

The symptoms have been found to follow administration of certain drugs such as the phenothiazine group, and in poisoning by copper, manganese and carbon monoxide. Provided damage is not too great the symptoms can be relieved by stopping the use of the drugs and removing the patient from the source of toxic substances.

Head injuries

The parkinsonian syndrome has been found to follow some severe head injuries and similar symptoms have been observed in boxers (the punch-drunk syndrome).

TREATMENT

Treatment of the parkinsonian syndrome as in all neurological disorders involves teamwork. Therapy may include skilled advice, the use of drugs, surgery, speech therapy, physiotherapy and occupational therapy. The pharmacologist, the nurse, the medical social worker, the welfare officer and disablement resettlement officer will also be needed.

DRUG THERAPY

A disturbance in the balance between the chemical transmitters in the basal ganglia in the direction of cholinergic dominance exists in parkinsonism. This could therefore be corrected either by blocking cholinergic activity with anti-cholinergic drugs such as benzhexol (Artane) or by raising the level of striatal dopamine by the administration of a precursor of dopamine, able to cross the blood-brain barrier, L-dopa. In many cases these two types of drugs are used together. Levodopa is now very widely used and many patients have obtained really impressive results from the use of this drug.

Prolonged treatment by L-dopa may possibly achieve its effect either by assisting regeneration in damaged, but not destroyed neurones, or by converting non-dopaminergic neurones into dopaminergic neurones (Wieringen 1971).

The greatest improvement is in the hypokinesia and bradykinesia. The facial movements improve and the mask-like expression disappears, walking is greatly improved, writing becomes larger, speech clearer and the patient can carry out fine movements of the hands which were previously impossible. Rigidity is reduced but tremor responds less well and occasionally as rigidity is reduced tremor increases (this can sometimes be dealt with by stereotaxic surgery). Spectacular improvement may take a considerable time – three months or more – to achieve, and some patients do not appear to benefit at all.

Side-effects can be a problem. Anorexia, nausea and vomiting can be a nuisance, but are usually avoided by a slow rate in increase of dosage, by anti-emetic drugs and by taking L-dopa after food. L-dopa tends to produce a fall in the systolic blood pressure and the patient may complain of giddiness. This can be dealt with by rest in bed for a few days and temporary reduction in dosage. Occasionally involuntary movements (dyskinesia) appear. There may be grimacing and choreo-athetoid movements of the face and limbs. Respiratory rate is sometimes increased. Treatment is then usually stopped for a day or two and then re-started at a lower dosage. One of the most serious side-effects is psychiatric disturbance, and this may require stopping the treatment and using tranquillizing drugs. The patient may be anxious, depressed, confused and restless. Some have markedly increased energy. Granulo-cytopenia, glaucoma, headaches and cardiac arrhythmia are occasional side-effects. Myocardial infarction and psychiatric disturbance are usually taken to be contra-indications to the use of L-dopa.

It is important to note that some patients on L-dopa feel so much better that they may undertake heavy physical exertion for which their cardio-vascular system is not suitable, and a watch should be kept on this problem.

Recent developments have resulted in the production of drugs containing a substance which inhibits the breakdown of levodopa outside the brain and therefore makes proportionately more of it available for transport to the brain and conversion there into dopamine. One such drug is Sinemet, which combines carbidopa with levodopa to achieve its effect. When such a drug is used it need contain only about 20 per cent of the normal levodopa dose to have an equal effect, and thus the side effects normally produced by levodopa will be mini-mized. However, if the dosage of Sinemet is high, side effects may occur and are similar to those produced by levodopa alone. As in all cases where drug therapy is first used or changed, dosage is increased cautiously, and in patients who have atrial, nodal or ventricular arrhyth-mias particular care must be taken.

Further pharmaceutical work is in hand in the effort to combat parkinsonism, and this includes work on a drug designed to act on the higher centres to encourage the release of an enzyme needed to produce dopamine in the appropriate areas. The drug amantadine is also in use as a result of the work of Schwab and his colleagues who used the drug to treat a type of influenza. It was found that patients who had parkinsonism (in addition to influenza) showed an improvement in their neurological symptoms when receiving this drug. How this effect was achieved is not known but it has been suggested that it may either have a central alerting effect or augment the action of dopamine.

SURGERY

Surgical procedures for the relief of the parkinsonian syndrome have been used for many years. Earlier methods were to divide dorsal nerve roots and to interrupt corticospinal pathways. Later the method has been to make destructive lesions in the basal ganglia and the thalamus. These lesions reduce or abolish tremor and reduce rigidity but they do not influence hypokinesia so that often the functional ability of the patient is not improved. With the excellent results obtained by the use of L-dopa surgery is now less commonly used. Its present role is probably likely to be to relieve tremor or deal with the dyskinesia produced in some patients by L-dopa, which otherwise limits the dosage which can be used.

GENERAL CARE (see also Chapters XX and XXI)

These patients are often elderly and are in danger of accepting their limitations, thinking that they are 'stiff' because of their age. Unfortunately relatives are also inclined to accept this situation and may encourage the patient to 'rest' or to sit down 'for safety'. Because the patient is slow in carrying out everyday activities, he is often assisted when he could manage quite well by himself if allowed to do so at his own pace. All of this sheltering may contribute to the patient's immobility and be, in fact, detrimental to his welfare. It is quite possible to make the symptoms worse than the disease process warrants by offering too much assistance and encouraging dependence on other people. The correct balance of assistance and independence is vital, and the patient should be encouraged to retain his independence for as long as possible. Movement is indicated in preference to static posturing, and participation in communal activities should be encouraged so that the patient does not become withdrawn from society and so feel valueless as a person.

If the patient is unable to remain at home and needs institutional care, it is particularly important that he is encouraged to help himself and others as much as he can without allowing him to suffer undue fatigue. In this way he will help to maintain his own physical condition and may also help avert the feeling of being virtually placed on a 'scrap-heap'.

Day hospitals and day centres are excellent for these patients since they can meet other members of the community, carry out useful activities and follow their own hobbies in sheltered circumstances. The advice and services of occupational therapists and physiotherapists are often available at these centres, and social service workers may visit the patients as necessary.

The help of the occupational therapist is of particular value with difficult activities of daily living and in the use of essential gadgets such as zips, Velcro fastenings, elastic shoelaces, eating utensils, etc.

In the more severe cases who may be more confined to wheelchair or even bed, careful nursing is needed to prevent respiratory complications and pressure sores. Patients at this stage will also probably have mastication, deglutition and speech problems and relatives or nurses may require help to manage these. The reader is referred to Chapter VI as well as to the next part of this chapter for further details on this aspect.

PHYSIOTHERAPY

Physiotherapy may be required for the patient who is also receiving drug therapy or who has undergone surgical intervention or, in fact, for the patient who is having no other form of therapy.

It is important to appreciate that the patient should be given help and advice by the physiotherapist as early as possible. Many patients are given a diagnosis of parkinsonism while in its very early stages, and may be given no help at all because they are considered 'not bad enough' to warrant drug therapy, physiotherapy or surgery. This may be true of drug therapy and surgery but it is not true of physiotherapy. The sooner the patient can be seen by the physiotherapist the better, because it is easier to prevent loss of normal movement patterns than it is to regain them after they have apparently disappeared and abnormalities have become a habit. Less time is required for the initial treatments and a few more months or years of relative independence may be gained by the patient.

If the patient has had surgery or is receiving drug therapy, he may still benefit from the help of the physiotherapist. By this time he may well have had the disease for several years. The onset tends to be gradual and the patient adapts to his symptoms, so that the various movement problems become a habit to such an extent that he is unaware of the true degree of his abnormality. Drugs and surgery may dramatically change the situation and make more normal reactions fairly readily available. However, the patient may have 'forgotten' the patterns and then will never realize his full potential without some help.

It is important to appreciate that physiotherapy cannot bring about a reversal of the changes which have occurred in the central nervous system as a result of the disease process. It is only possible to help the patient to minimize the effect of these changes by encouraging activities to remain as normal as possible. The patient's nervous system can only do its best in the circumstances, and the physiotherapist can only help it to exploit its full potential.

ASSESSMENT

All patients should be assessed carefully, since symptoms will vary according to the stage of the disease and the effect of other therapy being used. Assessment procedures should follow the lines indicated in Chapter IV and a functional assessment for daily living activities should preferably be conducted in the patient's home surroundings.

TREATMENT PROGRAMME

When the assessment has been carried out, a treatment programme can be planned. As the patient will never recover from his illness, it is important that an initial intensive treatment programme should be succeeded by checks and 'booster' programmes at intervals as befits the individual patient's needs.

RIGIDITY AND BALANCE REACTIONS

Treatment will almost certainly need to include activities to minimize rigidity and to improve the quality of balance reactions. The reader is referred to Chapter VI which emphasizes these activities. The patterns used in the proprioceptive neuromuscular facilitation techniques may be used to facilitate both limb and trunk activities and may be started through small range reversals with assistance, and gradually increased in range and speed so that the physiotherapist is ultimately only guilding the activity and encouraging more functional use of the pattern. The patient is often said to need 'pumping up' into an activity, by being prepared for it with much assistance and later taking over the activity himself. He may ultimately learn to prepare himself by carrying out repeated, simple swaying movements until he is sufficiently loosened to be functionally effective.

Static posturing and stabilizations are not usually suitable for such patients since they tend to be 'static' anyway as a result of the disease process. Thus the approach offered in stabilization techniques may only be suitable if the patient's response to drugs or surgery has produced symptoms of instability.

CONTROL OF HEAD AND NECK ACTIVITIES

In the parkinsonian patient there is a tendency for the head to drop forwards and for the thoracic spine to show an exaggerated primary curve of flexion (see Plate XVI/1). This is not good for the respiratory movements, makes equilibrium reactions even slower and inhibits speech, mastication and deglutition. Such patients may also complain of pain and discomfort in the neck and shoulder regions which is due to irritation of the cervical nerve roots. Conservative physiotherapy may help to relieve this pain, and the general activities already mentioned may well have the effect of automatically improving the functional posturing of the head and thorax. Far-reaching effects are often achieved by using trunk and balance activities without the need for specific head and neck activities. However, if automatic improvement of the head and neck posturing does not occur, some emphasis may be put on the cervical spine by giving assisted active head movements, suitably co-ordinated with the movements of the body as a whole. The patient should be encouraged to lead the upper trunk by using head and neck movements, and if upper limb reversals are used the patient should follow his hands with head and eye movements. Specific proprioceptive neuromuscular facilitation techniques may be used for the redevelopment of head and neck patterns, and the methods used are similar to those advocated for the limbs. Guided reversals through increasing ranges should be encouraged and stabilizations avoided. In addition, respiratory exercises should be encouraged so that the danger of chest complications is minimized.

Many people advocate the use of cervical collars for advanced cases and they may, indeed, be necessary if there is a danger of peripheral nerve root compression or cord damage. However, collars will inhibit movement and should only be used if absolutely necessary.

Parkinsonism

PROBLEMS OF MASTICATION, DEGLUTITION AND SPEECH

These are present in many patients demonstrating parkinsonism, and are particularly obvious in the more severely affected patients and those who have difficulty in controlling the position of the head.

Inactivity of the facial muscles and, in particular, of buccinator allows food and saliva to escape from the mouth and collect in the area between the cheeks and the teeth. This results eventually in distressing and unsightly dribbling at mealtimes and even at other times during the day. The patient becomes very embarrassed by this and feels socially unacceptable, which in fact he is, particularly to people who do not fully understand his condition. The tongue and supra- and infrahyoid muscles will also present problems, and difficulty with deglutition will be experienced. Speech is affected by the inactivity of all of these muscles and also by difficulty in vocalization due to respiratory impairment.

Stimulation of the tongue, facial muscles and hyoid muscles may be brought about by icing inside the mouth, the surface of the tongue, face and anterior aspect of the neck. Light stimulating massage may help to activate the facial muscles whilst respiratory exercise and chest percussion may help vocalization. Great attention must be paid to head posture, since deglutition and tongue movements can be severely impaired if the neck is in a non-functional position. For this reason it is important to see that the patient with poor head control is upright and well supported at mealtimes, with the head and neck in a good position for performing the functional movements associated with eating. Icing the tongue, cheeks, face and neck prior to attempting to eat may help the patient to cope with the problem and make mealtimes more enjoyable. Inexperienced nurses and relatives often need help on these matters if undue distress to the patient is to be avoided.

ADVICE AND ASSISTANCE FOR THE PATIENT AT HOME

Relatives and the patient should understand that prolonged periods of inactivity are detrimental to the patient. There are many ways in which help can be given. One of the worst times for the patient is on waking in the morning, because he has probably retained one sleeping posture all night and become genuinely stiff and immobile by the morning. If the problem is severe the relative may be required to loosen the patient passively by helping him to rotate his trunk. The less severe patient can help himself by turning over a few times before trying to get out of bed and by sitting on the edge of the bed.

Clothing can be made easy to fasten and of materials which are not too resistant to stretch. Clothes can be placed on both sides of the patient so that he has to turn and therefore rotate his trunk to pick up each article.

The patient can learn to help to loosen himself by swaying his body-weight in different directions before he stands up and attempts to walk. Any job he does about the house should be as active as possible, and sedentary work should not be carried out over long periods. Such patients are often unable to detect fatigue in themselves, and whilst encouraging movement it is important to avoid overdoing any one activity. Frequent changes of activity are helpful.

A few weeks of intensive physiotherapy and advice to both the patient and those with whom he lives will help him to realize his full potential. Thereafter the management should be restricted to check-ups and occasional 'booster' periods of treatment. It is useful to occasionally visit the patient at home to see him in his own surroundings and relatives will, in this way, be kept fully in the picture regarding his capabilities.

Occupational therapists and physiotherapists need to collaborate closely, since many patients can retain their functional independence with the help of some simple gadgets and instruction from the occupational therapist. The help of the social worker may be needed in certain circumstances, and the local authority can be approached if alterations to the home are required.

For references and further reading see end of Chapter XVIII.

CHAPTER XVII

Acute Infections of the Nervous System

by UTA GREINER, DIP.P.T.(BERLIN)
and SUSAN NOSWORTHY, B.PHTY(QUEENSLAND),
M.A.P.A.

Out of a great variety of acute infections of the nervous system, two main groups predominate. These are bacterial infections and viral infections.

BACTERIAL INFECTIONS

Bacteria enter the central nervous system in two distinct ways. Firstly, through emboli of bacterial or infected thrombi, travelling through the bloodstream from a primary septic focus in the body (e.g. lung). Secondly, through an extension of an infectious lesion adjacent to the brain (e.g. otitis, sinusitis, pyogenic cranial injuries, and osteomyelitis of the skull).

The most common bacterial infection is leptomeningitis, which is caused by the meningococcus. Other causative agents may be the pneumococcus, streptococcus or staphylococcus.

Meningitis

Meningitis always involves the pia mater and the subarachnoid spaces of the brain and spinal cord, including the ventricles. The inflammatory process involves the tissues lining these spaces and, therefore, can affect the cranial and spinal nerve roots. In some cases even the subpial white matter can be affected.

The inflamed lining of the spaces produces pus and this invades the cerebrospinal fluid and may cause obstruction leading to hydrocephalus or, possibly later, subdural effusions.

The clinical picture is usually one of violent headache, vomiting, neck stiffness and pain, high temperature and clouding of consciousness. If the bacterial action is not arrested quickly, delirium, focal fits and all the signs of cranial nerve involvement may be seen.

Early diagnosis and treatment is essential as delay often causes death or residual brain damage. Lumbar puncture is performed in order to culture the bacteria and thus determine its type, so that a heavy dosage of suitable antibiotic therapy can be administered. Where meningitis is caused by a primary infection somewhere else in the body, this source should be eliminated.

Anticonvulsants may be necessary to control fits as well as any other symptomatic treatment which is required.

Intensive nursing care in an isolation ward, as long as the causative agent remains infectious, is necessary. During this time physiotherapy is given in the form of chest care. Where motor dysfunction exists, or where consciousness is depressed, then the patient must be put through all ranges of joint movement. In the later stages any residual damage must be treated accordingly.

Brain abscess

A brain abscess is a focal infection which occurs in any part of the brain. It is secondary to a primary source of infection, usually from the ear, the sinuses or the lung.

The onset is always acute and signs depend on the actual site of the lesion in the brain, e.g.:

Temporal Lobe – dysphasia
Cerebellum   – nystagmus and cerebellar ataxia
Frontal Lobe – impairment of mental function.

In all cases, headache, raised temperature and all the signs of increased intracranial pressure exist.

As soon as possible intensive broad-spectrum antibiotic medication is begun. Intravenous urea (e.g. mannitol) is used in an attempt to lower the intracranial pressure.

When the abscess has become localized and encapsulated, surgical intervention in the form of burr-holes, drainage and aspiration, or total excision is indicated.

368

Physiotherapy is usually given as routine pre- and postoperative measures. After surgery full recovery is common. Any residual signs of hemiplegia, ataxia etc. should receive physiotherapy treatment as described in Chapters 5 and 6.

The brain, meninges, blood vessels, and cerebrospinal fluid are contained within a rigid 'box' which, except in childhood, cannot expand. A space-occupying tumour will therefore cause a rise in pressure within the 'box' and consequently affect all the other contents. Infiltrating neoplasms will have an effect less early than those which form masses.

The first structures to be affected by the rise in pressure will be the soft-walled veins and venous sinuses. Venous flow will be impaired and oedema result. Back-pressure in the veins will increase the formation and decrease the absorption of cerebrospinal fluid, resulting in hydrocephalus.

The outstanding symptoms of raised intracranial pressure are headache, papilloedema and vomiting. In addition there are sometimes giddiness, epileptiform convulsions, mental symptoms and disturbances in respiration, pulse and blood pressure.

Headache may be due to the tension in the blood vessels and stretching of the dura. It is usually described as throbbing or bursting and characteristically comes on at night and in the early morning. It may last only a short while, though later it may be continuous. Lying or anything which raises intracranial pressure such as straining or coughing increases the pain, which may be so intense that the patient sits up, holds his head, and is afraid to move it at all.

Papilloedema is swelling of the retina and optic disc. It is especially found when the pressure rises rapidly and in tumours of the temporal lobe, cerebellum and fourth ventricle. Its explanation lies in the fact that the optic nerve is surrounded by the same three membranes as the brain. It has therefore a subarachnoid space in continuity with that of the cerebral subarachnoid space. Rising pressure obstructs venous and lymphatic drainage from the retina and oedema results.

Vomiting often occurs with the headache and so takes place at night and in the early morning, often preceded by nausea and retching.

If pressure rises rapidly *pulse and respiration* become slow and blood pressure rises.

Mental symptoms vary. Chronic raised intracranial pressure is likely to cause progressive dementia with deterioration of intellect and personality. A fairly rapid rise causes confusion while with a sudden high rise the patient sinks into a coma.

VIRAL INFECTIONS

There are innumerable viruses which can affect the central nervous system. Due to this ability they are called neurotropic viruses. In many cases the origin of a viral infection of the central nervous system can be established through the presence of a previous viral infection, such as chickenpox, mumps and measles, while in other cases it is very difficult to identify the causative agent and to ascertain the nature of the disease.

Viral infections may produce one of three main syndromes. These are:

1. Encephalitis and encephalomyelitis
2. Herpes zoster
3. Poliomyelitis

All three categories are distinctly different in their clinical picture and accordingly treatment varies widely.

Encephalitis

The most common of the viral infections of the central nervous system is encephalitis. In this the virus attacks the nerve cells, the grey matter and/or the white matter.

Encephalitis may be due to direct viral infection such as is seen in epidemic form and may vary according to geographic and seasonal incidence, e.g. Eastern and Western equine encephalitis in the U.S.A.; lethargic encephalitis in Europe in the nineteen-twenties; Japanese B encephalitis; Australian X disease (Murray Valley encephalitis) and Russian Spring-Summer encephalitis. These viruses are thought to be transmitted by mammals and anthropoids as well as man.

The pathological process is usually one of direct neuronal destruction with phagocytosis of nervous tissue. Depending on the type of virus, different areas of the brain may be predominantly affected. This will consequently change the symptomatology which is then of great interest to the physiotherapist. The patient can present with pyramidal, extra-pyramidal or, most commonly, mixed types of neurological disorder.

Assessment and treatment as discussed in Chapters 4, 5 and 6 should guide the physiotherapist when confronted with an encephalitic patient. The early treatment will be similar to that discussed below.

Encephalomyelitis

This has not been proved to be a viral disease in itself because it usually follows as a complication after specific vaccinations (e.g. anti-rabies) or after acute viral infections such as measles, mumps, chickenpox and smallpox. It is commonly seen in teenagers or young adults, but it is not restricted to these age groups.

Pathologically the primary attack seems to be upon the myelin sheath of the nerves. This produces a focal demyelination whereas the encephalitis mentioned above acts more directly on the neurone. Because of this, differentiation between the two conditions can be made.

The onset of the illness usually occurs some weeks after the primary disease. Encephalomyelitis may be more 'encephalitic' or more 'myelitic' (i.e. 'spinal') in distribution. The encephalitic type presents with a return of fever after the original viral infection has subsided. Restlessness, headache, neck stiffness, drowsiness, and in some cases convulsions or even coma are seen. The 'myelitic' type shows mainly signs of flaccid paraplegia, sphincter involvement and symptoms of an acute upper motor neurone lesion.

The duration of the illness varies greatly from rapid recovery to lengthy periods of acute illness followed by a slow rehabilitation. The patient may show residual signs of limb paresis, speech disturbances, dystonia, and extrapyramidal symptoms.

Medically the condition is sometimes treated with steroids, often ACTH gel.

Physiotherapy treatment is begun from the earliest stages of the illness to prevent complications such as chest infections and pressure sores. Loss of joint mobility may also occur due to spasticity, lack of power, or gravitational effect due to poor positioning of the body. Loss of muscle and tendon elasticity and deep venous thrombosis can also occur.

Thus treatment depends on assessment of the individual's unique clinical picture. It may be necessary to build up, or inhibit, postural tone. Often the patient needs selective sensory stimulation to give him more 'feel' of normal postures and body movements.

It is essential from the earliest stages that careful handling and positioning of the patient is practised by everyone, thus the physiotherapist may have to advise the nursing staff on correct positioning. The use of bed cradles, pillows, bed boards, sheepskins, ripple mattresses should not be overlooked.

As the patient improves, active movements should be facilitated so that the patient retains the idea of movement and spatial awareness, both of which are so important to full recovery.

Herpes zoster (herpes encephalitis, shingles)

Herpes zoster is an acute infection of the nervous system characterized by the formation of skin eruptions in the course of peripheral or cranial nerves. It usually affects the posterior root ganglions in their segmental distribution on one or more levels, or the extramedullary roots of the cranial nerves (in particular the trigeminal nerve).

Herpes zoster is most frequently unilateral as the virus localizes in a section of the posterior horn. Then the disease often spreads along the sensory fibres of the involved segmental nerve and finishes off in a 'girdle-like' pattern, hence its name. Involvement is most frequently between the second thoracic and the second lumbar regions, or the fifth cranial nerve.

There is a serologic identity between herpes zoster and the varicella (chicken pox) virus.

Although this is a febrile illness, often patients first present with pain, making diagnosis difficult. After two to four days the typical vesicular rash appears in the affected dermatomes. These vesicles are at first oedematous, resolving after five to ten days and leaving a scale.

The whole course of the disease can vary from ten days to five weeks. The older the patient, the longer the course and the more disabling the post-herpetic complications. These may be in the form of neuralgic pains and to some extent, in cephalic or cervical types, paralysis.

The pain felt in the acute stages is not identical with that of post-herpetic neuralgia. The latter is of such intensity that patients may not be able either to rest or to sleep, and it may persist for weeks or months. Consequently, depression is often an associated feature.

Treatment in the acute phase consists of the administration of mild sedatives, aspirin or codeine for pain and calamine lotion for the skin lesions. Antibiotics are given only to prevent secondary infections.

Once the patient suffers from post-herpetic neuralgia the management of pain is much more difficult. It has been suggested that this pain is of thalamic origin. Various procedures such as injection of the dorsal root ganglion with alcohol, radiotherapy, dorsal rhizotomy or cordotomy have been attempted but with little success in the majority of cases.

Physiotherapy in the acute stages is only indicated when paralysis is present and this should be dealt with accordingly.

It is mainly in post-herpetic neuralgia that the physiotherapist plays a part in relieving the pain. Pain is transmitted through large and small fibres, the large, fast-conducting fibres being mainly inhibitory while the small, slow-conducting fibres are pain facilitating. In herpes zoster the large fibres are damaged, and the balance is upset, so the inhibitory component is decreased or absent. The authors have found that certain measures such as vibration, gentle clapping, electrical stimulation, and massage can stimulate the large inhibitory fibres and so restore their function. In our experience gentle percussion by hand or by rubber hammer, or else with the application of a mechanical vibrator, has been most effective. In the beginning it is often too painful to attack the affected dermatomes directly, thus the therapist has to work from the less hypersensitive areas to the centre.

Preferably the treatment should be given at frequent intervals – three or four times a day for a short duration as this increases the patient's tolerance more quickly.

Ultrasound and ultraviolet light are still used in the treatment of this condition.

Poliomyelitis

Poliomyelitis has undergone many changes in the last four decades. Before World War II the disease mainly affected children – hence the term 'infantile paralysis' – and virtually only the lower limbs. Today it is well known that poliomyelitis affects all age groups. Paralysis is not confined to just the lower part of the body, although ascending involvement of the spinal cord and brainstem is seen more commonly with respiratory paralysis becoming the main cause of death.

In the 1950s, there were world-wide epidemics, which occurred mainly in the three hottest months of the respective countries. It usually affected communities with lower hygiene standards.

The virus is transmitted by personal contact and through contamination of food and water.

In 1955 Salk developed a serum of dead viruses which after three injections built up immunity. However, the attenuated live type vaccine administered orally has proved to be the more effective.

As a result of vaccination the disease now occurs only sporadically and is much less virulent in the acute stage. Immunization is still of great importance as with mutations of the virus fresh epidemics may occur, hence leading to poliomyelitis in a new form.

The authors feel, therefore, that as so few cases are seen today it is misleading to over-emphasize poliomyelitis as a viral disease.

The virus attacks the anterior horn cells or grey matter of the brain stem, causing a flaccid paralysis. There are, however, various sites of neurological manifestation. Three main types have been established:

1. Spinal type – weakness and pain in the muscles of the trunk, extremities and respiratory muscles.

2. Bulbar type – brain stem involvement means respiratory and swallowing difficulties or failure.

3. Encephalitic type – drowsiness, unconsciousness and delirium are the main symptoms.

All types can overlap.

The clinical course of the disease has been divided into four stages:

1. Pre-paralytic
2. Acute paralytic
3. Convalescent
4. Residual

Pre-paralytic. Nine out of ten cases recover completely after the early symptoms of fever, nausea, muscle fatigue, muscle tenderness and headache. Treatment consists of bed rest to avoid fatigue and isolation to prevent spread of the disease.

Acute paralytic. In this acute stage paralysis occurs with different degrees of severity and distribution. Passive movements are necessary but overstretching of the muscles and undue pain must be avoided.

In cases of respiratory involvement different types of ventilators are used. Incidentally many types of respirator have been developed solely due to the great epidemics of the past (iron lung; rocking bed; cuirasse). Chest care is of utmost importance. Care must be taken in positioning during postural drainage because the patient is fully conscious in this acutely painful stage.

As we have the picture of a flaccid paralysis, positioning of the affected parts of the body in the midline position is necessary to prevent

374

over stretching of tendons and capsules, residual deformities and contractures.

Careful active movements should be commenced as soon as possible. Most of the recovery is expected to occur during the first month.

Convalescent stage. When the virus is no longer active, rehabilitation is begun in earnest. Many options are open to the physiotherapist depending, of course, on the degree of disability of the patient.

Independent respiration should be achieved as fast as possible. Active and passive treatment in bed should rapidly progress to mobilization in the gymnasium. During this stage hydrotherapy is of great benefit, physically and emotionally.

Recovery is thought to be completed after two years with most of this occurring in the first six months.

Residual stage. In this stage improvement of affected muscles is no longer aimed for. Maximum compensation by the unaffected muscles is desirable to achieve the maximum functional level of the individual. Surgical procedures such as muscle transplants and arthrodesis of joints in functional positions may be warranted.

Continuous check-ups are essential in paediatric cases to prevent deterioration during growth.

REFERENCES

Brain, R. (1955). *Diseases of the Nervous System*, Oxford Medical Publications, 5th ed.

Carini, R. N. and Queens, S. (1974). *Neurological and Neurosurgical Nursing*, The C. V. Mosley Company, 6th ed.

Chusid, J. G. and McDonald, J. J. (1976). *Correlated Neuro-anatomy and Functional Neurology*, Lange Medical Publications, 16th ed.

Harrison, T. R. (1974). *Principles of Internal Medicine*, International Student Edition, McGraw-Hill, 7th ed.

Matthews, W. B. and Miller, H. (1975). *Diseases of the Nervous System*, Blackwell Scientific Publications, 2nd ed.

Walshe, F. Sir. (1970). *Diseases of the Nervous System – Described for Practitioners and Students*, Churchill, 11th ed.

CHAPTER XVIII

Polyneuropathies

by UTA GREINER, DIP.P.T., and
SUSAN NOSWORTHY, B.PHTY.(QUEENSLAND),
M.A.P.A.

The term 'polyneuropathy' covers all diseases of the peripheral nervous system, no matter what the cause. Its usage is synonymous with 'polyneuritis' and 'multiple peripheral neuritis', but the authors feel it is preferable to use this term, as 'neuritis' might mislead the reader into thinking that the diseases are only inflammatory in origin.

As the causes are so diverse in nature, it is necessary to have a good knowledge of the functional anatomy of the peripheral nervous system in order to appreciate the clinical picture.

The peripheral nervous system covers all nervous structures outside the pia-arachnoid membrane of the spinal cord and brainstem. Hence the spinal and cranial nerve roots belong to the peripheral nervous system although they still lie inside the spinal canal. The afferent sensory and efferent motor fibres extend for a variable distance within the spinal canal, not yet being covered by their protective layers (epineural and perineural sheaths). These only commence where the nerves exit from the intervertebral foramina. Thus for a short distance these fibres are very vulnerable (e.g. to toxic agents). Consequently the first obvious signs of disability are seen peripherally, i.e. at the end organ of the respective affected, or destroyed, nerve cell.

Pathologically, degeneration of the myelin sheath and axis cylinder takes place leading to destruction of the myelin sheath, Schwann cells, axons and nerve cell cylinders. Breakdown of axons causes fragmentation of myelin into blocks, thus causing disruption of nerve conduction.

According to the degree of nervous tissue destruction, two types of lesions are differentiated:

1. Gombault's periaxial degeneration which involves the myelin sheath.

2. Wallerian degeneration where destruction of the axons takes place as well as of the myelin sheath.

This classification thus gives us an indication of the type, cause, and potential for recovery of the different peripheral nervous system diseases. Other very important criteria are the actual pathological changes in and around the nerve fibres.

The classification of the principal causes of peripheral neuropathies as outlined by Harrison in his text *Principles of Internal Medicine*, gives a clear indication of the magnitude of aetiology underlying the peripheral nervous system diseases.

TABLE I

Principal causes of Peripheral Neuropathy

I. POISONS
A. Metals: arsenic, lead, mercury, antimony, bismuth, copper, phosphorus, thallium.
B. Organic substances: carbon monoxide, carbon disulfide, trichloroethylene, methyl alcohol, triorthocresylphosphate, immune serums, benzene and derivatives.

II. DEFICIENCY STATES AND METABOLIC DISORDERS
Chronic alcoholism, beriberi, pellagra, combined system disease, pregnancy, chronic gastro-intestinal disease, carcinoma of lung, diabetes mellitus, porphyria, amyloid disease.

III. NON-SPECIFIC INFLAMMATORY STATES AND INFECTIONS
A. Acute idiopathic polyneuritis (acute febrile polyneuritis of Osler, Landry–Guillain–Barré syndrome).
B. Polyneuropathy complicating acute or chronic infection: diphtheria, Boeck's sarcoid, infectious mononucleosis.
C. Local infection of nerves: leprosy.

IV. VASCULAR DISEASE
Polyarteritis nodosa, arteriosclerosis.

V. FAMILIAL POLYNEUROPATHY
Progressive hypertrophic polyneuropathy, peroneal muscular atrophy.

VI. POLYNEUROPATHY OF OBSCURE ORIGIN
Chronic progressive or recurrent polyneuropathy.

A multiplicity of symptoms is possible due to the fact that there may be partial or total disruption of any of the fibres of the nerves affected, motor, sensory or trophic. It is not, therefore, really possible to describe a picture of all polyneuropathies though it is common to find that distal portions of the extremities nearly always are affected first (usually starting in the lower limbs). The spread of the disease is frequently upwards along the nerve trunk. In most neuropathies the trunk is spared and the sphincter function preserved. This leads to the conclusion that the longest and largest nerves are the most vulnerable.

Characteristic lower motor neurone lesion signs are usually common where the motor component is affected, i.e.:
1. flaccid paralysis
2. muscle wasting
3. loss of deep reflexes.

Sensory symptoms vary greatly in degree and distribution and may, or may not, precede the onset of paralysis. Hyperaesthesia, tingling, numbness, anaesthesia, and muscle tenderness are all well known in conjunction with various peripheral nervous system syndromes.

Trophic changes are seen more commonly in the later stages of these diseases and may be in the form of changes of skin or nail texture, or bone strength.

The remainder of the clinical picture may involve ataxia, vasomotor changes, high-stepping gaits, pain and an endless list of other signs and symptoms.

Because of this complicated mass of factors the physician usually carries out a number of diagnostic tests in order to determine the true diagnosis. Amongst the laboratory tests he has at his disposal are:
1. Nerve conduction tests. It is usual to find the conduction velocity of the nerve impulses lowered in chronic nerve diseases, but not in spinal cord or muscle disease (see Chapter IV).
2. Electromyography used to determine whether the muscle is primarily affected due to muscle disease, denervation of the muscle or a blockage of the neuromuscular junction (see also Chapter IV).

3. Cerebrospinal fluid examination.

4. Nerve and muscle biopsies.

It may be helpful for the physiotherapist to note how Harrison (1966) classifies the principal neuropathic syndromes as this gives a sound basis upon which to compare and contrast the groups of neuropathies that are most commonly seen.

TABLE 2

PRINCIPAL NEUROPATHIC SYNDROMES

I. Syndrome of acute ascending motor paralysis with variable disturbance of sensory function

A. Acute idiopathic polyneuritis (Landry–Guillain–Barré syndrome)

B. Infectious mononucleosis and polyneuritis

C. Hepatitis and polyneuritis

D. Diphtheritic polyneuropathy

E. Porphyric polyneuropathy

F. Toxic polyneuropathies (triorthocresylphosphate poisoning, Jamaica ginger)

II. Syndrome of sub-acute sensorimotor paralysis

A. SYMMETRIC POLYNEUROPATHIES
1. Alcoholic polyneuropathy and beriberi
2. Arsenic polyneuropathy
3. Lead polyneuropathy
4. Furadantin and other intoxications

B. ASYMMETRIC POLYNEUROPATHIES
1. Diabetic
2. Polyarteritis nodosa
3. Sub-acute idiopathic polyneuritis
4. Sarcoidosis

III. Syndrome of chronic sensorimotor polyneuropathy

A. ACQUIRED
1. Carcinoma, myeloma and other malignancy
2. Uraemia

3. Beriberi
4. Diabetes
5. Connective tissue diseases
6. Amyloidosis
7. Leprosy

B. FAMILIAL
1. Peroneal muscular atrophy (Charcot–Marie–Tooth disease)
2. Hypertrophic polyneuropathy (Déjerine–Sottas disease)
3. Polyneuritiformis hereditans (Refsum's disease)
4. Portuguese amyloidosis (Andrade's disease)

IV. Syndrome of chronic relapsing polyneuropathy

A. Idiopathic polyneuritis
B. Porphyria
C. Beriberi or intoxications

V. Syndrome of mono- or multiple neuropathy

A. Pressure palsies
B. Traumatic neuropathies
C. Idiopathic brachial and sciatic neuritis
D. Serum neuritis
E. Zoster
F. Tumour invasion with neuropathy
G. Leprosy
H. Paratubercular (polyneuritis cranialis multiplex)

Due to limitation of space the authors have decided to discuss in more detail those forms of polyneuropathies the physiotherapist is most likely to assess and treat in the physiotherapy department.

Acute ascending motor paralysis with variable sensory loss

The most frequent syndrome in this category is that of acute idiopathic polyneuritis. Other terms for this syndrome are Landry's paralysis, Guillain-Barré syndrome and acute infective polyneuritis. All the terms remain inadequate as they leave no clue as to the aetiology of the disease, while the last term implies that the illness is due to an 'infective' agent which remains unproven, to date. Therefore, perhaps a better name for this syndrome is acute idiopathic polyneuritis.

Polyneuropathies

This group of syndromes, while diverse in severity and symptoms, covers most of the severe, rapidly advancing polyneuropathies. The common picture is one of paralysis in the feet and legs, ascending over a period of days to involve the trunk, arms and sometimes the cranial nerves (facial diplegia dysarthria). Sensory symptoms often accompany this weakness in the form of hyperaesthesia, especially on touching the soles of the feet and palms of the hands; loss of vibratory sense; and loss of joint position sense.

The patient thus presents as a case where rapidly increasing paralysis may cause respiratory and cardiac difficulties which emphasizes the need for immediate, correct treatment. Intensive care facilities must be available in case of sudden crises while the disease is still spreading.

Death occurs in approximately 10–25 per cent of the cases in this category and is usually within two to three weeks of the onset of the illness, or occasionally later due to chest infections.

Sometimes the disease begins with the cranial nerves, or arms, and descends, causing increasing difficulty with respiration and locomotion.

Of the six polyneuropathies listed in Table 2 above, the authors propose to discuss only the Landry–Guillain–Barré) syndrome in greater detail as this is the polyneuropathy most commonly encountered. For all syndromes in this group the physiotherapy treatment will be along the same lines.

ACUTE IDIOPATHIC POLYNEURITIS

(Landry's ascending paralysis, Guillain–Barré syndrome, acute infective polyneuropathy)

In this syndrome there appears to be no seasonal incidence and cases occur sporadically. All ages and sexes are equally affected.

History of vaccination or illness seems unusual although most authorities on the subject report some significant incidence of mild respiratory or gastro-intestinal infection prior to onset. The aetiology remains a puzzle with no virus or microbial agent having yet been isolated.

The symptoms are generally as outlined above. Paralysis of the trunk and distal and proximal parts of the limbs also occurs. Sometimes in this kind of neuropathy, in contrast to many of the others, paralysis may be more marked proximally than distally.

Tingling, numbness and tenderness of muscles are common. Pain usually is present on full passive movement and stretch of the muscles.

Also hypersensitivity of hands and feet is often experienced when the physiotherapist handles the limb during treatment. Stiffness and cramp-like feelings are frequently described.

Hypotonia and areflexia are marked with headache and meningism being reported in some cases. Cranial nerve involvement may mean facial weakness, ptosis, loss of the convergence reflex, dysphagia, and dysphonia. At this stage the patient may be in respiratory difficulties due to additional involvement of the intercostals and diaphragm.

Sensory deficit is variable. In some cases only superficial sensation is affected, in others only deep sensation is lost. However, in some cases all modalities may be impaired. According to Professor J. Marshall (from the Institute of Neurology and National Hospital for Nervous Diseases, London), in his survey of 35 patients with this syndrome, the extent and severity of the sensory loss was paralleled by its persistence. In those patients in whom several modalities were affected over a considerable area, sensory loss persisted over many days or weeks.

In many cases both bladder and anal sphincter function will be affected. This is due to the nearness of the autonomic pathways to the actual site of the lesion (i.e. where the anterior and posterior roots fuse).

Usually the temperature remains normal, the cerebrospinal fluid is under normal pressure and is acellular. The pathology is a combined picture of Gombault's and Wallerian degeneration discussed previously (see page 377). Infiltrates in the liver, spleen, lymph nodes, heart and other organs reflect the systemic nature of the disease, but usually are not accompanied by parenchymal damage.

TREATMENT

When the patient enters hospital he usually presents with considerable weakness and is unable to walk. At this stage he is kept under constant observation for his respiratory function, pulse rate and cardiac involvement. The patient must remain very quietly on bed rest and provision is made for immediate intensive care treatment should it become necessary. Respiratory crises can happen very suddenly. With the increasing inability to move and communicate, due to weakness of the laryngeal and intercostal muscles, the patient is naturally very anxious. In this stage of complete helplessness there is a need for constant supervision and reassurance.

Medical treatment is aimed at stabilizing the organic functions and metabolism, as the course of the disease appears not to be influenced by medication such as steroids.

All the medical team, including the physiotherapist, are involved in continually assessing the progression of motor and sensory dysfunction. Use is made of a spirometer to ascertain the vital capacity at regular intervals. Should this fall below 800 ml then the patient will require urgent artificial ventilation. The only sensible way to do this is by performing a tracheotomy which prevents build-up of secretions and makes the physiotherapist's job much easier in keeping the airway clear.

In the acute progressive stage, treatment is mainly posturing and passive movements to prevent contractures, protect pressure points and avoid chest complications. The patient should be nursed on a firm mattress. Cradles may be necessary to take the weight of the bedclothes. Ankles, hips and shoulders seem to stiffen up more readily than other joints. Pillows, hand rolls and foot-boards are used to position the patient with sufficient shoulder abduction to allow adequate costal breathing and to maintain functional position of the hands and feet.

Passive movements should be done at least twice a day, not forgetting that attention should be given to the intercarpal, intertarsal, scapular and mandibular joints, as well as the usual gross range of joint movements.

Spread of the disease is variable from days to weeks. Once improvement starts then more active treatment is indicated. This follows along the lines of the patient with poliomyelitis, but it is important to remember there is often an additional sensory deficit. As a consequence of this the patient may lose his body image and appear to be ataxic.

Motor improvement usually occurs more quickly than sensory recovery. In most cases normal function is achieved within a few weeks, but some cases may take from six to eighteen months.

Once the patient is able to sit up for most of the day, ball-bearing arm supports should be attached to his wheelchair to assist arm function and prevent fatigue and overstretching of connective tissues. Temporary springs can be fitted to shoes to help dorsiflexion which, if weak or lost, usually takes longest to return.

The use of a pool, if available, is of great value. Care should be taken not to overheat the patient as there is a tendency to oedema formation which will be encouraged by heat. On the other hand, in cases of contractures heat may assist manual stretching as the collagen fibres are more elastic at 40–43 °C.

The innate potential of the patient with the Guillain-Barré syndrome to regain full function makes it one of the most satisfactory conditions treated by the physiotherapist.

Sub-acute sensorimotor paralysis

I. SYMMETRICAL FORM

This, too, is a fairly symmetrical polyneuropathy usually beginning in the feet and legs and later spreading to involve the hands and arms. The syndrome of pain, hypersensitivity of skin, and the tenseness of muscles, usually develops over a few weeks. The most common cause is vitamin B deficiency (beriberi), or in alcoholism, where the vitamin B balance is also disturbed. Toxins from arsenic, lead and mercury can also lead to this syndrome.

Alcoholic polyneuropathy and beriberi. As already mentioned above, disturbed and deficient vitamin B metabolism is the cause of both syndromes. These syndromes usually start after three months of dietary inadequacy. Motor weakness is most commonly preceded by sensory symptoms of numbness, tingling, tenderness of the feet, and in addition diminished touch, joint position sense and vibration. As is typical of polyneuropathies in this category, the symptoms spread from distal to proximal, first involving the legs, then the arms, but sparing the trunk and cranial nerves. Without medical treatment, weakness and sensory loss progress until the patient is confined to bed. By this time the disease has become chronic.

Pathologically both Gombault's and Wallerian degeneration are seen in the longest and largest fibres of the crural and brachial nerves. At any stage vitamin B therapy and adequate diet will arrest the syndrome. Prognosis for full functional recovery is quite good in the early stages, but where paralysis has occurred recovery may take up to six months or more and may never be complete.

The physiotherapist will usually have to treat a form of ataxia which is due to loss of sensation accompanied by muscular weakness. Should the patient become bedridden and go untreated, then contractures, severe muscular atrophy and pressure sores may be the result. At this stage there will often be mental confusion (e.g. Korsakoff's psychosis in alcoholics) which hampers the patient's recovery. Where pain and tenderness are acute, analgesics may be indicated.

Arsenical polyneuropathy. This syndrome progresses as in beriberi. A special feature is arsenical encephalopathy in which mental disturbances, convulsions and coma precede the polyneuropathy. A typical sign of this syndrome is white transverse banding of the nails (Mees lines). Poisoning due to mercury presents a similar picture.

Lead neuropathy. After chronic exposure to lead, a polyneuropathy may be seen in which the most prominent characteristics are motor weakness of the upper limbs with few or no sensory signs, producing wrist and finger drop (bilateral radial nerve palsy). This syndrome is confined to adults and affects the most used muscles. In children the same exposure leads to lead encephalopathy, a syndrome of increased intracranial pressure, convulsions, blindness, mental deterioration in some cases, and coma.

The only treatment is to remove the patient from exposure to lead and to initiate measures to eliminate it from the bloodstream. According to the severity of the syndrome, good motor recovery is to be expected. In the more chronic cases it may take a longer time. Hence physiotherapy can be of great value in overcoming the existing paralysis.

2. ASYMMETRICAL FORM

Mainly patients with diabetes mellitus and polyarteritis nodosa show this form of peripheral nerve involvement. Another such syndrome is sub-acute idiopathic polyneuritis, which as the name indicates has an unknown cause, but where symptoms and signs tend to appear and disappear over a period of months.

Diabetic polyneuropathy. In a high percentage of diabetic sufferers, especially those with untreated diabetes, involvement of the peripheral nervous system may lead to several clinical syndromes such as diabetic ophthalmoplegia, sudden or acute mononeuropathy and painful asymmetric polyneuropathy.

In the latter two syndromes, proximal weakness may predominate. Hip and pelvic muscles as well as sphincter involvement may lead to a syndrome called 'diabetic amyotrophy'.

Pain and muscle weakness are usually features, one making the other difficult to assess. If pain is present, it is of a severe lancinating, tearing, pulling type. Often vibration sense, proprioception and touch are diminished. Sensory ataxia will then be the result.

Physical treatment will only be effective if the diabetes can be controlled and gradual recovery may take several months.

Polyarteritis nodosa. While this on its own is actually a vascular disease, it can also lead to involvement of the intraneural vessels. However, in only a small percentage of patients with polyarteritis nodosa does a neuropathy become apparent. This might then lead to the actual diagnosis of the primary condition (i.e. polyarteritis nodosa) which has only shown itself before in a variety of obscure organic disorders, e.g. haematuria, fever, abdominal and vague limb pains and hypertension.

This polyneuropathy follows no definite lines being acute or subacute, symmetrical or asymmetrical in distribution, spinal and cranial nerves being affected alike.

No medication has changed the course of the disease but remissions and arrests of the polyarteritis are known. In these cases the polyneuropathy will also recede, but usually the disease is fatal.

Physiotherapy is aimed at maintaining the patient's function as long as possible, thus making him more comfortable and less depressed.

Chronic sensorimotor polyneuropathy

As indicated in Table 2 (see page 379) the chronic polyneuropathies fall into two distinct groups, one being acquired, the other having a familial or hereditary component. Both groups, however, tend to develop and progress over a number of months or years and often the exact time of onset is never established.

In general the syndromes can be asymmetrical or symmetrical. In many cases little is known of the pathology behind the lesion. It is interesting to note, however, in many of these syndromes the nerves may be enlarged and thus palpable.

The authors intend to discuss only the two main syndromes of the acquired form of polyneuropathy in more detail, as the others are rarely seen by the physiotherapist. However, it is worth remembering where chronic kidney disease, other connective tissue diseases e.g. rheumatoid arthritis, amyloidosis, and nutritional deficiencies (which are often unchecked in the underdeveloped countries of the world) exist, then slowly developing sensorimotor polyneuropathies may also occur. The treatment usually consists of controlling the underlying disorder. The prognosis and treatment are interdependent.

Physiotherapy may play a role in restoring or just maintaining the patient at his highest functional level. Often, however, paramedical treatment may be greatly limited by the chronic state of the patient's health in general and thus treatment is symptomatic, along the lines of that already discussed in the previous section covering sub-acute polyneuropathies.

ACQUIRED POLYNEUROPATHIES

There are two main forms of acquired polyneuropathies, carcinomatous or myelomatous polyneuropathy and leprous polyneuropathy.

Carcinomatous or myelomatous polyneuropathy. This occurs insidiously with the growth of a tumour or myeloma. The development of severe sensory loss, paralysis, muscle atrophy and ataxia often progresses to the state in which the patient is completely chair or bed-bound. This may happen before the primary tumour has been diagnosed.

The outlook is gloomy, but early diagnosis with excision of the tumour and control of the neoplasm may give temporary relief to the neuropathy. Considering the prognosis, the medical team should aim for the individual's comfort, giving him and his relatives as much psychological, social and physical support as is necessary.

Leprous polyneuropathy. Leprosy (Hansen's disease) has for many years been a medical backwater and thus only recently has more specific treatment been evolved.

It is caused by the *Bacillus leprae*, and is the least infectious of all infectious diseases. While it seems to thrive in unsanitary and over-populated communities, the particular feature responsible for the persistence of the disease is still unknown. Thus, for example, leprosy is found in the United States of America where high living standards are present on the whole.

Against all popular beliefs, this disease has not been proven to be contagious. People develop it without previous contact with carriers. Likewise a proportion of people in a contaminated community will never contract the disease. This leads many to believe that a predetermining, genetic factor may exist.

The bacillus is unique in its predilection for the peripheral nervous system and here the clinical manifestations are infinite. There are two forms of leprosy:

a. Lepromatous leprosy
b. Tuberculoid leprosy

Lepromatous leprosy. In this form there is little or no resistance to infection. The bacilli spread widely throughout the body causing damage to skin, hair follicles, cutaneous nerves and elastic connective tissue. The bacilli are detected by examination of skin scrapings. Once the diagnosis has been established, drug therapy may be successful in some cases, while others remain incurable.

Many patients exhibit 'glove and stocking' anaesthesia due to the destruction of peripheral nerve endings. No regeneration of these nerves occurs, early treatment only arresting further spread of the disease.

Tuberculoid leprosy. Here the patient has a high resistance to infection and may only present with a single hypopigmented, anaesthetic patch. This form is often self-healing and curable if treated early and correctly with drugs.

Geographically the two groups are seen in different incidence. In Asia the majority of patients are lepromatous, but where darker pigmented skins are found (e.g. in New Guinea) the disease tends to become more tuberculoid.

Pathologically, where the major nerves are affected the inflammatory reaction leads to extensive scar formation which restricts, or even strangles conduction along the nerve fibres.

Curiously, the bacilli attack certain nerves at definite levels, e.g. the ulnar nerve at the elbow, the median nerve in the forearm and the radial nerve in the radial groove of the humerus. In the leg, the usual nerves affected are the lateral popliteal at the knee, and the posterior tibial at the ankle, giving a foot-drop with stocking-like anaesthesia.

The facial nerve is also often damaged and with corneal anaesthesia the eyes are at considerable risk from exposure keratitis. These nerve lesions occur over months, even years, after the first cutaneous signs.

Due to severe sensory loss and motor weakness, the patient is exposed to repeated trauma. Continuous bruising leads to necrosis. The so-called 'shedding of fingers and feet' occurs due to this mechanism.

PHYSIOTHERAPY

After drug therapy, physiotherapy is the most important aspect of treatment. As this is a very specialized field and much has been published about it, the authors intend to give only a very brief outline of the basic factors of treatment. For further reading, references have been included at the end of this chapter.

388

Each treatment begins with a detailed assessment of hands and feet. All sensory and motor deficiencies are charted. This makes control and management for the future easier. It is also helpful to the surgeon in determining what reconstructive surgery is indicated. Wax baths are given and exercises to strengthen weakened muscles are taught to the patient. In cases of septic fingers or feet, splinting and rest are necessary. To prevent trauma in the first place, special footwear (e.g. sandals with thick synthetic inlays) is supplied. The patient must be taught to watch his limbs carefully during daily activities.

Where muscle and nerve transplants are to be performed, physiotherapy will be of great importance in the pre- and postoperative stages. Pre-operatively, maximal correction of contractures through passive movements and serial splinting ensures the best functional results. Postoperatively, a repetitive scheme of exercises is desirable for the teaching of new abilities in a patient.

The most important aspect is teaching the patient the general facts about leprosy; early signs, hand care, foot care, eye care, first aid treatment of wounds and general hygiene. Only with this knowledge will the patient benefit from treatment and be able to protect himself from further damage. This teaching programme should also include the patient's family as well as the community in which leprosy is found, thus the patient will find understanding acceptance and helpful co-operation when re-entering the workforce.

It is preferable to have an occupational therapist in any treatment centre for leprosy, though where this is not the case, therapeutic treatment by the physiotherapist must cover adaptation of tools (e.g. farming equipment), advice about new work habits (e.g. use of protective gloves, pads, tongs, handles, etc.), and instruction and supervision in doing simple daily activities (e.g. gardening, cooking, wood-carving, weaving and needlework).

FAMILIAL POLYNEUROPATHIES

Familial polyneuropathies are divided into three categories:
1. Peroneal muscular atrophy (Charcot–Marie–Tooth disease).
2. Progressive hypertrophic polyneuritis (Déjerine–Sottas disease).
3. Chronic polyneuropathy with deafness and retinitis pigmentosa (Refsum's disease).

All start in childhood or early adolescence and are slowly progressive.

All usually begin in the lower limbs. Both motor and sensory modalities are affected to a greater or lesser extent.

Charcot–Marie–Tooth disease may arrest at any stage, but it never progresses beyond the mid-thigh and elbow regions.

Déjerine–Sottas disease is usually diagnosed by palpable enlarged ulnar and peroneal nerves in contrast to Refsum's disease where the nerves are not enlarged. Nystagmus and kyphoscoliosis are a common feature in the latter condition.

PHYSIOTHERAPY

The treatment is always symptomatic. The physiotherapist will be presented with a variety of handicaps to treat. The aim will be to prevent undue deterioration and make maximum use of latent potential.

Relapsing polyneuropathies

It is worth mentioning two forms of polyneuropathy that commonly relapse. The first is porphyria which can be induced through administration of certain drugs like barbiturates to people with an existing metabolic deficiency and who may relapse each time these drugs are given again. The other is chronic idiopathic polyneuritis – a condition so far not pathologically understood. Like the previously discussed chronic sensorimotor polyneuropathies, thickening of the nerves may also occur, and treatment is along the same lines.

Mononeuropathies and multiple neuropathies

This section is devoted to discussion of neuropathies caused by a pathological process in one or more of the peripheral nerves. It is appropriate to include this subject here as, although quite distinct from the polyneuropathies so far described, all afflictions of the peripheral nervous system have in common some aetiology, pathology and symptomatology.

Mononeuropathies are due to disease of the nerve roots, the nerve trunks or the nerves themselves and exhibit characteristic lower motor neurone lesion signs:-

1. Segmental or peripheral distribution of weakness.
2. Decreased tonic stretch reflexes, i.e. flaccid paralysis.
3. Diminished or absent tendon jerks due to decreased phasic stretch reflexes.

4. Marked wasting of muscles (atrophy).

5. Sometimes, fasciculation of muscles.

6. Impaired co-ordination due to weakness.

7. Eventual postural changes determined by distribution of weakness.

8. Sensory changes including joint position sense, temperature, vibration, stereognosis and pain, including causalgia and neuralgia.

9. Vasomotor, trophic and secretory disturbances – cyanosis, oedema, discoloration, nail changes and trophic ulcers.

10. Electrical changes in the conduction velocities along the nerve fibres. Nerve conduction tests, strength-duration curves and electromyographic studies are often used to assess the state of injury and subsequent recovery of the nerve (see Chapter V).

There are basically four types of injury to the peripheral nerves which sometimes overlap:

Trauma.

Mechanical – non-traumatic.

Infection.

Idiopathic.

Traumatic type

This is extensively described in Chapter XIX.

Mechanical – non-traumatic type

This category broadly covers a whole variety of injuries produced by compression of the nerve fibres, lack of blood supply and tumours. The most commonly seen peripheral nerve lesions probably are due to pressure either acting directly, or indirectly on the nerve thus affecting the functioning of the nerve.

Direct compression may be seen in the following examples. It is, however, wise to remember these are only a very few illustrations of peripheral nerve injuries resulting from pressure.

Spondylosis (osteoarthritis of the spine)

This is a degenerative affection of the spine usually precipitated by previous injury, repeated minor traumas and increasing wear and tear. The central intervertebral joints are first affected. Degeneration and subsequent narrowing of the intervertebral disc takes place. The bone reaction of the joint margins leads to osteophyte formation. Secondly, changes, as seen in any osteoarthritis of a diarthrodial joint, occur in the posterior intervetebral joints, and osteophytes (spurs) form at the joint margins (see Fig. XVIII/1).

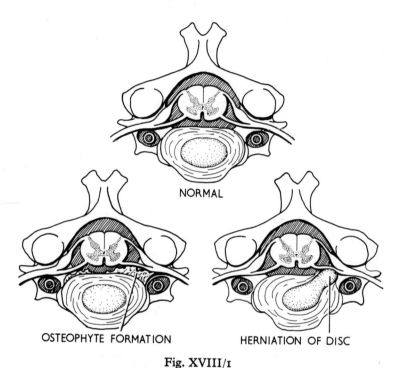

NORMAL

OSTEOPHYTE FORMATION

HERNIATION OF DISC

Fig. XVIII/1
Top. Normal disc – no pressure on nerve
Bottom left. Disc compressed and protruding, space limited – nerve touched by osteophyte formation
Bottom right. Disc herniated – space so limited that nerve is compressed

With this disease process, the intervertebral foramen becomes narrowed and thus compression of the nerve root and the nerve passing through it will occur on movement of the segments of the spine. Should this degeneration be severe, or trauma be superimposed on this already abnormal state causing oedema of soft tissues, then all the manifestations of neuropathy may be seen. Naturally the symptomatology will depend on the degree of severity and of the level of the lesion within the spinal column.

The commonest site of involvement is in the middle of the cervical spine. It is the point of greatest mobility coinciding with the smallest diameter of the intervertebral foramina of the spine.

As innumerable articles have been written on this subject, we will not dwell too explicitly on the exact nature of this condition. It is, however, seen clinically as a variety of pain, weakness, loss of spinal movements, decreased reflexes, wasting of muscles and sensory signs in the distribution of the affected nerves. Occasionally vertebro-basilar artery insufficiency and postural changes are observed.

PHYSIOTHERAPY

Treatment is of a very individual nature, assessment and treatment being almost inseparable. Many tools are available to the physiotherapist but the most important are her hands to 'feel' and her eyes to 'see' how the patient moves and reacts to various movements.

Heat, ice, traction, collars, corsets, mobilization, manipulative techniques and remedial exercises are all of value in different cases. A detailed and continual assessment is paramount to success. Maitland (see references) or Cyriax (see references) assessment and treatment procedures have proved to be of great therapeutic benefit in many cases. But in spite of conservative treatment, surgical decompression of the foramina or spinal fusion may be necessary.

Disc lesions

Prolapse or herniation of an intervertebral disc is a common cause of peripheral nerve injury. The prolapse is traumatic but where degenerative changes of the spine are present, there is a higher risk of herniation.

The most frequently affected discs lie between C_5 to C_7 and L_4 to S_1. Commonly the gelatinous nucleus pulposus protrudes through the annulus fibrosus at its weakest part (postero-lateral). This causes the nerve root to be compressed back into the vertebral canal or the nerve to be compressed in the intervertebral foramen (see Fig. XVIII/1 and Fig. XVIII/2).

There is often a history of some sudden injury followed within a few hours or days by pain, restricted movements and some or all of the neurological manifestations of lower motor neurone lesions. Often pain

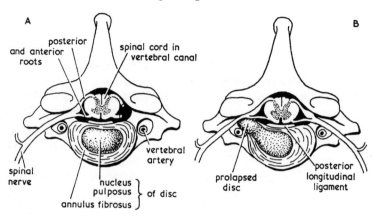

Fig. XVIII/2
A. Position of issuing nerve
B. Prolapsed disc compressing nerve

and sensory signs (paraesthesia, numbness, unpleasant burning feelings) are more marked than paralysis.

TREATMENT

Treatment is symptomatic and usually conservative. Bed rest, or immobilization in a collar or corset, analgesics, and physiotherapy are prescribed. If these measures are unsuccessful, excision of the herniated disc material or epidural block and manipulations may be necessary.

PHYSIOTHERAPY

Again the physiotherapist needs to assess the patient very carefully and record the results accurately. Depending on the clinical picture, heat, traction (continuous or intermittent while still on rest) and mobilization may be indicated. Where there are signs of root compression, manipulation is contra-indicated except by a very experienced manipulator.

Once the acute stage is past, exercise to strengthen paralysed or weakened muscles and postural correction should be begun. It is extremely important that the physiotherapist assesses the strength of the abdominal muscles which provide the ventral support for the spinal column. Advice should also be given on home and work conditions as a prophylactic measure to prevent further injury.

Carpal tunnel syndrome

This is a compression of the median nerve in the carpal tunnel, i.e. where the nerve passes beneath the flexor retinaculum at the wrist. The compression appears to occur most commonly in middle-aged to elderly women. It may be due to any abnormal condition occurring in this confined space, e.g. osteoarthritis of the wrist, thickening of the tendon sheaths from a chronic inflammation or following fractures of the lower end of the radius. In many cases no cause for compression can be found.

The patient complains of paraesthesia (tingling 'pins and needles') which wakes the patient at night, a burning pain in the hand and later numbness in the radial three and a half digits (median nerve distribution). The patient complains of clumsiness and 'dropping things' when lifting heavy objects or carrying out fine movements. If the compression becomes severe, then wasting or weakness of the median innervated small muscles of the hand, especially abductor pollicis brevis and opponens pollicis, results. Sensory deficiency is confined to impairment of pinprick discrimination.

At first conservative treatment by hydrocortisone injections and immobilization of the wrist for two to three weeks may be tried. If the symptoms recur then surgical division of the flexor retinaculum will be necessary to relieve the pressure.

PHYSIOTHERAPY
Postoperative physiotherapy is valuable in reducing oedema, maintaining joint movements and re-educating to full functional recovery of the hand. A home programme should be instituted and checked.

Thoracic outlet syndrome

Under this terminology come a number of clinical conditions which the physiotherapist may be asked to treat. Anterior scalene syndrome, claviculocostal syndrome, cervical rib syndrome and other congenital abnormalities may be seen with symptoms of neurovascular compression. With all of these, the nerve trunk and artery are compressed between soft or bony tissues due to abnormal alignment of the anatomical structures. They all present with pain and paraesthesia in the hand but these do not often correspond to any one individual nerve. They may be the result of compression of part of the nerve plexus. Rarely are weakness or trophic and reflex changes of any importance (see Fig. XVIII/3).

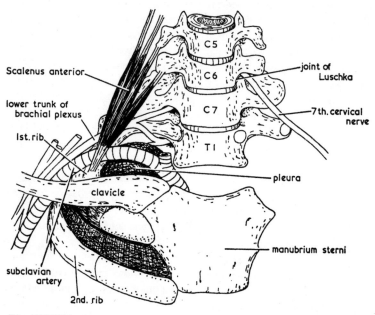

Fig. XVIII/3 Artery and trunk in angle between scalenus and first rib

The patient may be sent for postural correction exercises, traction, a collar and general advice about the condition. If the compression is enough to cause unbearable pain, paralysis, disruption of function, or if the symptoms continue to increase in severity, then surgical procedures may be instigated to release the nerve and artery from pressure. The physiotherapist may then be involved in postoperative care in the form of breathing exercises, general mobility, strengthening and postural exercises.

Postural compression neuropathies

Under this heading come a variety of conditions due to compression of some peripheral nerve because of faulty posture. The reasons for this happening may be unconsciousness, coma and states of intoxication.

Where warning does not exist due to lack of sensation and where generally bad postural habits exist, then syndromes like these can occur.

It is wise for the physiotherapist to consider this section with care as it is often her role to check on the positioning of patients in beds and chairs. It is also necessary to look for neuropathies following splinting of limbs, and last, but not least, it is often within the realm of the physiotherapist to improve on poor postural habits and thus prevent further peripheral nerve involvement.

The peroneal, axillary and ulnar nerves are frequently at risk but other conditions such as posterior tibial nerve entrapment (causing severe burning pain in the forefoot) or poor shoe design causing anterior tibial nerve compression may be seen. Another syndrome is the scapulocostal syndrome where local tenderness and pain at the insertion of the levator scapulae muscle are felt. All these may be improved by mobilization, postural training, and advice about factors such as fatigue and emotional stress.

Ischaemia

Deprivation of the blood supply to the peripheral nervous system may be due to trauma, compression, vascular malformations or injury during surgical procedures. Here the surgeon will need to restore a good blood supply to the affected segmental nerves as soon as possible. Recovery will depend upon the extent of damage to the nerve cells.

The physiotherapist will need to treat the patient for any resultant disability along the lines of a traumatic peripheral nerve lesion.

Tumour

Nerves may be the seat of tumours, known as neuromata. These exist in two forms. Firstly, ganglio-neuroma (true neuroma) in which the nerve fibres and ganglion cells form part of the tumour's structure. This type of neuroma is very rare and seen only in the thoracic and abdominal cavities.

The neurofibroma (false neuroma), however, is not an uncommon tumour. Its origin is in the connective tissue of the nerve and it may be found adhering to the side of the nerve trunk, or arising from the centre of the nerve fibres. It may be confined to one nerve or plexus, or widely scattered throughout the body (Recklinghausen's disease). Neurofibromas vary in size from small nodes to large masses of several inches in diameter.

It is usually the single neurofibroma which causes discomfort in the form of pain along the course of the nerve.

Neurofibromas tend to attack certain nerves more than others. One of the commonest sites is the *acoustic nerve* (the eighth cranial nerve). This nerve acquires the quality of a peripheral nerve within the internal auditory meatus and it is here that a fibroma occurs. Due to spatial confinement in this area, any growth causes structural displacement of the surrounding tissues. The trigeminal, facial, glossopharyngeal and vagus nerves all pass through the cerebello-pontine angle and thus may also suffer from compression.

The symptoms vary, but often present as progressive deafness, tinnitus, and vertigo, followed by a stiff neck and postauricular or suboccipital pain. There may also be spasms or twitching and facial palsy. Dysphonia, dysphagia and homolateral cerebellar ataxia of arm and leg may be seen in the later stages.

Surgical excision is indicated, after which many of the symptoms disappear, but invariably the patient will suffer from an acoustic nerve palsy through irreparable damage. Besides routine pre- and postoperative care, the physiotherapist may need to treat residual disabilities. Frequently deafness, facial palsy, vertigo and ataxia are encountered, and exercises to restore balance and confidence are mainly necessary.

Infection

This has already been discussed under other headings, e.g. leprosy, diphtheria, herpes zoster and sarcoidosis.

Bell's palsy may also fall in this category but is more commonly idiopathic in nature, and will be discussed under that heading.

Idiopathic

As the name implies this group of syndromes has no known aetiology but comes possibly into the category of mechanical compression, as in fact any inflammatory process around the nervous tissue will result in pressure symptoms. Bell's palsy and brachial and sciatic neuritis all come into this group of idiopathic conditions.

Bell's palsy

As this is a common condition, frequently treated by the physiotherapist, it is advisable to have a good understanding of its clinical
features.

There is usually a sudden, unexplained onset of unilateral facial
paralysis. It may be due to exposure to cold or draught; after a blow
close to the stylomastoid foramen; after 'flu; but in most cases the
palsy just develops without obvious reason. The symptoms are thought
to be due to compression of the facial nerve in the long, bony, narrow
canal where it lies before leaving the skull via the stylomastoid foramen.

The paralysis is of a lower motor neurone type and should be dis-
tinguished from the upper motor neurone variety of facial palsy as seen
in the hemiplegic patient.

The patient characteristically cannot close the eye and on attempting
to do so the eye will turn up and outwards (Bell's phenomenon).
Through the sagging of the eyelid, tears cannot be drained and will
run down the cheek. The forehead cannot be wrinkled, the patient
cannot frown, nor can he show his teeth as the lips cannot be separated
on that side. Food and saliva may dribble from the corner of the mouth
as this is drawn downwards through the sagging of the cheek. Sensation
is left intact except for a small area near the ear. Thus the picture is
one of loss of all expression on one half of the face.

Prognosis depends on the causative agent, and as this is not often
known only time will tell. Usually recovery begins in two to three weeks
and is complete in six weeks. Sometimes recovery may be very slow
and never complete.

Electrical testing, as described in Chapter IV, p. 88, can be of use
in assessing the state of the nerve and its conductivity. ACTH has been
advocated by some in the early treatment of these patients in an attempt
to reduce inflammation.

PHYSIOTHERAPY
The physiotherapist must instruct the patient carefully in facial movements to be practised in front of a mirror at least a few times each cay.
Most patients are highly motivated as the face is of such cosmetic
importance to us all. The patient should be told about postural effects
on the muscles and the need to prevent contractures and loss of elasticity
of the muscles.

Heat, ice, massage and tapping may be used to stimulate the circulation. Electrical stimulation is of doubtful benefit to the patient (see also Chapter V, p. 111).

Splinting in the form of adhesive strapping from above and below the lips to the front of the ear can help prevent the postural sagging of the flaccid muscles. The patient must also be instructed in care of the eye and mouth, as the functions of these are often impaired as well.

Brachial and sciatic plexus neuritis

Brachial plexus neuritis presents with severe pain in the shoulder and down the arm. Weakness and numbness of the arm and hand may also be seen. Treatment is to support the arm in a sling to prevent traction on the nerve plexus. It also includes strengthening of the affected limb once the pain subsides.

Sciatic neuritis is characterized by pain in the lumbar area and down the back of the leg from the buttock to the ankle. It is of a burning or persistent, aching quality which is aggravated by movement or straining. Stretch or palpation of the sciatic nerve causes tenderness. Motor weakness in the sciatic nerve distribution and absence of the ankle jerk are often accompanying features. Sensory loss is variable but usually minimal.

A differential diagnosis must be made between compression (spondylosis or disc lesions) and neuritis. The former often shows more progressive symptoms of motor and sensory involvement and the nerve is less tender on palpation.

Symptomatic treatment by rest, heat, massage and exercise often provide relief as the syndrome recovers with time.

REFERENCES

Atkinson, H. W. (1969). 'The Neuromuscular System and the Re-education of Movement'. Physiotherapy, Vol. 55, No. 4.

Brain, R. (1955). *Diseases of the Nervous System*. Oxford Medical Publications, 5th ed.

Bobath, B. (1969). 'The Treatment of Neuromuscular Disorders by Improving Patterns of Co-ordination'. Physiotherapy, Vol. 55, No. 1.

Cailliet, R. (1966). *Low Back Pain Syndrome*. F. A. Davis Company, Philadelphia, 3rd ed.

Cailliet, R. (1967). *Neck and Arm Pain*. F. A. Davis Company, Philadelphia, 3rd ed.

Polyneuropathies

Cailliet, R. (1967). *Shoulder Pain*. F. A. Davis Company, Philadelphia, 2nd ed.

Cailliet, R. (1968). *Foot and Ankle Pain*. F. A. Davis Company, Philadelphia, 1st ed.

Carini, R. N., and Owens, G. (1974). *Neurological and Neurosurgical Nursing*. The C. V. Mosley Company, 6th ed.

Chusid, J. G., and McDonald, J. J. (1976). *Correlated neural anatomy and functional neurology*. Lange Medical Publications, 16th ed.

Clezy, J. K. A. (1967). 'Leprosy and the Physiotherapist'. The Proceedings of the Fifth Congress, Melbourne, May, 1967.

Crawford Adams, J. (1967). *Outline of Orthopaedics*. Churchill Livingstone, 6th ed.

Cyriax, J. (1947). *Rheumatism and Soft Tissue Injuries*. Hamish Hamilton Medical Books.

Dyck, P. J., Thomas, P. K., Lambert, E. H. (1975). *Peripheral Neuropathy*, Vols. I and II. W. B. Saunders Co., Philadelphia.

Goff, B. (1969). 'Appropriate Afferent Stimulation'. Physiotherapy, Vol. 55, No. 1.

Goodwin, C. S., and Watson, J. M. 'Neuritis and Paralysis in Leprosy'. Physiotherapy, September 1968 pp. 327–332.

Harat, S., and Furness, M. A. 'Reconstructive Surgery and Rehabilitation in Leprosy'. Physiotherapy, September, 1968, pp. 317–322.

Harrison, T. R. (1974). *Principles of Medicine. International Student Edition*. McGraw-Hill, 7th ed.

Kendall, K. (1970). 'Facial Paralysis'. Practitioner, No. 1222, Vol. 204.

Lance, J. W. (1970). *A Physiological Approach to Clinical Neurology*. Butterworth and Co. London, 1st ed.

Maitland, G. D. (1973). *Vertebral Manipulation*. Butterworth & Co., London. 3rd ed.

Marshall, J. 'The Landry–Guillain–Barré Syndrome'. The Institute of Neurology and National Hospital for Nervous Diseases, Queen Square, London, W.C.

Matthews, W. D., and Miller, H. (1975). *Diseases of the Nervous System*. Blackwell Scientific Publications, 2nd ed.

Rehabilitation Journals, July–September and October to December, 1969. Third International Seminar Papers.

Walshe, Sir F. (1970). *Diseases of the Nervous System. Described for Practitioners and Students*. Churchill Livingstone, 11th ed.

Ward, D. J., and Neville, P. J. 'Anaesthesia in the Hand and Foot in Leprosy'. Physiotherapy, September 1968, pp. 323–6.

Wilkinson, N. (1970). 'Cervical Spondylosis'. Practitioner, No. 1222, Vol. 204.

CHAPTER XIX

Peripheral Nerve Injuries

by MAUREEN I. SALTER, m.c.s.p.
and BARBARA J. SUTCLIFFE, m.c.s.p.

Structure

A peripheral nerve is composed of sensory, motor and autonomic fibres collectively known as the nerve trunk. These trunks contain a variety of fibres, afferent ones carrying impulses into the spinal cord and efferent ones outwards towards effector organs and muscles. This trunk of nerves is surrounded on the outside by a loose construction of connective tissue making up the epineurium. Contained within are the bundles of individual nerves further encased in a strong sheath, the perineurium. Each of the individual nerves is again enclosed by a layer known as the endoneurium. Individual nerve cells of the trunk are called neurones (see Fig. XIX/1). Each consists of a cell body and its projections, the dendrites, and the axon or nerve fibre. The nerve fibre is the long process of the neurone with the properties of excitability and conductivity. The sensory and motor fibres are myelinated nerve cells which consist of the following structures from within outwards: a central core that is semi-fluid, the axoplasm, which is thought to flow from the cell body to the periphery; separating the axoplasm from the surrounding structures is a cell membrance, the axolemma; wrapped around this are rings of insulating myelin sheath consisting of Schwann cells (see Fig. XIX/2). This sheath is interrupted at intervals by the nodes of Ranvier. These nodes are important in conduction. As the impulse travels down a fibre it 'leaps' from node to node, a process known as saltatory conduction (*saltare*, Latin, to leap).

The speed of conduction varies with the diameter of the nerve and

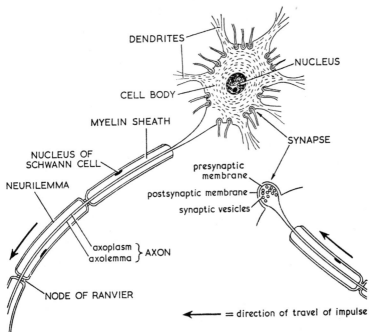

Fig. XIX/1 Neurone

distance between nodes (less resistance is offered with larger diameters and therefore the impulses travel faster). The speeds range from 2 to 120 metres per sec. i.e. 270 miles per hour. If this mechanism was not present the impulses would travel directly along the nerve i.e. by 'cable conduction', at a speed approaching 5 metres per second instead of the normal 50 metres per second. Very slow velocities are in fact found in diseases which attack the myelin sheath causing segmental demyelination (e.g. infective polyneuritis and diabetes).

The motor unit consists of one anterior horn cell, its peripheral

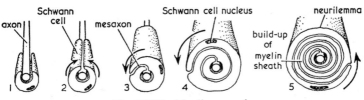

Fig. XIX/2 Myelinogenesis

403

axon and many muscle fibres, the number varying with the precision of the muscle concerned. The sensory fibres convey impulses from the skin, muscles, joints and other deep structures to the posterior root ganglia and then to the spinal cord. The sympathetic fibres of the autonomic nervous system are post-ganglionic from the sympathetic ganglia. These fibres innervate involuntary structures such as blood vessels and sweat and sebaceous glands.

Causes of injury

Peripheral nerves are frequently injured by laceration, particularly the median and ulnar nerves which are susceptible to damage at the wrist where they may be divided by glass or by knives. They may also be damaged by pressure following a fracture of the humerus which may cause a radial nerve lesion, or the nerve may be trapped in the callus formation as the fracture heals. In rheumatoid arthritis inflammation of the synovial sheaths of the flexor tendons as they pass under the flexor retinaculum may lead to compression of the median nerve in the carpal tunnel. Pressure from tourniquets and badly applied plasters may also lead to interference in nerve conduction. Industrial and traffic accidents and gunshot wounds may cause both the division of a peripheral nerve and widespread soft tissue damage.

Stretching of a nerve can occur with an increasing cubitus valgus deformity following an elbow injury and may produce a delayed paralysis of muscles supplied by the ulnar nerve. Traction injuries can cause brachial plexus lesions, these commonly occurring in motor cycle accidents, because the head is forcibly side flexed and the shoulder depressed when the victim hits the ground, whilst still holding onto the handlebars of the machine.

Types of injury

The three main classifications are neurapraxia, axonotmesis and neurotmesis.

Neurapraxia is defined as a non-degenerative lesion. Electromyographic studies may show slight evidence of degeneration suggesting a mixed lesion. It is possible to stimulate the nerve electrically below the site of the lesion but not above it. There is a total motor paralysis but sensation is frequently normal and recovery usually occurs within six weeks.

Axonotmesis. The term axonotmesis is used when the axon degenerates but the nerve sheath remains intact. The nerve fibres mostly regenerate to their original end organs. Recovery should be good if muscles, joints and skin have been maintained in good condition.

Neurotmesis. The term neurotmesis is used when the lesion affects both the axon and the sheath. Nerve suture must be carried out to allow the regenerating axons to grow down the sheaths to their peripheral end organs. Motor and sensory fibres rarely regrow to their correct end-plates, so that there will be incomplete restoration of power and faulty localization of sensory stimuli. Therefore re-education is essential if a good functional result is to be obtained.

DEGENERATION

Following an axonotmesis or neurotmesis retrograde degeneration occurs proximally for 2 to 3 cm, and changes also occur distally. The process whereby the axis cylinder breaks up and the myelin sheath gradually turns to oily droplets, is known as Wallerian degeneration. The debris is cleared away by macrophage activity, and Schwann cells fill the endoneurial tubes within three months.

In the muscle fibres changes also occur, and the coarse striation becomes less apparent. Muscles are gradually replaced by fibrous tissue, this fibrosis being complete within two years if regeneration does not occur.

REGENERATION

If the nerve ends are in apposition, sprouting axons will regenerate down the endoneurial tubes. Several fibres may grow down each tube, but after two to three weeks all degenerate except one which continues to grow to the periphery. The myelin sheaths begin to develop after fifteen days, and these take a long time to mature. When the axon reaches the nerve ending it may establish a connection, but the end-plate formed depends on the function of the parent cell, so may not be appropriate to the structure re-innervated.

The rate of recovery depends on the age of the patient and the distance between the lesion and destination of the regenerating nerve fibres. The average rate of peripheral nerve recovery is 1.5 mm per day in the early stages, but these rates decrease later, and are also slower in elderly people.

If accurate alignment of the nerve ends is not achieved by the surgeon, many of the sprouting axons will be unable to regrow down their endoneurial tubes, and a neuroma will form.

Effects of peripheral nerve injuries

The effects are motor, sensory and autonomic.

MOTOR

Interruption of a motor nerve produces a lower motor neurone paralysis with loss of reflexes, of tone, and of any active contraction of the muscles which it supplies. There is atrophy of muscle and soft tissue. Patients should be made aware that even with intensive treatment wasting will occur. Deformities are caused by the unopposed action of the unaffected muscles, e.g. the claw hand of the ulnar nerve lesion. The strong pull of the long finger flexors and extensors is unopposed by the interossei, and clawing occurs.

Due to lack of movement, adhesions may occur between tendons and sheaths and fibrous tissue may form in muscles and joints. These complications can be prevented by maintaining full range of movement and a good circulation.

SENSORY

The sensory effects are loss of cutaneous and proprioceptive sensations. The initial size of the anaesthetic area will decrease around its periphery, due to adjacent sensory nerves taking over. Loss of temperature sensation means that patients are liable to burns. Repeated warnings should be given to remind patients of the dangers of cigarettes, kettles, radiators, and hot plates, and even hot soup has been known to cause a burn. Similarly, intense cold, as from refrigerators and ice boxes, can cause blistering of the skin.

AUTONOMIC

Damage to sympathetic nerves causes a loss of sweating and the skin tends to become first scaly, and later thin and shiny. The nails become brittle and the skin is more liable to pressure sores. If trophic lesions occur these will be slow to heal. The limb will take on the temperature of its surroundings and so to maintain an adequte circulation it is essential to keep the hand or foot in a warm glove or sock especially in cold weather.

Operative treatment

A divided nerve must be sutured if it is to regenerate. If the patient is seen within six hours, and the wound is clean and the patient fit, an experienced surgeon may perform a primary suture immediately. Otherwise the nerve ends are approximated and secured to prevent retraction and the suture delayed for two to three weeks. At the secondary operation the scarred ends are resected and, with the aid of microscopic equipment, accurately aligned. Resection and transposition of the nerve may be necessary to prevent tension of the sutured nerve ends, e.g. the ulnar nerve may be transposed to the anterior aspect of the elbow and the adjacent joints immobilized by a plaster slab.

OTHER SURGICAL PROCEDURES

Provided they are not too extensive, gaps can be bridged by a nerve graft, when the sural or medial cutaneous nerve of the forearm may be used. If a nerve is compressed by scar tissue, a neurolysis is performed to free it.

If nerve repair is not feasible, or regeneration does not occur, then reconstructive surgery of joints and tendons should be considered. For example, in non re-innervation of opponens pollicis, the tendon of flexor digitorum superficialis to the ring finger is transferred to the base of the proximal phalanx of the thumb, to restore opposition.

Useful motor function is regained only if there is sufficient return of sensation. In special circumstances, where there is permanent loss of cutaneous sensation of median distribution, neurovascular skin island transfers may be carried out from the ulnar side of the hand. An area of skin from the ring finger plus its neurovascular bundle is transferred to the thumb and index finger to provide the sensation necessary for precision grip. Results, however, are not as encouraging as preliminary reports suggested.

POST-OPERATIVE CARE

To prevent undue stretch of the nerve ends, a Plaster of Paris dorsal slab is applied for two to three weeks with the adjacent joints positioned to reduce tension, and the limb is supported in elevation to prevent oedema. Care must be taken not to put any passive stretch on the nerve for at least eight weeks. In the upper limb shoulder exercises are given to maintain joint mobility.

Physiotherapy treatment

The treatment of peripheral nerve injuries involves a team led by the surgeon or physical medicine specialist and backed by the skill of the physiotherapists and occupational therapists. In a peripheral nerve injury the loss of movement and sensation, particularly in the upper limb, may have a profound effect on the patient's personality and outlook and this should be considered when planning treatment. It has been found that a programme of physiotherapy and occupational therapy four times a day for a short period is more effective and economical than less intensive treatment over a long period. The doctor and therapists should see the patient together to plan and to integrate treatment. The patient should be given a full explanation of the reasons for treatment so that he will co-operate and work hard both in the department and at home. The social worker may need to be involved at an early stage so that support may be provided for the patient and his family. Prospects of future employment should be considered and discussed. Unless the patient is co-operative and well motivated the most skilled therapy is unlikely to be successful.

STAGE OF PARALYSIS

The principles of treatment whether surgery has been performed or not are as follows:

1. To maintain and improve the circulation and reduce any oedema.
2. To maintain or obtain full movement.
3. To correct deformity.
4. To encourage function.
5. To increase the power of the unaffected muscles.

A thorough assessment should be made prior to treatment. It is easy to be confused by trick movements and variations of nerve supply in the upper limb. One person in five has an anomalous nerve supply in the hand, and this can be confirmed by electrical stimulation. If the muscles of the thenar eminence are contracting in a median nerve lesion, it may be a partial lesion, or the muscles may be supplied by the ulnar nerve. Range of movement should be measured and recorded. Both extension and flexion of each joint is measured with a goniometer to indicate deformity; the distance of finger tips towards and away from the palm is measured with a ruler. These measurements are repeated weekly. They can also be used to show the patient that progress is being made, and to encourage him to continue working at home. Muscle power is recorded by using the 0-5 Medical Research Council Scale, and sensory charts showing the areas of diminished or absent sensations are made periodically.

First priority of treatment must be given to reducing oedema. If the limb is allowed to remain oedematous, fibrin is deposited, and the tissues become bound down, causing permanent stiffness.

The upper limb should be supported during the day in a sling, with the level of the hand above that of the elbow, and the fingers free to move. At night the arm should be supported in a roller towel slung from a drip stand or other suitable means, until the oedema is controlled.

In the lower limb, oedema should be controlled during the day by the use of an elastic bandage, and a well-fitting shoe is essential. The bed should be elevated at night. Massage should be given in elevation to reduce the swelling, using oil to improve a dry, scaly skin. A warm water or saline soak may be given prior to this, and the patient encouraged to move the limb in the water. This is found preferable to wax baths. If wax is used great care must be taken to lower the temperature to 115°F (45°C) maximum or burns will occur.

The use of cold is contra-indicated for peripheral nerve lesions, as the limb remains cold for a long time after this form of treatment. It is essential to maintain a good circulation by keeping it warm, and a glove or warm footwear should be worn out of doors in cold weather.

Active movements are encouraged where possible, otherwise joints must be moved passively to maintain or increase the range. When passive movements are given the joint range of the sound side should be compared so that joints are not over-mobilized. Facilitation techniques are used to maintain or increase available muscle power, to increase range of movement by use of relaxation techniques and as a means of maintaining the pattern of movement in the patient's mind. Trick movements are taught, as they are useful for maintaining function, particularly when lively splints are provided. Lively splints may be used to correct or prevent deformity and to increase function. Details are given later in the chapter under the individual nerve lesion.

STAGE OF RECOVERY

Motor and sensory re-education begins at this stage. As re-innervation occurs a muscle will be found to contract first as a synergist and later as a prime mover. Muscles should be re-educated by facilitation techniques, springs, hydrotherapy, games and activities in occupational therapy. Sensory re-education details are given under treatment of a median nerve lesion.

As the patient's ability to work increases, a functional assessment should be carried out by the occupational therapist. Results of this are valuable in giving guidance about future employment prospects.

Throughout treatment the physiotherapist must check that the patient is carrying out treatment on his own, particularly if he is unable to attend the physiotherapy department regularly.

PERIPHERAL NERVE INJURIES IN THE UPPER LIMB

TREATMENT OF SOME SPECIFIC NERVE LESIONS
The methods already outlined apply to the following injuries, but some specific points will be discussed.

Brachial plexus lesions

Injuries to the plexus may be partial or complete, and may combine the three types of lesion, neurapraxia, axonotmesis and neurotmesis. Upper trunk lesions are more common than lower.

The plexus may be damaged by traction as in motor cycle accidents, by gunshot or stab wounds, by fractures of the clavicle, dislocation of the shoulder and by carcinoma of the lung. The motor and sensory changes will vary according to the site of the lesion.

COMPLETE LESIONS
All the muscles of the upper limb are involved except trapezius, and there is complete anaesthesia apart from a small area on the medial side of the arm which has T2 root supply. The limb hangs limply in medial rotation, the head of the humerus may subluxate due to the lack of tone in the deltoid, the elbow is extended and the forearm pronated. The hand loses its normal contour and becomes blue and swollen when dependent.

PARTIAL LESIONS
Upper trunk lesions affect the muscles round the shoulder and the

elbow flexors. Causalgia is a feature of partial lesions. It is an intense burning pain which radiates down the limb and may be precipitated by sudden noise and shock. Only drugs such as chlorpromazine (Largactil) are likely to be of any use in relieving this pain. If these are not effective then a stellate block or sympathectomy should be tried but sometimes as a last resort a cordotomy has to be performed.

SITE OF LESION

It is important in complete lesions to diagnose whether the damage is pre- or post-ganglionic, as recovery cannot occur if the injury is proximal to the dorsal root ganglion. The following methods are used to indicate the position of the lesion.

A sensory conduction test is carried out by electromyography. If a sensory action potential is obtained from a digital nerve, then the peripheral axons are in continuity with the posterior root ganglion, so that the lesion is pre-ganglionic. It is usual to wait ten days after injury before performing these tests to allow Wallerian degeneration to occur, otherwise inaccurate results may be obtained.

If the results of the previous test are negative, the lesion may be distal to the posterior root ganglion, and recovery might occur. However, there may be a pre-ganglionic lesion also, and a myelogram should therefore be carried out in all cases. Meningoceles will indicate that the dura has been torn and therefore the prognosis for that root is hopeless.

SURGICAL TREATMENT

In complete pre-ganglionic lesions it is often recommended that the arm should be amputated above the elbow and the shoulder arthrodesed as soon as possible. The patient is fitted with a prosthesis, which he learns to use before he has time to adapt to life with only one arm.

In partial lesions time should be allowed to see how much recovery is going to occur before embarking on reconstructive surgery. Lively and supportive splints should be worn during this waiting period (see Plate XIX/1). If regeneration does not occur, a variety of muscle and tendon transfers are available which can restore function, e.g. strong wrist flexors may be transferred to the wrist and finger extensors, if these are paralysed, to restore wrist and finger extension.

PHYSIOTHERAPY

Passive movements to the affected joints should begin as soon as possible, but delay may be unavoidable if there are un-united fractures. A full range of movement should be given twice a day, and the patient taught to carry this out for himself. Lateral rotation of the shoulder with abduction and supination of the forearm quickly become limited in range of movement, and the thumb web becomes tight and the metacarpophalangeal joints very stiff if not regularly mobilized. If stiffness occurs it takes weeks of intensive treatment to rectify. Hydrotherapy techniques are used to increase the range of stiff joints, and progressive resisted exercises in water are introduced when recovery occurs.

Compensatory movements should be encouraged. It is possible to re-educate shoulder abduction while lying down if the joint is fully mobile and biceps and infra-spinatus are contracting. With the elbow flexed to a right angle, the shoulder is laterally rotated, allowing the long head of biceps to abduct the arm to a right angle. This also enables the clavicular head of pectoralis major and serratus anterior to help complete the movement. As the patient's ability to make this movement improves, the back of the plinth is gradually raised until he is vertical, and able to perform the movement without support.

Axillary nerve injury

This nerve supplies deltoid and teres minor and may be injured with fractures of the surgical neck of the humerus and in dislocations of the shoulder. There is marked flattening of the contour of the shoulder and there is an area of sensory loss on the lateral side of the upper part of the arm. Powerful abduction can be restored if compensatory movements are taught. Some patients teach themselves this movement, whilst with others it may take some weeks of intensive rehabilitation. When re-innervation occurs and deltoid regains strength, the trick movement will disappear.

Ulnar and median nerve injury

The ulnar and median nerves are frequently divided at the wrist as the result of putting the hand through a window. Tendons and arteries are usually damaged at the same time. The tendons of flexor pollicis longus and flexor digitorum superficialis are often divided at the same time as the median nerve, and flexor carpi ulnaris with the ulnar artery and ulnar nerve. It is usual for primary tendon suture to be performed. Both nerves may be involved in elbow injuries, more commonly the ulnar nerve with the medial epicondyle. The median nerve may be compressed in the carpal tunnel, but this can be relieved by surgical division of the flexor retinaculum.

The deformity of an ulnar nerve lesion is the claw hand. There is hyperextension of the metacarpophalangeal joints of the ring and little fingers, due to action of extensor digitorum being unopposed by the paralysed medial two lumbricals, and the interossei. There is flexion of the interphalangeal joints of these two fingers, due to the strong pull of the long flexors unopposed by the paralysed interossei.

If the lesion is at the elbow there will be paralysis of flexor digitorum profundus to these two fingers also.

The sensory loss does not impair the patient's function severely though burns may result on the affected fingers and ulnar border of the hand.

The deformity of a median nerve lesion is the monkey hand. The thumb is held alongside the index finger by action of extensor pollicis longus, unopposed by the paralysed abductor pollicis brevis and opponens pollicis. The thenar eminence becomes flattened due to atrophy of the underlying muscles. The sensory loss is a severe disability, as sensation is lacking over the thumb, index and middle fingers and a large area of the palm. The patient is therefore unable to recognize objects, and the lack of cutaneous sensation and proprioception greatly impairs motor function, especially precision grip (see Plate XIX/2 and Plate XIX/3).

PROGRESSION OF TREATMENT FOLLOWING SECONDARY
SUTURE OF MEDIAN AND ULNAR NERVES

If the suture is at the wrist, this joint is usually immobilized in flexion by a plaster splint for three weeks. If at the elbow an extensive resection has been necessary, then a turnbuckle plaster may be applied to maintain the elbow in flexion. After three weeks the elbow is gradually extended by use of the turnbuckle, which allows flexion, but controls extension. Full movement is regained within three to five weeks.

One to three weeks
Active movements of the unaffected joints of the upper limb are
encouraged.

Three to five weeks
The daily treatment follows the routine for a peripheral nerve lesion,
avoiding tension on the sutured nerve ends. Patients must be warned,
for instance, not to allow the hand to hang palm uppermost over the
edge of the table thereby applying tension on the sutured ends. The
nails should be cut by the physiotherapist to prevent the patient
damaging his anaesthetic skin. If there are unhealed areas, or if trophic
lesions have occurred, saline soaks are used and the wounds cleaned
with half-strength Eusol.

Treatment should be repeated three to four times daily and alter-
nated with periods of occupational therapy. If this is not possible the
patient must be made aware of how important it is to carry on his own
treatment.

Six to eight weeks
Deeper massage with lanolin is given to help free adherent scars, and
soften indurated areas.

It is essential to differentiate between deformities caused by overaction of the antagonists, those caused by joint stiffness, and those
caused by tendon adherence. In the contracture following laceration of
the flexor aspect of the wrist, flexor digitorum superficialis may become
adherent at the scar and the proximal interphalangeal joints will be
held at 90° flexion. This deformity will disappear if the wrist and
metacarpophalangeal joints are flexed and the tension on flexor digitorum superficialis is released. It reappears as the wrist and metacarpophalangeal joints are extended. Graduated resistance is introduced and
facilitation techniques are used. The flexion abduction pattern encourages wrist and finger extension. If these movements are limited,
strengthening and relaxation techniques may be employed in bilateral
and unilateral patterns. Games such as table tennis and darts progressing to badminton, are useful and encourage the patient to use his
whole arm, but volley ball, where the hand may be forcibly extended,
is not suitable. Precision movements may be encouraged, by playing
with such things as cards, matches and Pik-a-Stik.

When full passive mobility has been restored, lively splints are needed to prevent stretch of ligaments, capsules and muscles, and to improve function.

The aim of the ulnar lively splint is to correct the hyperextension of the metacarpophalangeal joints when the patient extends his fingers, and to give support to the proximal phalanges so that the long extensors may extend the interphalangeal joints. The splint should also maintain the palmar arch and allow full flexion and extension of the fingers. Shaped bars are fitted over the dorsum of the hand and over the proximal phalanges, with a pad under the palm. A coil of wire, in line with the metacarpophalangeal joints, acts as a spring and maintains these joints in slight flexion while the hand is at rest as shown in (Plate XIX/4 (b)).

The aim of the median lively splint is to place the thumb in a functional position of palmar abduction, rotation and opposition, and to prevent permanent flattening of the thumb. A pinch grip to the index and middle fingers can then be made by using flexor pollicis longus. A strip of rubber is looped round the metacarpophalangeal joint of the thumb and taken across to the ulnar side of the wrist where it is fixed by a leather cuff, and so maintains the thumb in the functional position (see Plate XIX/4 (a) and (b)).

Eight weeks onwards
More vigorous resisted exercises are now introduced. Passive stretching is required if full mobility has not been regained. The stretch should be slow and steady and combined with relaxation techniques to avoid stimulating the stretch reflex. Serial stretch plasters are necessary in stubborn cases, and this is a skilled technique which must be applied with care and under medical supervision.

The plaster is applied by the physiotherapist who treats the patient so that no more than the correct amount of stretch is given. Twelve layers of 4 inch Plaster of Paris are used with a crescent cut out to allow free movement for the thumb (see Plate XIX/5). Vaseline Petroleum Jelly is applied to the skin if it is hairy, to prevent adherence. The layers are soaked in warm water, squeezed out and smoothed well so that no wrinkles remain. They are placed directly onto the skin of the palm and forearm, and held so that the maximum extension of the wrist and fingers is obtained. Care is taken to prevent both hyperextension of the metacarpophalangeal joints, and ulnar deviation of wrist and fingers. The position is held until the plaster has set. When dry the plaster is lined with cotton-wool and the forearm placed on the plaster. The fingers are then extended into position and a thin layer of cotton-wool placed between each to prevent friction. The splint is held in position by a crêpe bandage, keeping the fingertips free so that the circulation may be checked. The splint should be worn for about one hour only during the day, and a check made by the physiotherapist on its removal. As soon as the patient has increased his range of movement and is able to lift his fingers from the splint, a new one must be made. The splint should only be worn at the allotted times so that function is maintained. Plasters must be used with extreme care where there is complete anaesthesia especially in combined median and ulnar nerve lesions, as trophic lesions can easily be caused by a badly applied splint. In-patients should, at night time, wear the splint made the previous day, so that any correction obtained during the day is not lost. This, however, may need to be modified for out-patients who have sensory loss.

Special care must be taken to assess the patient's suitability to wear these splints. He must be sufficiently intelligent to understand the significance of the instructions concerning the circulation, to observe that the limb remains warm and the colour normal. If he is an out-patient he must be able to attend the hospital for the splint to be checked regularly. Contra-indications to the use of stretch plasters include oedema and circulatory impairment, and infections and un-healed areas. Their use when there is intracapsular joint damage is necessarily limited in value and they should be used with great care. If the nerve is unlikely to regenerate the use of passive stretches and serial plasters must be limited to prevent the joints from becoming hypermobile. When the optimum degree of mobility and function has been achieved the patient should be able to care for his hand at home and may be able to return to work.

The doctor checks his progress at intervals and treatment is resumed when re-innervation takes place.

In an ulnar nerve lesion, the first muscle to recover is abductor digiti minimi, on average 90 days after a suture at the wrist, and it will contract first as a synergist in opposition of little finger and thumb. It is easy to be misled by the tightening produced by the pull of flexor carpi ulnaris onto the pisiform bone or onto an adherent wrist scar.

In a median nerve lesion flexor pollicis brevis is the first muscle to recover followed shortly by abductor pollicis brevis, the average of the former being 80 days and of the latter 90 days. Before a contraction can be felt, there is an improvement in the position of the thumb due to increasing tone.

Intensive rehabilitation is essential and should include individual and group re-education of muscles and functional activities. Facilitation techniques should be used as the threshold of the anterior horn cells is high following a nerve lesion and maximum excitation is necessary to produce a contraction.

SENSORY RE-EDUCATION

Motor function is dependent on sensory feed-back of cutaneous and proprioceptive sensations. When there is some return of sensation to the fingers, sensory re-education is started so that the patient may use any altered sensation for stereognosis, i.e. recognition of objects.

Large blocks of wood of differing shapes, weights and sizes are used at first. The patient, with eyes shut, is asked to describe the blocks, and also coins, materials and everyday objects (see Plate XIX/6). An assessment is made, with a reappraisal every month on the same objects. Training on similar items, looking if necessary and feeling before closing the eyes again, helps to build a visual-tactile image.

Any incorrect localization caused by crossed re-innervation, can be improved by localization training. The patient is asked to point, while his eyes are closed, to the place where he is being touched. If incorrect he is told to look so that he may learn to interpret his altered localization correctly. Gradually he will say that it feels in one position but that he knows it is elsewhere, until he eventually points directly to the correct spot.

Radial nerve injury

The radial nerve is most frequently damaged where it winds round the humerus, as a result of fractures or by pressure from callus formation. It may also be damaged in the axilla by pressure from an axillary crutch.

Complete interruption of the nerve in or above the axilla causes paralysis of the extensors of elbow, wrist and fingers. If the injury is below the axilla the triceps will not be affected. Although there is inability to extend the wrist or metacarpophalangeal joints, the interphalangeal joints can be extended by the interossei, and the thumb by abductor pollicis brevis, as it has an insertion into the extensor expansion of the thumb.

Damage to the posterior interosseus branch will spare the brachio-radialis and extensor carpi radialis longus muscles. A simple lively splint of wire should be worn with a pad under the palm and a coil acting as a spring on either side of the wrist which will allow the fingers and wrist to be flexed and then return the hand to a functional position. Leather loops suspended from wires should not be used as these tend to hyperextend the metacarpophalangeal joints. The patient sometimes finds, however, that the addition of a spider splint is useful for finger release in precision movements. This consists of four plastic-coated wires, fixed by a cuff round the base of the proximal phalanx of the thumb, spread out and looped under the proximal phalanges of the fingers (see Plate XIX/7 (a) and (b)). This allows full flexion of the fingers and holds the metacarpophalangeal joints in slight flexion when relaxed. A light splint is required at night to support the wrist in slight extension until there is a return of activity in the muscles.

Reconstructive surgery may be carried out if regeneration of the nerve does not occur, by transferring one or more flexor tendons into the extensors, to restore active extension of wrist and fingers.

PERIPHERAL NERVE INJURY
IN THE LOWER LIMB

The sciatic nerve may be severed by wounds of the pelvis or thigh, and quite commonly is damaged either completely or partially by dis-location of the hip. In a complete lesion there is paralysis of the ham-strings and all muscles distal to the knee, and sensory loss also which is extremely disabling. The common peroneal branch may be damaged by fractures of the neck of the fibula or by pressure from a badly applied plaster cast. A foot-drop occurs as there is paralysis of the anterior tibial and peroneal muscles. The sensory loss is over the dorsum of the foot and lateral side of the leg. The patient walks with a high-stepping gait to clear the floor when gravity and the unopposed calf muscles cause the foot to drop into equinovarus. This can be corrected by the use of a toe-raising spring, or a foot-drop device fitted into the heel of the shoe.

Passive movements should be given daily to prevent contracture of the calf muscles and clawing of the toes. The patient can carry this out for himself by standing with the affected foot on a low step and pushing his body weight forward over his foot. A night splint should be made to support the foot at 90° dorsiflexion and in the mid-position between inversion and eversion. The splint should extend for an inch distal to the toes to keep the weight of the bed-clothes off the foot, and should be lined carefully to avoid causing pressure sores. If contractures have developed, correction is necessary by passive stretching and the use of serial stretch plasters. Particular care must be taken however when using these plasters if there is total anaesthesia of the skin. During the recovery stage, facilitation techniques are used for re-education. Balance reactions are effective for stimulating the peronei and anterior tibials and a balance board is also useful. The board may have a rocker underneath or a rounded shape which allows it to roll in all directions. Balance boards are also valuable forms of equipment for re-educating proprioception in the lower limb.

As the power of the dorsiflexors increases, the strength of the toe-raising spring is reduced. Postural re-education and correction of gait is important throughout treatment.

Lesions of the tibial branch of the sciatic nerve may occur in supracondylar fractures of the femur. There is paralysis of the calf, posterior tibial and plantar muscles. Contracture of the plantar fascia may follow paralysis of the short muscles of the foot.

Trophic lesions are liable to occur on the sole of the foot, due to lack of sensation and vasomotor changes. It is therefore essential that shoes fit well. A well-fitting Plastazote insole will help to prevent these lesions. During sensory recovery, hyperaesthesia may be severe. This may be relieved if the patient is encouraged to walk barefooted on different surfaces such as linoleum, carpet and tiles and in summer out of doors on the grass.

Lesions of the femoral and obturator nerves are rare. With paralysis of the quadriceps the knee gives way and the patient cannot lift himself up on the affected leg to climb stairs. However, he quickly learns to compensate by hyperextending the knee and achieves a surprisingly good walk. Paralysis of the hamstrings proves a greater disability than paralysis of the quadriceps. There is inability to extend the hip and a loss of stability of the thigh on the lower leg, and the patient has difficulty in walking.

Surgical procedures may be indicated, if there is irreparable nerve damage, or the distance from site of lesion to the paralysed muscle is too great. With lack of dorsiflexion or plantar flexion the ankle joint is arthrodesed. With lack of eversion a triple arthrodesis is performed.

Electrical stimulation

Electrical stimulation is believed to maintain protein metabolism and to preserve the bulk of muscle fibres if carried out regularly. To be effective, though, it must be maintained daily for a considerable period of time. Results from intensive rehabilitation, which maintains the circulation and function, have been so good that routine stimulation has been stopped. Patients with brachial plexus lesions who have received no electrical stimulation have been seen with worthwhile recovery in the hand two to three years after injury.

Stimulation is useful for detecting anomalies of nerve supply, and for re-education in the stage of recovery if the patient is having difficulty in relearning the feel of a muscle contraction.

FURTHER READING

Nathan, Peter (1969). *The Nervous System*. Penguin.
Wynn Parry, C. B. (1973). *Rehabilitation of the Hand*. Butterworth.

CHAPTER XX

Growing Need for Community Care

by ANN COMPTON, M.C.S.P.

In Great Britain as in other developed nations, there is a rising proportion of elderly to young and an increasing number of younger people identified as being appreciably handicapped. The majority of these people are living in the community, cared for by their families, friends and neighbours, with varying degrees of support from health and social services.

The cost of residential care, and to an even greater extent of hospital care, is rising continuously. For this and other reasons, early discharge after surgery has become more common, the mentally handicapped are being moved from the hospitals into hostels and lodgings, and there is increased use of day hospitals for the treatment and care of the mentally ill and the elderly. These factors, and the small number of qualified physiotherapists relative to the demand make it imperative that professional expertise is used to the best advantage.

This can often better be achieved by giving treatment in the home instead of in a busy outpatient department because for many people, particularly the elderly and those from rural areas, outpatient treatment can mean:

1. Long tiring journeys.

2. Difficulty in entering and leaving vehicles and often long waits.

3. Some degree of stress due to such factors as incontinence, travel sickness, and increased pain from vehicle motion.

4. Problems in making alternative arrangements for dependents in the family who cannot always be left.

5. During the wait for outpatient treatment, acute conditions may well have become chronic and time in which useful help and advice could have been given has been wasted.

6. Patients cannot relate treatment and functional retraining given at the hospital to the home situation, because of different facilities, thus wasting the time and skills used.

7. The patient's family have been unaware of new abilities or have misunderstood home programmes, so that the patient has not been allowed to, or encouraged to do things himself.

8. Reliance on the hospital with an inability to cope when treatment is discontinued.

In some, but by no means all districts, physiotherapists attached to schools, paediatric units, geriatric units, day hospitals and intensive rehabilitation units are already visiting patients at home to improve liaison with their families and to explain the purposes of treatment.

VALUE OF PHYSIOTHERAPY IN THE HOME

1. The physiotherapist is likely to see the patient much earlier, and the latter can benefit from her knowledge and skill before bad habits become ingrained and difficult to eradicate, and before lack of progress produces apathy and low morale.

2. Often members of the family can be taught to carry out basic procedures, so saving skilled time and leaving the physiotherapist free to deal with more patients.

3. It is often possible for those patients suffering from deteriorating conditions to stay in their own homes longer if they are visited by community workers who can teach members of the family such things as lifting, transferrals, positioning and functional maintenance.

At present, community physiotherapy services vary greatly; in some districts, physiotherapists are based on health centres or group practices; in others they are organized as a team covering a whole Health District serving different sectors and groups of patients. Other Districts have hospital-based physiotherapists coping with different aspects as they are able, while others have no service and general practitioners can only obtain physiotherapy by referring their patients to hospital consultants first, thus causing delay in obtaining help.

VALUE OF PHYSIOTHERAPY IN THE COMMUNITY

The real objectives of the physiotherapist working in the community are as follows:

1. To improve physiotherapy services by making them as comprehensive and flexible as possible.

2. To reach all patients as early as possible.

3. To use staff as efficiently and economically as possible.

4. To relate the treatment and management as much as possible to the patient's daily life.

With the trend towards community care, and the changes precipitated by both Health Service and Social Services reorganization, the remodelling of the training curriculum, and closer liaison between remedial professions, the opportunities to establish physiotherapy in the community are many.

If the physiotherapist is to work well in the community she has to realize that she is part of a team all working to achieve the same end. She must, therefore, have some knowledge of the responsibilities and functions of each member of the team.

In the community there are two teams of people who work closely together, those in the Social Services and those in Community Health.

SOCIAL SERVICES DEPARTMENT

The main services provided by the Social Services team are:

(a) FOR CHILDREN
    i. Preventive work for children at risk.
    ii. Protection of children whose families are unable to care for them, and those in private fostering.
    iii. Supervision of children who are 'boarded out'.
    iv. Provision and supervision of 'community homes'.
    v. Provision of intermediate treatment facilities.
    vi. Day-care for pre-school children, including registration of child-minders and playgroups.

(b) FOR THE MENTALLY ILL AND MENTALLY HANDICAPPED
    i. Provision of social work services, preventive work and after care.
    ii. Provision of adult training centres, adult and junior hostels.

423

    iii. Liaison with education, employment and other departments.

(c) FOR THE PHYSICALLY HANDICAPPED
    i. Estimation of numbers and need, including the keeping of registers.
    ii. Provision of day and occupational centres.
    iii. Provision of supportive services at home and residential accommodation if necessary.

(d) FOR THE ELDERLY
    i. Provision of residential accommodation.
    ii. Provision of meals, domestic help and recreational facilities (day centres, clubs and holidays).
    iii. Provision of social work services.

(e) MISCELLANEOUS
    i. Registration of voluntary and private homes.
    ii. Registration of charities for the disabled.
    iii. Registration of blind and partially sighted people.

The Social Worker

The Social Worker is mainly concerned with the provision of these statutory services, and with helping people who have requested advice over personal and family problems.

To assist in some of this work the Social Services provide Home Helps and staff for residential homes.

Home Helps assist those people physically unable to maintain their homes, and give help and guidance to families needing their support; for example, a home help will run the home, taking over any or all of the household duties normally done by a housewife, such as cleaning, cooking, shopping, caring for the children, essential washing, ironing and mending. The hours spent in the home are decided by the Home Help Organizer, taking into account supply and demand and the presence of other family members who could assist in household duties. The service is free to those below a certain income level, but those with incomes above this may be asked to contribute towards costs.

Residential Homes Staff. Local Authority Old People's Homes are part of the Social Services Department's responsibilities. The staff usually have some basic training in helping and caring for the elderly, while the Matrons are usually State Registered nurses. (Wardens of elderly persons' flats are attached to the Housing Department and may not have had any basic training).

Children's Homes staff have similar training in the care of the young.

To carry out these obligations the Social Services are organized in a similar way to the Health Service, with Areas and Districts. Unfortunately the Social Services District boundaries are not always the same as the Health District boundaries although the original intention in re-organization was that they should coincide. In some cases, therefore, Health Personnel are working with Social Services Personnel in more than one District.

The Occupational Therapist

Most Occupational Therapists working in the community are attached to the Social Services. Their role varies a little according to the District, but the majority are involved in assessing people for aids and housing adaptations, while others are concerned with day centres for the elderly, handicapped or mentally ill. When an occupational therapist is not available it is common to find one particular social worker designated for aids and adaptations.

The General Practitioner

The patient usually gains access to health care via his general practitioner who, in addition to having the usual medical qualifications will often have completed a further course to prepare him for the special problems of general practice.

He is contracted to undertake basic medical care of his patients, covering all hours, and may work single-handed, in partnership, in a group practice or from a health centre. The demands placed on him are varied. Much of his work will be very different from what he has seen in hospital before entering general practice in that up to one in five people visiting him have complaints of 'nervous' origin, while minor acute, transient infections and diseases such as laryngitis and measles, and chronic incurable diseases such as arthritis and bronchitis make up most of the remainder of his work-load. Major acute incidents such as a stroke, coronary thrombosis or an acute abdomen are rare, perhaps seen once a month, and he will probably only see major congenital abnormalities and conditions like multiple sclerosis a few times in his working life. Minor casualty work and work injuries needing physiotherapy occur regularly. It is always the doctor's decision, taking into consideration local circumstances, as to which patients he refers to hospital for second opinions, treatment and investigations.

A general practice is organized in different ways according to the the area and its need, some having the advantage of their own qualified nurses on the premises able to cope with dressings, injections and medical enquiries and perhaps help with 'well-baby' clinics. In addition, in most districts, health visitors, community nurses and midwives from the community nursing service are attached to these general practices, so that doctors and staff are able to work together and have better knowledge of their patients.

COMMUNITY HEALTH SERVICES

These services complement and support the hospital services by providing primary care, terminal care, preventive medicine and health education. (The hospitals are used for crises, specialized aid and investigations beyond the scope of the average surgery.)

District Community Physician

Heading this department is the District Community Physician, an experienced doctor who co-ordinates the health care within the district with the assistance of various administrators, in order to balance the needs of acute, chronic and preventive medicine.

Attached to this department are a number of medical officers whose work is mainly preventive medicine, health education and liaison. It includes:

1. Running clinics for under-fives to check developmental progress, carrying out vaccination and immunization programmes, and taking any action necessary if abnormalities or incipient problems are noted.

2. Carrying out school medical examinations and liaising with school authorities, general practitioners and paediatricians over any medical problems that arise within the schools.

3. Liaison with Education Authorities and hospital consultants over

426

school placements for children with conditions which make attendance at their local school difficult or impossible.

4. Health education on all aspects affecting a person's way of life, such as birth control, effects of smoking, alcohol, diet, sexually transmitted diseases and mental health.

5. Medical liaison with Social Services and Housing departments.

6. Ensuring that necessary precautions are taken during outbreaks of infectious diseases.

7. Checking immigrants' health at entry points to the country.

The Health Visitor

The Health Visitor is an important member of the Community Health Team who provides a continuing health advisory, educational and counselling service to families and individuals. She is a State Registered nurse with midwifery or obstetric training who has taken a one year post-registration course to obtain the Health Visitor's Certificate.

She is probably the best-known member of the team since she has contact with every family after the birth of a new baby. Since the National Health Service Act of 1946 the local health authority has been obliged to send a health visitor to every home in which there is a new baby. In general her duties are:

1. To give advice,
    i. on the care of young children, persons suffering from illness, and expectant and nursing mothers.
    ii. as to the measures necessary to prevent the spread of infection.
2. The prevention or alleviation of the consequences of mental and physical ill-health.
3. Early detection of ill-health through surveillance of high-risk groups.
4. Health teaching.
5. Provision of care, support and guidance.
6. Recognition and identification of need.
7. Mobilizing appropriate resources when necessary
8. Work in 'well-baby' clinics.
9. Hold antenatal classes and visit mothers with children under five.
10. Visit the physically and mentally handicapped and the elderly at risk.

Most health visitors are attached to general practices and work closely with the doctors concerned as well as with Community Health Services, medical officers, and social workers and voluntary organizations.

Community Nurse (*District Nurse*)

The Community Nurse is a State Registered nurse who has taken a further sixteen weeks' training for the National Certificate in District Nursing. In addition a State Enrolled nurse may qualify for the National Certificate in District Nursing (S.E.N.).

The community nurse works in close liaison with the health visitor, domiciliary midwife and doctors in the general practice to which she is attached. She provides clinical nursing care either in the patient's home, the doctor's surgery or the health centre, where she may hold 'dressings' clinics and deal with minor injuries when no separate practice nurse is employed. Apart from clinical nursing care the nurse is responsible for the general rehabilitation of recovering patients.

Since many patients who in previous years would have been treated in hospital are now treated at home, the community nurse is usually very busy and may be assisted by nursing auxiliaries who work under her guidance. In most districts, a Hospital Liaison Sister visits each hospital ward daily to collate information on patients being discharged and this gives continuity of nursing supervision. In addition she may be able to pass on useful information such as how to gain entry to the home where a patient lives alone, or information about any other handicap relevant to the patient's care. In some places there is a 24-hour service, but the length of time covered varies throughout the country.

Community nurses have available on loan or supply a variety of nursing equipment such as incontinence pads, protective sheets and clothing, commodes, bath seats, ripple beds, sheepskins, bed cradles, hoists and Zimmer walking frames.

The Domiciliary Midwife

Domiciliary Midwives, the majority of whom are State Registered Nurses, have qualified as State Certified Midwife in maternity hospitals, and this includes twelve weeks spent in the community. Although the majority of babies are born in hospital nowadays, midwives will have assisted in the antenatal care and taken relaxation and parentcraft classes, either with or instead of health visitors. In general practitioner units the mother may well have been delivered by her own domiciliary midwife, as happens at home confinements. The midwife also visits mothers who are at home in the immediate postnatal period, including those who are admitted for 48 hours or less to hospital units. In most Districts, midwives are attached to particular general practices.

The School Nurse

Other nursing staff attached to the Community Health Team are school nurses who, in conjunction with the appropriate medical officers, provide health education in some schools and assist the medical officers at school medical examinations. (Assistants provided to assist handicapped children placed in ordinary schools work with the Education Authority.)

The Chiropodist

Chiropodists find that their main responsibilities are to pensioners and the physically handicapped. They hold clinics, visit Local Authority homes for the elderly, the housebound, and in some places community and geriatric hospitals, treating feet and making appliances to help keep people mobile. Chiropodists also do preventive work through health education on the care of feet and choice of footwear.

Speech Therapy Service

In many Districts the speech therapy service in the community and hospitals is integrated, as is the case with the chiropody services, so that speech therapy started in hospital can be continued after discharge where this is appropriate. The whole age range is treated with families being offered advice after assessment of the patient as well as treatment sessions for the patient.

Other Community Health Staff

Dietitians may be found in some Districts giving advice to individuals and to groups on special dietary requirements. There is also a dental service which provides treatment and undertakes health education in

429

schools, at homes and in various sheltered workshops and training units.

THE FAMILY COMMITMENT

The final and most important members of the caring team in the community are the patient's family. It is not only necessary to gain the patient's co-operation, as in the hospital situation, but also that of the family. For some patients the family may be replaced by a friend, a neighbour or residential care staff, but for treatment purposes these people are considered as family.

After nearly 30 years of responsibility for total health care being with professionals, some of that responsibility is now being returned to the family who have grown unused to this role.

Important points to bear in mind are that:

1. The family understand the importance of each part of the treatment, its purpose and its aims.

2. The achievements which can be expected by the patient are explained and understood by all members of the team.

3. The family help to plan the treatment programme so that it fits in with the other members of the household.

4. Both the patient and his family should be able to see that the treatment is actually effective. This may be noted in the form of improvement of mobility and function, a slowing down in the rate of deterioration, or in coping with practical difficulties more effectively.

5. If ultimate aims are broken down into lesser targets which are within the patient's abilities to reach step by step, and which the family can see are realistic, incentive and encouragement to continue are gained as each of the lesser targets is achieved.

6. Throughout, clear indications should be given of how much or how little assistance is necessary and at what times it should be given.

7. The family, who are in the dual roles of pupils to the professionals and operatives to the patient, need clear and purposeful instruction, constant praise for effort and achievement, encouragement and reassurance that they are capable of doing as asked, and gentle correction which does not destroy their confidence in their ability to cope with a handicapped member successfully. For true rehabilitation to take place, the education of those who live with the patient is as important as the education of the patient.

CHAPTER XXI

Physiotherapy in the Community

by ANN COMPTON, m.c.s.p.

The physiotherapist in the community health team will not only need to fulfil the same basic role as other members of the team in primary and terminal care, but she will also need to do preventive work and health education. She must liaise with other community health staff and co-operate with the social services staff. It is also very necessary that she/he works in conjunction with the hospital physiotherapist so that smooth transitions are effected when patients move between hospital and home.

To function most effectively in this setting the physiotherapist needs to be familiar with the roles and services commanded by the various community personnel, hospital staff and voluntary agencies. She also needs to be aware of the social and occupational milieux from which her patients come. Sound basic knowledge, good general hospital experience, an ability to consider the whole patient and the effect of his disability on him and his family are essential. An ability to mix confidently with people in a variety of surroundings and an adaptability within her own role are the other assets which stand her in good stead.

Physiotherapists are not alone in being concerned with physical activity, and many organizations and professions are concerned with the physical care of people of various age groups suffering from different illnesses; much of the work referred to in this context is preventive rather than curative. Static and moving posture, the capabilities of people with various handicaps and their actual occupations are of interest to schoolchildren and 'lay' organizations as well as other professionals.

431

To achieve all this the community physiotherapist needs to be able to:

1. Assess a patient's physical condition.
2. Assess his and his family's ability to carry out instructions.
3. Advise the patient, his family and other workers involved in physical management.
4. Teach lay and professional people different aspects of physical care.
5. Co-ordinate her work with that of other community workers and, if appropriate, with the family.
6. Give some continuity of treatment, to the point where professional help is no longer needed, to those patients discharged from hospital.

Referrals and liaisons

As is the case with other community health workers, referrals come to the community physiotherapists from general practitioners, or from hospital consultants either direct to her care or as a progression from hospital treatment. It is essential to maintain contact with the physician and other staff who are treating the patient so that all are aware of what action is being taken.

In most practices there is a regular time each day when staff either meet or are available to discuss the patients' condition, medication, nursing treatment or problems. They pass on useful information on gaining entry to homes, particularly where people live alone, or on coping with pets who regard all visitors either as trespassers or in need of energetic welcomes.

It is helpful to the physiotherapist to have an arrangement with the hospital consultant connected with the hospital rehabilitation unit, so that necessary calipers and other appliances can be ordered without delay, as it is not possible for general practitioners to order these at present. Occasionally an underlying condition may be suspected which may influence treatment, and if a general practitioner requests further investigation or the physiotherapist requires further advice, quick access to consultants is required so that treatment is not delayed or prolonged.

PHYSIOTHERAPIST'S ROLE IN HEALTH EDUCATION

The physiotherapist's role in health education is three-fold. *Firstly*, he or she has to teach both professionals and members of the public aspects of health care related to physiotherapy. These may include teaching the safest and most effective way of lifting and moving things for people at work or at home, or how best to assist people with different disabilities. This may well include the correct use of different types of walking aids and wheelchairs.

Secondly, she deals with requests for lectures, discussions and demonstrations which can come from allied therapists, schools, women's organizations, old peoples' groups, slimming clubs, various nursing groups, parents' groups or organizations for the disabled.

Thirdly, she should take a keen interest in the work done by other therapists in such matters as the care of people of all age groups suffering from different illnesses, much of this work being preventive. She has also to know something of the many occupations patients are likely to have been engaged in.

It is most important, if possible, to join discussion groups on different aspects of rehabilitation with other professional groups, to exchange information and learn new techniques.

The conditions with which the community physiotherapist is involved are the same as those seen in most hospital departments and cover the same wide range. Neurological, arthritic and chest conditions are the most common, and she will see relatively more very young and elderly patients.

When treating these conditions the basic assessment, aims and principles are the same whether the patient is seen at hospital or outside; however, the method used may need slight modification for it to be understood and applied by a lay person. A functional approach is often that most readily followed, but it is important to emphasize that the method being used is only for the patient who has been assessed, and that it should not be applied to a friend who appears to have a similar condition.

Assessment

When assessing the patient, care should be taken to be thorough,

433

particularly in checking for sensory defects, for it is rare to be given more than a record of medical treatment and a diagnosis. When checking functional ability the quality of movement may be poor, but careful consideration should be paid as to whether improving the quality of movement will improve functional ability.

Where the family is to be involved, family relationships should be noted, as it may be necessary to devise a programme in which different members of the family share in the tasks of supervising or helping the patient, and this can be arranged to fit in with the capabilities of the various members and their relationships with each other and the patient. In a home the layout, floor coverings, space and arrangement of the furniture, its sturdiness and whether it could be rearranged, should all be borne in mind so that exercise can be planned around the available facilities. If it is anticipated that the patient will be going out, the local terrain, such as pavements, steps and levels, and the whereabouts of amenities, such as the postbox, bus stop and shops, in relation to the house, should be noted.

PLANNING A PROGRAMME

People are usually very willing to help in the treatment of a member of their family, but if they are to do so effectively they need to be shown how to help and also to be told why such help is needed and when, where and by whom it should be given. In order to be able to do this the physiotherapist needs to be aware of the patient's daily activities and of the family's commitments. It is probably easiest, having decided what needs to be done, to go through the day with those involved, fitting in the programme where it seems most appropriate. As conditions alter so the programme can be modified.

Children are often very helpful, particularly if the patient is another child or grandparent, and most take very seriously any duty or task which is allocated to them. The contribution which children can make should not be overlooked if they show an interest, for even young children will 'play games' with the patient if suggestions are made.

Making shift

Since basic treatments are the same whether carried out at home or in the hospital department, thought has to be given to substitutions for common apparatus which cannot be supplied in the home, or to temporary solutions which are safe, readily available and easily managed. This may involve the use of special apparatus, a change of method or a homely substitute. In deciding what is the best solution, consideration must be given to the time needed to set up the equipment each time it is used, as few people can be bothered with time-consuming or complicated procedures.

APPLICATION OF HEAT

Heat to help relaxation and to relieve pain can be applied by the patient sitting by the fire or taking a hot bath. For hands and feet a soak in a deep bowl or sink of hot water will often suffice. If the skin is very dry or eczematous and immersion would be detrimental, wearing a polythene bag will keep the immersed part dry while still allowing all-round warmth. If recommending a bowl, it should be checked that the patient can fill, lift and empty it safely or that someone else is easily available to do it.

If the patient owns a lamp it is safest to check its output before making any recommendation, as it is not unusual to find that both ultraviolet and infra-red elements are fitted.

For knees, backs, hips, shoulders and necks, electric pads, over-blankets or small underblankets pre-heated and disconnected, can be placed round the joint, provided that this can be done without creasing the blanket. A hot water bottle half-filled with very warm water and with the air excluded, and then wrapped in a cloth and placed around the affected part, can be very comforting. For those unable to use any of these methods, a warmed towel on the painful area can be just as effective and is often preferred. With any method for applying heat or cold, all the usual precautions should be taken, adequate instruction should be given and the patient should be supervised when first using the method.

USE OF COLD TREATMENT

Where cold packs are preferred, and a refrigerator is available, the patient can be shown how to make ice-packs, or a damp (not wet) towel can be left in the refrigerator for an hour or so, the time depending on the refrigerator setting, and then applied to the treatment area. Ice cubes can be used for stroking or rubbing if careful instruction is given.

PULLEYS

Pulleys for shoulder exercises can be made from a length of sashcord or similar smooth rope run over a coathook on the back of a door or a padded S hook suspended from the picture rail or top of a door. A folded teatowel, scarf or wide tie laid across the back of a hemiplegic hand, the ends taken round into the palm, leaving the thumb free, crossed, then taken to the back of wrist and securely knotted to the pulley cord, makes a satisfactory hand support which can be removed by easing the hand out, and re-used by slipping the hand in to wrist level, twisting the cloth and sliding it over the fingers.

An old scarf or tie can be used to help lift a hemiplegic leg forward when stepping, or to make a temporary footstop if it is looped under the sole of the shoe and secured there with adhesive tape and the ends pinned securely to strong trousers.

NEWSPAPER USES

Newspapers have many uses: they can be folded lengthwise as a splint or collar; they can be bundled and securely tied to make back rests, seat raises, foot-blocks in bed or footstops when sitting to stop a foot sliding forward. They can be opened to make a flat bundle and securely tied for use as a step to practise individual steps, or several bundles can be placed side by side under a mattress to firm a bed. Bundles suitably made up can be used to elevate a leg or arm or to stop a leg rolling.

WORKING SURFACES

Working heights or floor space will not be ideal, and thought must be given to the most suitable surface to use or to possible modifications of what is available. A low bed and tall helper may mean teaching the helper to work from the kneeling position. The settee may be more suitable than the bed for some activities, and the hall passage the best place for walking practice. No furnishings, fixtures or household items should be overlooked when improvising or suggesting alternative places to carry out activities.

POSITIONING

In conditions where positioning is important, be it in lying, sitting or standing, it should be remembered that neither patient nor his family will know the correct position, as comfort comes to mind first. Positioning should be taught carefully and help given in finding suitable pillows, cushions or other means of maintaining it when support is required. Rolled blankets, towels and old curtains make good substitutes for pillows until the nursing service can lend more, and they may in fact make a more suitable support than pillows. Foam off-cuts are very useful for positioning as well as for use as hand exercisers. If a bed cradle is needed but not available, a strong cardboard carton will serve.

CLOTHING AND ATTITUDES

Similarly, guidance on suitable clothing and footwear can be important, as few people wear 'walking shoes' indoors or realize the change of attitude brought about by getting dressed or the amount of exercise involved. If the patient has been in bed, getting dressed indicates 'getting better', and similarly the first time out of doors points to 'almost fit'.

From choice, the physiotherapist works closely with the occupational therapist, and there are situations where the help needed can be given by either therapist, such as when functional independence is the major aim, and in linking the purpose of advised activity to occupation. A joint approach may be indicated where aids, adaptations and retraining are required.

Efforts should be made to encourage contact with old friends and the social worker can be asked to introduce the patient to a suitable club or visitor.

ASPECTS OF TREATMENT

Particular aspects of treatments need consideration. The neurological conditions will be taken first and the assumption made that the reader is conversant with the rest of this book. For other conditions it is assumed that there is a familiarity with standard treatment required.

Head injury, neuroviral infection and neurosurgery

Patients who have suffered head injuries, neuroviral infection or who have undergone neurosurgery are usually referred when a check is required by hospital staff that the patient is maintaining or progressing in abilities achieved while undergoing intensive treatment, or to advise families on the maintenance of joint mobility, transfers or lifting. It is essential that the community physiotherapist is conversant with the patient's abilities before visiting the home, as otherwise a very different impression can be gained and time be wasted assessing true potential.

Spinal cord lesions

Similarly the majority of contacts with patients who have spinal cord lesions are to check that maintenance programmes are being carried out properly, that relatives can cope with lifting, turning and transfers without undue strain, and that they are positioning and doing movements or chest care correctly. Occasionally assistance is requested in rebuilding strength and regaining mobility if prolonged bed rest has been enforced for some reason, or if spasticity is increased. If this is so a check on bladder drainage and kidney function should be initiated via the general practitioner or supervising consultant. On any contacts with these patients, a check should be made that the 'reminders of care' (see page 232) are being observed, and the patient should be reminded that he himself must play the major part in his own rehabilitation and maintenance programme. Help should be withdrawn as soon as the family is coping as there is otherwise a risk that dependence can develop which can be detrimental to both patient and family.

Spina bifida and hydrocephalus

The community physiotherapist will need:

a to help the family to accept the child as normal but born with a disability which needs treating so that its effects are reduced. Emphasis on a child's abilities and efforts to improve on problems help to lay the foundations for a practical and realistic outlook for both family and child.

b to pay special attention to hips and feet, and, if the orthopaedic surgeon agrees, prone play and regular hip stretching should become part of the child's life, as should checking the child's skin for pressure marks, and his shoes for abnormal wear, so that prevention of damage becomes a habit.

c to encourage the child to attend a play-group. Usually she will need to contact the health visitor or Playgroups Adviser to obtain for the child a place in such a group, and to liaise with the playgroup leader over activities to be encouraged.

d to make contact with the local school teacher, where the child attends school. It is necessary to ensure that teachers and pupils understand the child's capabilities so that he is not left out of activities because he is too slow, might get hurt or might catch cold. Assistance in adapting physical education activities is usually required to prevent the child being excluded from these, and suitable protective clothing should be suggested.

e Sometimes problems can be eased by the physiotherapist giving advice when necessary. For example toileting may be a problem if the child does not have a special assistant and has difficulty in balancing while adjusting clothing, or if he needs to be reminded to go to the toilet at regular intervals. Potential problems often can be resolved if the situation is fully explained and if detailed instructions are given about the amount and kind of help which the child needs. For those children with ileostomy or colostomy bags, 'matron' should have knowledge of basic care so that she can cope with any emergency.

Cerebral palsy

Children with cerebral palsy are seen from a very early age, often when only a few weeks old and when the parents need support in regaining confidence in coping with their child. They need to be taught basic handling, positioning and developmental exercises to instil patterns of movement. The importance of giving the child stimulation and sensory experience and of involving him in situations can be taught while helping the parents to adjust to a way of life which gives equal importance to other members of the family.

Many of the less severely affected children go to local schools for normal children, although the incidence of cerebral palsy is higher in schools for educationally subnormal children. As with spina bifida children, the teaching staff need to understand the child's physical capabilities and difficulties so that any failure is not automatically ascribed to his condition. Suggestions for physical education and classroom activities to overcome or minimize hand difficulties are welcomed. (Nancy Finnie's *Handling the Young Cerebral Palsied Child at Home* is very helpful here.)

CLUMSY CHILDREN
'Clumsy' children are frequently minimal cerebral palsy cases and may

not be recognized as such until they start school. If parents and teachers introduce, with help from the physiotherapist, appropriate measures to improve spatial awareness, body image, sensory awareness, balance and movement patterns, many of the problems are overcome and the clumsiness diminishes.

Other children with mild cerebral palsy are first seen when development is delayed or when parents notice abnormal or deficient movement.

Mental handicap

Some of those children who present with developmental delay are mentally handicapped, while others have Down's syndrome. The parents of these children often need more support than the child's physical condition would appear to warrant, but the time is well spent helping the parents to cope with their feelings and to see their child as a personality in his own right to be encouraged to develop to his full potential. Teaching the parents how to handle their child and demonstrating those abilities he has in common with other children can often do more than words.

Multiple handicap

With the multiply handicapped child with any combination of physical, mental, speech, sight or hearing handicap, much can be done to encourage a positive attitude on the part of the parents and to help them with the management of the child. It is an asset to the physiotherapist to have acquired some knowledge of the teaching skills used with the deaf and the blind so that appropriate stimulation can be included to aid overall development. At all times treatment should be planned in conjunction with other professionals involved so that no aspect of handicap is omitted from correction in the daily management.

Cerebrovascular accidents – hemiplegia

Fifty per cent of cerebrovascular accidents are not admitted to hospital, and this figure is likely to rise with an ageing population, since the majority of such cases are over 60. Some do not recover, but for those who do, help is required as soon as possible so that the family do not regard the patient as a permanent invalid and are helped to think in terms of rehabilitation from the start.

At this stage the patient may well be confused and the family may be uncertain how to care for him and how to handle the affected limbs. They are, therefore, willing to accept instruction on correct positioning, movements, encouraging the patient to help wash, feed and dress himself, transferrals, and helping him to stand with a tripod. They also appreciate help in sorting out a daily routine of 'little and often', in knowing when to help and when to let the patient 'have a go'. If speech is affected they will welcome help in establishing a communications system until the speech therapist can give more expert advice.

Loss of sensory input and rejection of affected limbs are difficult for many people to understand, and this should be explained to both the family and the patient, and help should be given to make the patient aware of the affected arm and leg.

The community nurse and physiotherapist should both stress the need for getting the patient out of bed, and they should explain that temporary incontinence will often gradually come under control as the patient is mobilized.

The occupational therapist should be contacted early if it is apparent that aids or adaptations will be necessary. Social worker support may not be required at the early stage but should be requested without hesitation if problems arise or if social re-integration will require help.

It is important to avoid the use of the term 'walking' as this gives a visual picture of the normal gait pattern; the term 'getting about' overcomes the problem and does not lead to false expectations. Similarly 'being able to get your clothes on' overcomes the difficulty of the patient who feels that he cannot 'dress' because he has only one good arm. It avoids misunderstandings and loss of trust on the part of people who may well not have seen a hemiplegic person before.

It has been found that particular attention needs to be paid to positioning and movements of the head, shoulder girdle and shoulder to prevent later 'shoulder-neck' pain and stiffness. Frequent assisted exercise, the use of pulleys and encouragement to look round, together with adjustments to the viewing height and angle of the television screen all help.

As the patient becomes fitter and if it is thought that he would benefit both physically and socially, rehabilitation at a nearby rehabilitation department or day centre should be arranged.

With patients in some modern houses the question often arises of whether the patient is better upstairs near the toilet but isolated, or downstairs in the hub of the house with a commode and perhaps less chance to rest. Often the place of collapse and lack of help for the patient decides where he is to remain, but if the physiotherapist is asked it is best to point out the pros and cons of each situation and leave the final decision to the family, aiming to teach the use of the stairs as soon as it is practical.

Multiple sclerosis and Friedreich's ataxia

Those patients who have multiple sclerosis or Friedreich's ataxia usually fall into one of two levels of disability: those who are still working or running their own homes and need advice in maintaining a good pattern of rest and exercise and those who are severely affected. With the less affected, good movement patterns should be maintained provided that they do not detract from safety and function. The occupational therapist can help many of these patients to minimize their disabilities.

The family of the patient severely affected by one of these conditions often needs help and instruction in lifting and transferrals, positioning, minimizing spasticity so that nursing care can be given and joint range maintained, turning to prevent pressure sores, and chest care to prevent respiratory complications.

For many families the contact with the physiotherapist is as important as what she can do, as many feel 'written off' by all except the nurse and do not always feel that the social worker understands their problems in the way a medical person does.

Parkinsonism

With parkinsonism, the main value of the community physiotherapist is in helping the family to understand the inherent need for the patient to remain active to realize his full potential, and in emphasizing to medical practitioners the benefit of early contact with patients to prevent loss of normal movement patterns, even before drug therapy is instituted. (See Chapter XVI).

Assistance in planning daily activity will encourage many families to learn to 'pump up' rather than to do things for the patient (see page 363), and to check head and neck posture when necessary. If similar instruction can be given to staff at a day centre or social group, regular attendance can be helpful to both patient and family.

Motor neurone disease

Patients with motor neurone disease are rarely seen, but for those who are referred efforts are directed towards preventing deformities and maintaining strength in unaffected muscles. In co-operation with the occupational therapist help is given to both patient and family in coping with a deteriorating condition by providing aid as required to maintain independence, and by teaching transferrals and lifting methods. The family do not feel neglected and gain a psychological boost, while moral support is given and contact maintained.

Arthritis

Arthritis in its various forms accounts for a large proportion of the physiotherapist's patients. It is helpful to explain the nature of the condition to the patient so that the purpose of the advice given is understood properly. A maintenance programme is taught for affected joints and advice on general physical management and daily routine is given. This includes ensuring that adequate rest is taken. This can best be done by going through the patient's daily activities and making modifications which eliminate unnecessary journeys on stairs, excess carrying and poor working positions. Seat heights should be checked to make rising simpler and chairs looked at as regards the sitting position they provide. The bed should be looked at, as a change of height board or cradle may be needed. With the occupational therapist, working heights and methods, kitchen layout, bathing, choice of clothing and fastenings including footwear, should all be checked. Resting positions should also be considered, as those chosen by the patient are not always those which prevent deformity or joint stress.

With this advice, any necessary aids and adaptations, and the services of a home help when household tasks become difficult, much can be done to improve life and maintain independence.

Geriatric patients

Elderly patients form the majority of referrals in community health care. Particular disabilities require treatment on the same basis as for younger people, but emphasis should be placed on maintaining independence and avoiding bed rest as far as possible.

443

When planning treatment and management which involves the family, care should be taken to include the patient in any discussion and not to 'talk down to' or 'talk across' him. All instructions should be given clearly and simply in terms which can be seen to be understood.

Many elderly people who live at home expect their relatives and friends to care for them, sometimes even when they are still capable of some activities themselves. After dealing with any problems in daily activities caused by poor balance, weak muscles, stiff joints or loss of confidence, considerable tact and diplomacy may be required to gain a gradual withdrawal of unnecessary support while maintaining essential assistance, so that the patient regains the independence he is capable of achieving, and thus can be maintained in his own home for longer with less stress on the family.

Close links with the local geratric unit and day hospital are essential for the patient to gain utmost benefit, and full use should be made of a team approach, incorporating all social services facilities and those of voluntary organizations as well.

Where people are resident in old people's homes, many become apathetic and prefer to sit all day doing nothing. Mental alertness and activity can be stimulated if care assistants are taught how to take short sessions of general exercise, perhaps to music, which include breathing exercises and posture. These can be very beneficial if the slower tempo and pauses on changing position to prevent loss of balance are remembered.

Further reading on this subject is recommended in order to gain more insight into the particular needs of the elderly patient. (See *Geriatrics for Physiotherapists and Allied Professions* by Margaret Hawker.)

Chest conditions

The community physiotherapist will also encounter the chest conditions of bronchitis and cystic fibrosis. Here her job will include working out the best positions for postural drainage, teaching percussion or shaking to relatives and teaching breathing exercises to the patient. She will look at the daily routine to ensure that there is time to carry out drainage properly and that exercise does not cause undue breathlessness through attempts to hurry. With the cystic fibrotic child at school the medical officer and physiotherapist should ensure that teaching staff are aware of the child's condition, his exercise tolerance and his need to keep his chest clear of secretions.

Asthmatics may need to be taught breathing exercises, and relaxation positions suitable to their circumstances should be worked out. Relatives need explanation of the need to remain calm when an attack occurs and can be shown how to be most helpful. With a school child, his teacher and school matron should also be advised if attacks are likely at school.

Orthopaedics

Orthopaedic patients who are seen are usually elderly, and either they have had some form of joint surgery to relieve an arthritic condition, or they are recovering from fractures such as those of the neck of femur. The community physiotherapist may be asked to supervise the final stages of rehabilitation at home, and to check the patient's safety and ability to cope with stairs and outside terrain, thus making rehabilitation more realistic and obviating the need for tiring journeys.

Occasionally children are seen at school and home if hospital treatment would entail much missed schooling and provided that adequate continuity of treatment can be obtained for a good result to be seen from the surgical intervention.

Cancer

Patients suffering from cancer are given help to maintain their mobility and to relieve any symptoms due to nerve involvement giving rise to spasticity or joint pain. Advice on chest care and breathing exercises is also useful. Patients show a wide variation in symptoms and effects, depending on the primary and secondary sites, the nature of the cancer and rate of progression, so support and instruction are given to the family as required, in close collaboration with other medical and social workers.

Other conditions

In some districts physiotherapists may be working in conjunction with health visitors or midwives at antenatal classes, and advising on post-natal exercises.

Various minor acute injuries will be seen if the physiotherapist has a session at a health centre or group practice. These may include back, shoulder and knee injuries, and advice and immediate care are given. These patients may need more intensive treatment with the use of electrical or other specialized equipment which can be arranged at a local physiotherapy department.

Requests for exercises to control stress incontinence or to help retrain incontinent patients may be received. It is advantageous to plan the patient's programme with other medical personnel involved, such as the nurse, preferably in advance, particularly if the patient is elderly, so that positive reinforcement is given by everyone involved.

The community physiotherapist may encounter various rare conditions and congenital malformations such as absence of a limb or arthrogryphosis. In all these cases the patient is given the same advice as he would receive in a hospital department, with any necessary adaptations to suit the home circumstances.

CONCLUSION

It seems likely that there will be an increasing demand for the services of community physiotherapists. The logical development would seem to be a community physiotherapy service closely integrated with the hospital physiotherapy team with free interchange of patients between the services as seems most appropriate to the physiotherapists. Under the co-ordination of a District Physiotherapist the hospitals would be undertaking intensive acute treatments and rehabilitation, while community staff deal with patients nursed at home or who require self-management programmes. The physiotherapist would be taking her place as another professional using her knowledge and skill in the expanding field of community care.

REFERENCES

Literature of the Open University course on 'The Handicapped Person in the Community'.

Wilkes, Eric, 'Community Care', *Physiotherapy*, December 1975.

Nursing and Midwifery in the Community. H.M.S.O. Publication No. NLO 28.

The Health Visitor, her Function and its Implications for Training. 5th report. Council for the Training of Health Visitors.

CHAPTER XXII

Applied Psychology for Physiotherapists

by DAVID HILL, B.SC., M.C.S.P., DIP.T.P.

The Behavioural Science Course Objectives for students of physiotherapy have recently been revised by a panel which has frequently sought advice from behavioural scientists. Final minor modifications were made in the light of comments from principals and teachers of physiotherapy schools and the result is a syllabus inspired by the expressed needs of physiotherapy teachers, and formally structured with the assistance of behavioural scientists. This chapter gives an interpretation of the agreed course objectives as best applied to students of physiotherapy. 'A good student will probably soon become a good physiotherapist, with or without a knowledge of psychology. But psychology may help her to become an even better physiotherapist even sooner.'[1]

Psychology defined

Psychology may be defined as the study of behaviour and experience. Consideration of this definition reveals that there are few, if any, areas of human activity without a psychological component. The scope of the subject necessitates division into areas, and some of these areas are now listed.

Physiological psychology deals with the relationship between physiological processes and behaviour. Activity within the nervous system is closely related to behaviour, and neuropsychology is an important area of physiological psychology.

Comparative psychology compares behaviour between different

447

animal species, and frequently correlates structural differences with differences in behaviour.

Social psychology studies the way in which members of a species, especially man, interact with each other.

Developmental psychology considers the changing processes in organisms as they mature, and whether such changes are due to inherited genetic factors or acquired environmental factors.

Educational psychology deals with those areas of study which have significant parts to play in the learning process, with some emphasis on children of school age.

Clinical psychology is concerned with the study and treatment of those members of society whose behaviour is abnormally undesirable, whether due to inherited or environmental factors.

Occupational psychology is the study of man in relation to his working environment, and deals with organizations in industry, hospitals, offices and the armed forces.

Human behaviour has attracted the attention of experts from many academic disciplines. Biologists, medical practitioners, philosophers, engineers, sociologists, physical scientists and mathematicians have all contributed to the fund of knowledge. It is not surprising, therefore, that various schools[2] of thought have arisen in attempts to explain and ultimately predict human behaviour. The hard scientific approach of the behaviourist school attempts to explain behaviour in strictly definable and measurable terms and is not much concerned by notions of mind and consciousness which are difficult to define and measure. At the other extreme are the analytical schools which are mainly centred on Freudian psychology. Although at first the conflicting schools appear irreconcilable, deeper study frequently shows that they are looking at similar problems from different view-points, and it is unwise to accept blindly the teachings of any one school to the exclusion of all others.

DEVELOPMENTAL PSYCHOLOGY

Literature dealing with anatomical and physiological development reveals that the differences between child and adult are more than differences in body dimensions. Differences in body proportions and composition also exist. Likewise, differences in the quantity and quality of behaviour and mental experience are extensive. The physiotherapist working with children schould be aware of these differences, and the approximate ages of transition of development from one stage to another, so that she can tell whether the child's failure to understand the world in adult terms is due to lack of maturity appropriate to the child's age, or due to genuine mental retardation.

The most valuable recent contribution to developmental psychology has come from Jean Piaget of Geneva. His work deals with the development of a child's understanding of the events which occur in the world around him. A brief description of the observed stages follows. For more detailed information the reader should consult suitable textbooks.[3, 4]

The sensory motor stage lasts from birth to two years. Early behaviour is mainly reflexive, and this implies that certain nerve pathways are innate, and the child arrives in the world with certain abilities, already well described by Helen Atkinson in the earlier sections of this book. These innate reflexes combine to give more complex, purposive movements during the first few months of life. The term, sensory motor, is self-explanatory. The child responds to sensory stimuli with fairly specific motor responses. Towards the end of this stage the use of language and the development of play and imitation reveals that the child is developing real understanding, and not just responding reflexly.

The pre-operational stage lasts from two to seven years. During this stage the child becomes increasingly skilled at handling objects in the material world, but his perception of these objects is still at a very different level from that of the mature adult. For example, if fluid from a container is poured into a container of a different shape, the child will state that the amount of fluid is either more than previously, or less than previously, but not the same. The conservation of volume with change of shape is not appreciated. Similarly it can be demonstrated that there is lack of appreciation of conservation of mass and number. The rules of simple arithmetic as we know them are just not accepted. Evidence to date suggests that practice and training have little if any effect in speeding up a child's progress through this stage. Presumably one has to wait for appropriate neurological maturation.

The concrete operational stage follows and extends to the age of eleven. The child now realizes that properties such as weight, volume, number, mass, and area are conserved, even though dimensions of objects may be changed. In this stage the child also learns to classify groups of objects according to colour, size, shape and other properties.

449

The formal operational stage starts at eleven years. The child learns to transfer his knowledge and skill from concrete objects to ideas and concepts of a more abstract nature. For example, practical experience with weights and volumes gives rise to the concept of density or specific gravity. Generalization of the properties of objects enables the child to appreciate scientific laws concerning such phenomena as buoyancy, the laws of reflection of light, and other laws of physics and chemistry.

The above stages demonstrate a progressive understanding of the properties of the physical world.

The development of moral and ethical values has also been studied by Piaget. He simply read stories to children in order to determine a child's sense of right and wrong.[4] Children under seven judged naughtiness by the consequences of an act while older children and adults tend to make moral judgements based on the intentions leading to the act. Thus a child who accidently broke fifteen cups was judged by young children to be naughtier than a child who broke one cup while stealing some jam. It is unlikely that a child possesses a conscience, or knowledge of right and wrong as understood by adults. He knows that certain acts will result in punishment if discovered. Distinguishing between different types of naughtiness is difficult for young children. They classify both swearing and the telling of untruths as lying. Both are undesirable forms of verbal behaviour, and therefore go together. As the child matures, the idea of reciprocity develops, in which the level of punishment is equated with the severity of the crime. By the time adolescence is reached ethical values are frequently well developed. Whole complexes of abstract ideas and concepts may be fervently advocated, and may be of a religious, political or social nature. Not only can the adolescent appreciate abstract concepts and laws concerning the material world, but he also feels strongly about how this material world should be manipulated for moral reasons in order to provide, for example, a socialist or a capitalist society.

Learning

Learning is the adaptive change in an organism as a result of experience. It is a change which is inferred because of changes in behaviour. The physiotherapist should be familiar with certain aspects of learning theory, since the majority of patients are required to learn at some stage in their treatment, whether it be breathing exercises, muscle strengthening, or re-education of walking. Some types of learning are more relevant to physiotherapy, and appropriate consideration of these types follows.

Classical conditioning was studied in great detail by Pavlov. His best-known experiment involved a bell repeatedly rung in the presence of a dog. Food was presented to the dog shortly after each bell ring. After several such episodes the dog salivated to the sound of the bell in anticipation of the food. Humans show evidence of classical conditioning. We may salivate at the sound of a dinner gong, or experience an increased pulse rate when we hear a police siren. We, in common with Pavlov's dogs, have learned to associate or pair stimuli and events, and the autonomic nervous system responds in a manner appropriate to the anticipated event. Many psychologists believe that classical conditioning plays an important part in attitude formation, and in this respect has some relevance to physiotherapy. Many patients are apprehensive, and a few are possibly terrified on their first visit to the department. The signs of stress will be demonstrated by the activity of the sympathetic nervous system. It is up to the physiotherapist to ensure that favourable attitudes are developed towards therapy. A friendly approach and a comfortable, effective treatment are essential in the early stages. Attitudes are rapidly formed and slow to decay. Imagine the attitude of Pavlov's dog if the bell had been followed by painful stimuli. Further sounds from the bell would have resulted in stress and anxiety.

Operant conditioning has been investigated by B. Skinner. In this type of learning the organism works for a reward. A rat may learn to press a lever and be rewarded by a pellet of food. A child may run an errand and receive a tip. An adult will work for a month to receive a pay cheque. Operant conditioning involves the use of the voluntary skeletal muscles to create the conditions in which a reward is earned. The therapist can train the patient by operant conditioning[5] to improve his skill level when voluntary movements are involved. The most effective rewards will probably be praise and encouragement from the therapist and a realization of improvement in the patient's condition.

Avoidance conditioning is a sophisticated term for punishment, and has little part to play in physiotherapy. The function of punishment is to suppress undesired behaviour, and although the therapist does not usually physically attack an unco-operative patient, it must be remembered that words and facial expressions of disapproval may act as avoidance conditioners, especially to sensitive patients. Punishment is unreliable as an avoidance conditioner,[6] whereas operant conditioning by rewarding a correct response is usually highly successful.

The three types of conditioning described are all examples of associative learning, in which specific stimuli are paired with specific responses. The timing of reward or punishment is critical. If presented long after the paired behaviour, the links may not be forged and learning will not occur. Consideration of conditioning processes in isolation gives the impression of man as a machine, responding when the appropriate button is pushed, but much evidence exists to suggest that man also learns with conscious understanding. Latent learning takes place when no apparent reward or punishment is involved. You probably know the make of your neighbour's car, the name of the pub at the bottom of your road, and the colour of the walls of the department in which you work. Such learning has gone in as an impression received and retained, simply by existing as part of your environment.

Insight learning occurs when the learner receives a flash of inspiration, which results in the solution of a problem. We all know the feeling when 'the pieces all fall into place'. Evidence exists to suggest that many higher mammals enjoy insight learning. Creativity is probably the most advanced form of mental activity, in which a series of mental processes result in a completely new solution to a particular problem in science, or a new form of expression in art, literature or music.[8] Because man is capable of the cognitive processes, the physiotherapist should explain in suitable terms the relevant details of the patient's pathology and the aims and objectives in treatment, in order to harness greater co-operation and higher motivation from the patient.

Habituation is a form of learning in which a repeated stimulus eventually produces a reduced response. For example, a doctor may take a patient's blood pressure two or three times, and the successive reductions in recorded pressures indicates habituation to the process of taking blood pressure. Patients will habituate to successive physiotherapy treatments and will co-operate more fully and perform at a higher level as their anxiety is reduced.

To return briefly to the theme of child development, we can now consider some of the learning processes involved during the process of socialization, when the child acquires the accepted values, traditions, and behaviour norms of the culture in which he is reared, and acquires what we loosely refer to as a conscience.

The American sociologist, Talcott Parsons, has called the birth of new generations a recurrent barbarian invasion.[4] Behaviourists claim that these barbarians become civilized by conditioning processes applied during maturation of the nervous system. Behaviour is shaped by various mixtures of rewards and punishment until culturally desirable behaviour is elicited. Love-oriented techniques, using the social rewards of praise and affection, and the withdrawing of these rewards for undesired behaviour, produce superior results to object-oriented techniques of tangible rewards and physical punishment. Superior, in that the children have fewer feeding and toilet training problems, and possess a stronger conscience, whereas physical punishment produces individuals low in self-esteem, aggressive and unfriendly.[7] Innate tendencies to certain forms of behaviour do exist, but they can be profoundly modified by conditioning processes.

Intelligence

It is a matter of common observation that some people are more clever than others. But when we attempt to define intelligence a hard-and-fast definition seems impossible. This is because intelligence is an abstract idea which is assumed to exist, and yet remains intangible. Such intangibles are known as constructs. We assess intelligence by observing intelligent behaviour. Hence the rather cynical definition that 'intelligence is what intelligence tests measure'. An intelligence test samples behaviour of individuals. Heim[9] defines intelligence as 'grasping the essentials in a given situation and responding appropriately to them'. The grasping cannot be assumed until the responding has been observed. Detailed consideration of intelligence testing and measuring is not appropriate in this chapter, and the interested reader should consult standard references.[10] One name which stands out in the history of intelligence testing is Binet, a Frenchman who devised test items which, with slight modifications, are still included in some current tests. Briefly, he identified abilities of average children of all age-groups. He then measured the abilities of individual children, and described their mental ages according to the level of test items they could pass. Thus a child of chronological age twelve years who performed at the level of an average nine year old would be said to have a mental age of nine. From this data the intelligence quotient could be calculated as

$$\frac{\text{Mental Age}}{\text{Chronological Age}} \times \frac{100}{1} = \frac{9}{12} \times \frac{100}{1} = 75$$

After the age of sixteen years intelligence does not increase in the same manner as during maturation, but the idea of a spread of ability among the population persists. The precise ranges of scores in a population varies with the type of test, but as a broad generalization two-thirds of the population have I.Q.s. between 85 and 115, the population mean being, by definition, 100. There is strong evidence indicating that intelligence is due to genetic, inherited factors to a much greater extent than environmental factors. For example, genetically identical twins reared apart have closer I.Q. scores than genetically different twins reared together.[11]

There is a general (g) factor in intelligence which was identified by Spearmen.[12] This g factor contributes to all areas of intellectual activity. The result is that the more intelligent the individual is, the more likely he is to be above average in all areas of ability. In addition to the g factor, possession of specific abilities raises one's performance to higher levels in some areas than in others, so that some excel in maths, others in history or art.

The trained physiotherapist should remember that her proven ability in passing the pre-entry requirements for physiotherapy training, plus her ability to pass the qualifying examinations indicate that, together with other professional people, she is of above average intelligence. Her colleagues at school, work, and in social contexts are also probably of above average intelligence. But if the patients she treats form a typical cross-section of the community, half of them must by definition be of below-average intelligence. They will less easily understand the pathology of their condition and the principles of treatment. It is easy to interpret this inability as stubbornness or lack of co-operation.

Personality

Personality is that area of psychology most concerned with individual differences. When an acquaintance is described as generous, aggressive, kind, greedy or sulky, he is being compared with some mythical averages of these qualities, or behaviour tendencies, which exist in varying degrees in all individuals. Not only do individuals differ from each other in the strength of these tendencies, but the strength varies from time to time within the same individual. The behaviour tendencies are referred to as *traits*, and one of the aims of students of personality is to identify and measure such traits. Each trait adjective has an opposite, so that a person's score for kindness would exist on a dimension between kindness and cruelty.

Eysenck[13] has developed tests which identify two important traits on the dimensions of extroversion-introversion and stability-neuroticism. He describes extroverts and introverts as follows:

'The typical extrovert is sociable, likes parties, has many friends, needs to have people to talk to, and does not like reading or studying by himself. He craves excitement, takes chances, often sticks his neck out, acts on the spur of the moment, and is generally an impulsive individual. He is fond of practical jokes, always has a ready answer, and generally likes change; he is carefree, optimistic, and likes to "laugh and be merry". He prefers to keep moving and doing things, tends to be aggressive, and loses his temper quickly. Altogether, his feelings are not kept under tight control, and he is not always a reliable person.

The typical introvert, on the other hand, is a quiet, retiring sort of person, introspective, fond of books rather than people; he is reserved and distant except with intimate friends. He tends to plan ahead, "looks before he leaps" and distrusts the impulse of the moment. He does not like excitement, takes matters of everyday life with proper seriousness and likes a well-ordered mode of life. He keeps his feelings under close control, seldom behaves in an aggressive manner, and does not lose his temper easily. He is reliable, somewhat pessimistic, and places great value on ethical standards.'

The behaviour patterns of these two groups may be broadly summarized by saying that the extrovert seeks continuous stimulation, variety, and change, while the introvert avoids these. Eysenck proposes a neurological explanation of these behaviour patterns which should appeal to physiotherapists with their background of neurophysiology. Briefly, the extrovert has an underactive ascending reticular activating system, and he is, therefore, continually seeking stimuli to arouse and alert the cerebral cortex to optimum efficiency. The introvert has an overactive reticular system, and surplus stimuli result in over-arousal of the cortex, with consequent discomfort and loss of efficiency.

A strong case can also be presented for an organic basis of the stability-neuroticism dimension, with manifestations demonstrated via the autonomic nervous system.

These two independent dimensions can interact to give four extreme types. Thus there are neurotic introverts, stable introverts, neurotic extroverts and stable extroverts. Before the reader tries to force himself into one of these categories, it is important to stress that these groups are extreme, and the majority of the population are near to the centre of the dimensions. When large specific groups are studied certain tendencies can be observed. Physiotherapists tend to be slightly extroverted and slightly neurotic when compared with the population mean.[14] Such a person prefers contact with people and is anxious to do a good job. Physical educationalists, on the other hand, tend to be stable extroverts, which equips them for the stressful conditions of competitive performance.[15] Other professional groups also display typical personality profiles.

The neurotic extrovert displays hysterical symptoms of a physical nature when under stress. Examples are functional aphasia, hysterical paralysis, and asthma of psychosomatic origin. Such symptoms provide the individual with an escape route away from the stress-producing situation. Thus a man who is required to talk in his job can escape by precipitating aphasia, while a clerk would develop hysterical paralysis of his writing arm.

The neurotic introvert under stress is more likely to develop obsessional neuroses, which consists of unnecessarily repetitive behaviour which is time-absorbing and takes his thoughts away from the stress- or anxiety-producing circumstances. It will be appreciated that a neurosis is not so much an illness as an individual's personal solution to a problem. Furthermore, cure of the symptoms without removal of the stressful cause may result in substitution by an even more severely handicapping set of symptoms. Much tact must, therefore, be employed when treating neurotic patients. When the stress is removed spontaneous recovery frequently follows, but the symptoms may persist as habits, in which case they may be cured without risk of substitution.

Sometimes whole clusters of personality traits appear together to form a personality type. Combinations or clusters of traits can be detected by special tests designed to measure personality types. For example the authoritarian type demonstrates a clustering of patriotism, conservatism, prejudice, tough-mindedness and rigid thinking.[4, 16]

Motivation

Without a motivating or driving force the human organism is totally inactive. Something has motivated the reader to cast his eyes across this page! Motivations or drives may be regarded as inner forces compelling us to action. The hunger and thirst drives compel us to eat and drink. Without such drives we would soon die from malnutrition or dehydration. Such physiological drives ensure our continued survival. The sex drive ensures the perpetuation of the species. Once the biological drives are satisfied we have time for drives ensuring safety and comfort, such as seeking a warm, safe place to live and suitable clothes to wear. Social drives compel us to seek companionship, to obtain a sense of belongingness, and to exchange love and affection with other people, and be respected by them. If the physiological and social drives are satisfied man can rise to higher drives in creative spheres and find satisfaction in art, music or other aesthetic or philosophical activities.

This brief description of drives suggests a hierarchical structure, and has been proposed by Maslow.[17] The higher drives are unlikely to receive attention unless the lower ones are satisfied. A man dying from starvation is unlikely to be appreciative of fine art or music. Similarly a patient deprived of the social satisfaction obtained from family and friends, and restricted to a ward bed, may show a regression in behaviour because his motivations have changed. If he is in pain his motivations may appear selfish, but will be concerned with escape from pain. When he is well on the way to recovery he may be more concerned with escape from hospital and the medical team can capitalize on the driving force. Most patients want to be breadwinners and home-makers, but the occasional patient finds life rather pleasant when the physiological drives of hunger and thirst are satisfied by the tender loving care of attentive young nurses. It is the task of the hospital team to shift his motivations higher up the hierarchical list. He should be encouraged to help in routine ward activites or sent to a convalescent or rehabilitation centre where a more independent life-style is possible and the circle of interests may be enlarged. It is imperative that during this stage the patient should experience feelings of success and achievement whenever progress is made towards greater independence. Praise should be meted out generously for each step forward, whether the patient is a young motorcyclist with a fractured femur, a middle-aged amputee or an aged hemiplegic. In many ways motivation is the core of psychology. Without it man is virtually lifeless. When present its nature determines our choice of behaviour.

THE ACQUISITION OF MOTOR SKILL

Definitions of skill are many and varied, some experts regarding almost every activity of any living creature as an act of skill. For the purposes of this chapter Guthrie's definition is the most suitable. Skill is defined as 'the learned ability to bring about predetermined results with maximum certainty, often with the minimum outlay of time or energy or both'.

If car driving is taken as an example of a skill, the highly skilled driver is more likely to complete the journey (predetermined result) in a relaxed manner (minimum energy) and shorter time than the learner driver.

Not all skills are 'learned' abilities in some senses of the word. A baby crawls and walks as a result of neurological maturation rather than learning but continued effort increases the ability level. We may, therefore, use the term maturational skill to describe crawling, walking or running as distinct from learned skills such as driving, cycling, swimming or using mechanical apparatus such as a camera or a piano.

The majority of students and practitioners of physiotherapy are more concerned with skill acquisition than with any other area of psychology. The student is required to learn to handle apparatus and equipment which is very unlike anything she has ever used before. In addition she must develop the skill of manipulating the body tissues of the patients in her care. The practitioner of physiotherapy is, in the vast majority of cases, concerned with encouraging the development of new skills, or reviving lost skills in her patient. The majority of treatment sessions include some form of exercise, and for this the co-operation and motivation of the patient are essential. But even with optimum motivation, much of the energy put into skill acquisition may be wasted if the therapist does not follow certain principles.

The first of the principles is *guidance* during the practice of the skill. Practice may be undertaken for one of three reasons – to acquire a new skill, to improve an existing skill, or to maintain an existing high level of skill. The student is concerned with the first two, the qualified therapist will be fulfilling the second throughout her daily routine, and may become involved with the first when new treatment techniques are introduced. The third reason concerns individuals at peak levels of performance of a skill, such as professional sportsmen or musicians. The patient may be concerned with the first two. Some patients may never have used the diaphragm correctly, and will, therefore, be concerned with a new skill, whereas other patients will be concerned with relearning (re-education) of existing skills such as walking.

Guidance of the learner is most important. Proper guidance results in quicker and more effective skill acquisition. Lack of guidance may mean that the skill learner will never realize his otherwise potential skill level.[18] Usually the initial guidance is verbal, that is an explanation of the nature and requirements of the skill. This should usually be followed by *visual guidance*, or demonstration, which will assist the learner by providing the opportunity of imitation. Finally, *manual or mechanical guidance* may be used, as when the teacher places her hands on the student's hands when teaching massage manipulations. Spring or weight-assisted exercises, and plaster slabs to enable patients to use their limbs, are all examples of mechanical guidance. Learning without guidance is learning by trial and error, and this is seldom satisfactory. The learning is slower and less effective, and the maximum possible skill level is seldom achieved. There is little to recommend 'being thrown in at the deep end'. Motivation will certainly be high, but the end result may be fatal!

Having got the learner practising with appropriate guidance, the teacher should provide a *continuous feedback of information* to the learner concerning progress. To modify a truism, 'practice with feedback makes perfect'. The patient learning to walk with crutches will require continual corrections in the early stages. Length of pace, timing of pace, position of head, general posture, weight on wrists, and many other points will need frequent attention. If the patient is sent to the far end of the gymnasium to practise on his own, the faults will become ingrained and may prove difficult to eliminate. The best feedback is praise for good performance whenever possible. Blame and criticism, if too frequent, are demotivating, and can cause the sensitive learner to give up completely.

The next considerations are *spacing, duration, and timing of practice sessions.* The optimum duration and frequency for maximum skill level may conflict with administrative desirabiliy. If a new skill is practised for ten minutes without a break the total gain in learning will probably be less than if the skill is practised for two sessions of five minutes. Learning by massed practice results in what is known as reactive inhibition, which reduces total learning.[13] Briefer periods of spaced practice suffer less in this way. Two five-minute sessions of diaphragmatic breathing, or quadriceps exercises, although inconvenient because of time spent travelling by the therapist to and from the ward, will result in more total learning than one ten-minute session. Perhaps a compromise could be reached by going round the patients in a ward twice during one visit, spending less time during each treatment.

Transfer of skill must be considered in most learning situations. Transfer is concerned with what happens when a skill is practised in a different context. Strictly speaking it is impossible to repeat a movement. Even a simple repetitive task, such as throwing darts at a board results in different scores with successive throws. The goal may be the same on each occasion, but success at approximating to the goal varies due to minor modifications in the interpreation of perceptual cues, and variations in muscle action. In skill-learning situations the aim is to achieve maximum positive transfer. This will mean that skill will bé performed at a high level even though the environment or stimulus situation is different. Many skill-training situations necessitate transfer. Air pilots are required to make their initial mistakes in a dummy cockpit before being trusted with a planeload of passengers. The extent to which the skills learned in the simulator can be utilized when placed in the real situation is a measure of the degree of positive transfer. Students practise massage and other therapeutic techniques on each other before they are allowed to treat patients. The greater the similarity between the practice environment and the treatment environment, the larger will be the amount of positive transfer. A student who has only practised a certain treatment technique on the left arm of a healthy, thin, young fellow student sitting on a chair will not enjoy much positive transfer when faced with treating the right arm of a sick, obese, elderly bed-ridden patient.

Transfer is also important from the patient's point of view. He may have learnt to walk up and down the gymnasium steps, which have a rise of five inches and a tread of ten inches, and a handrail on the right. Confident that he can manage stairs, he is discharged. He then realizes that his own stairs have a seven-inch rise, a nine-inch tread, a hand rail on the left, and a spiral at the top. The importance of students and patients practising skills in different contexts is obvious, but this aspect of skill acquisition is frequently neglected.

Perception

Perception is sometimes considered to be synonymous with vision, but this is a rather limited view of what is really a wide-ranging and complex area of study.

The author chooses to define perception as the organism's inter-pretation of the environmental stimuli impinging on its sensory receptors. Much laboratory work in perceptual research has been performed on animals and the word organism embraces them. The environment includes internal and external environments. One fascinat-ing area of perception deals with determination of innate perceptual abilities and acquired perceptual abilities. The nature-nurture contro-versy ranges throughout most areas of psychology. The philosophers Locke and James assumed that the neonate's perceptual awareness was analogous with a blank slate, waiting for impressions to be made by experience. 'A big, booming, buzzing confusion'[19] was how James described the infant's consciousness. Confusion was assumed to decrease as perceptual learning occurred. More recent work by skilled psychologists has demonstrated that the newborn infant possesses many perceptual abilities which earlier workers had been unable to detect. Recognition of human faces, distances, and other perceptual abilities either exist at birth or develop very rapidly.[20] Such abilities are rapidly lost if visual stimuli are absent or distorted, so an interaction between the organism and a normally stimulating environment is essential. There is also much evidence that cultural factors affect perception profoundly. Tribesmen reared in visually restricted jungle environments interpret small retinal images as being necessarily produced by small objects, instead of large distant objects. They are less susceptible to illusions involving straight lines typical of the Westerner's 'carpentered' environment.

The internal environment can also play perceptual tricks. Hungry

461

subjects perceive pictures of food as brighter than other equally illuminated pictures. This is known as perceptual set, and similar forms of set affect us all far more than we normally realize. Southerners have a stereotyped picture of Northerners and *vice versa*. Each will tend to perceive in the other that which they expect to perceive. A special form of set is perceptual defence. This occurs when we raise the threshold of perception to stimuli that we do not wish to be aware of, because we find them embarrassing or annoying. We turn a convenient subconscious blind eye if it suits us.

Emotion

Human emotions have interested man throughout history. The supposed anatomical sites of the origin of emotions have varied through the ages from the womb, heart, guts and spleen until present-day theories developed by electrical stimulation techniques point to the brain as the seat of emotion. The mid-brain and hypothalamus are the pleasure centres, while stimulation of discrete regions of the temporal lobe gives rise to feelings of anger and rage.

Brain-damaged patients frequently appear in the physiotherapy department and emotional disorders are sometimes present in a subtle form, and may even be wrongly attributed to distress concerning the accompanying physical symptoms such as those of hemiplegia or Parkinson's disease. But depending on the specific areas of brain involvement, signs of depression, anger, distress and weeping, euphoria and rapid swings of mood can be directly due to brain damage. To complicate the issue even further, the displayed behaviour may not even match the mood experienced. Some hemiplegics display uncontrolled weeping even though they report feeling quite cheerful. Close relatives will sometimes report changed moral values in the patient. He may have started telling lies or stealing. The therapist will tend to assume that the patient has always been so inclined unless informed to the contrary.

The physiotherapist is not concerned with treatment of the psychologically abnormal unless she is employed in a hospital unit which specially caters for such patients, in which case she would be well advised to attend courses and refer to books dealing with the psychologically abnormal. For those readers who are interested some suitable textbooks are recommended. Much controversy exists even between experts in the complex area of abnormal psychology. Analytic techniques aim at probing the mental life of the patient and restructuring the personality brick by brick, while behaviourists consider many behaviour disorders as consequences of faulty learning, and the treatment consists of eradication of such learning by avoidance conditioning and substituting correct learning by operant conditioning. The efficacy of treatment frequently seems to be more related to a satisfactory relationship between the patient and clinician than to any particular treatment technique!

With progress in neurology and biochemistry more and more mental disorders are being recognized as physiological in origin, and the controversy over cause and appropriate treatment recedes.

The day may come when it will be possible to explain all psychology in terms of physiology, but it may not prove to be the most useful and productive way of explaining behaviour. A multi-disciplinary approach to the study of man results in a balanced rounded view of homo sapiens, the organism at the top of the evolutionary tree.

REFERENCES

1. Hill, D. A. *Psychology Teaching*, Vol. 2, 1974.
2. Woodworth, R. S. *Contemporary Schools of Psychology*. Methuen, 1970.
3. Beard, R. M. *An Outline of Piaget's Developmental Psychology*. Routledge & Kegan Paul, 1969.
4. Brown, R. *Social Psychology*. Cassell Collier Macmillan, 1966.
5. O'Gorman, G. In *Physiotherapy*, June 1975.
6. Wright, D. S. & Taylor, A. *Introducing Psychology*. Penguin, 1972.
7. Hilgard, E . R., Atkinson, R. C. & Atkinson, R. L. *Introduction to Psychology*. Harcourt, Brace, Jovarovich.
8. Vernon, P. E. (ed.) *Creativity*. Penguin, 1970.
9. Child, D. *Psychology and the Teacher*. Holt, Rinehart & Winston, 1974.
10. Vernon, P. E. *Intelligence and Attainment Tests*. University of London Press, 1964.
11. Mittler, P. *The Study of Twins*. Penguin, 1971.
12. Wiseman, S. *Intelligence and Ability*. Penguin, 1967.
13. Eysenck, H. J. *Fact and Fiction in Psychology*. Penguin, 1967.
14. Child, D. In *Physiotherapy*, October 1974.
15. Kane, J. Ph.D. thesis, University of London, 1968 (Personal Communication).
16. Eysenck, H. J. *Uses and Abuses of Psychology*. Penguin, 1953.

17. Maslow, A. H. *Toward a Psychology of Being*. Van Nostrand Reinhold, 1968.
18. Knapp, B. *Skill in Sport*. Routledge & Kegan Paul, 1967.
19. Vernon, M. A. *The Psychology of Perception*. Penguin, 1962.
20. Gregory, R. L. *Eye and Brain*. Weidenfeld & Nicolson, 1970.

FURTHER READING

Gillis, L. *Human Behaviour in Illness*. Faber & Faber, 2nd edition 1972.
Holding, D. H. *Principles of Training*. Pergamon, 1965.
Shakespeare, R. *The Psychology of Handicap*. Methuen, 1975.
Singh, M. M. *Mental Disorder*. Pan, 1967.
Stafford-Clark, D. *Psychiatry Today*. Penguin, 1967.
Williams, M. *Brain Damage and the Mind*. Penguin, 1970.

CHAPTER XXIII

Physiotherapy in some Psychiatric Conditions

by JOAN M. DODGSON, M.C.S.P., O.N.C.

In the ever-changing field of psychiatry, the physiotherapist is taking an increasingly active part. The purpose of this chapter, however, is not only to be of assistance to the serious student of psychiatric physiotherapy, but, it is hoped, to be of some value to the physiotherapist in a general department.

We have all met the patient who, in spite of many courses of different types of physical treatment, fails to improve. There may, or may not, be obvious signs of tension or anxiety in the patient. After a while, when all investigations have failed to produce a physical origin for the complaint, the patient is labelled 'neurotic', or the condition labelled 'psychosomatic' and he is referred to the psychiatrist.

In the Physical Medicine Department, the therapist who can recognize and understand the underlying psychiatric problems at an early stage will be of much greater value to the patient than the one who is concerned solely with the physical problems. Persistence of symptoms of, for example, osteo-arthrosis may be due to over-anxiety caused by association of the term osteo-arthrosis with progressive and unavoidable crippling. Prolonged physical treatment, without the recognition and understanding of the underlying anxieties associated with any physical illness, can only be harmful. In fact, it has been said that 'the essential link between psychiatry, general medicine, surgery and obstetrics lies in the ultimate impossibility of treating states of mind apart from states of body, or states of body apart from states of mind.'

PSYCHOSOMATIC INTERACTIONS

The word 'psychosomatic' is used in various ways, commonly in reference to specific diseases, such as asthma, peptic ulcers, menstrual disorders etc., in which emotional factors are considered to be of definite aetiological significance; but sometimes as a synonym for psycho-neurotic.

Pearson in *Fundamentals of Psychiatry* defines it as representing a point of view on the study of disease as a whole. He says: 'The investigation of disease from the psychosomatic point of view is the study of illness in terms of the emotional factors (feelings, moods, conflicts, attitudes, interpersonal relationships and personality developments), as well as of the physical factors (constitution, immunity, bacterial or viral invasion, trauma, degeneration and neoplasm formation)'.

Man owes his survival and his power over his environment to the flexibility of his adaptive capacity. When the individual's mental resources are not enough to meet the demands on him, and adaptation is incomplete, a state of internal disharmony occurs. This manifests itself in symptoms of physical or mental dysfunction, or, more commonly, in both.

Thus, a psychosomatic illness is one in which psychological factors appear to play an important part in producing a disorder of the function or structure of the body. There are several types of psychosomatic disorders:

1. Where various physical symptoms exist, but no physical cause can be found.

2. Where physical disease exists, but the structural changes are a result of emotional factors.

3. Where actual organic disease exists, but some of the presenting symptoms arise not from this disease, but from mental factors. Here the disability is often out of proportion to the physical disease.

PHYSICAL CHANGES IN EMOTIONAL STATES

All emotions are expressed through physiological processes and all are accompanied by physiological changes. Thus we show sorrow by weeping, amusement by laughter and shame by blushing. Emotional situations arising from interaction with other people give rise to nervous impulses which influence the complex muscular interactions that take place in the body. Thus fear produces palpitation of the heart; anger produces increased heart activity, elevation of blood pressure, and changes in carbohydrate metabolism; and despair causes sighing (i.e. deep inspiration followed by deep expiration).

These changes in the body as reactions to acute emotion are of a passing nature and return to normal when the emotion disappears. If the emotion is repressed, however, or unduly prolonged, the functional disturbance produced in any organ may lead finally to definite anatomical changes, and to the clinical picture of severe organic illness. For example, hyperactivity of the heart may lead to hypertrophy of the heart muscles, or hysterical paralysis of a limb may lead to certain degenerative changes in the muscles and joints because of inactivity.

Two emotional states which commonly give rise to psychosomatic illness are anxiety and tension.

Anxiety

Anxiety in its simplest form may be considered as a normal reaction to danger, or the threat of danger. Biological changes occur in the individual which improve his responsiveness to external stresses. A small amount of anxiety increases alertness and efficiency of performance, but an increase in the amount of anxiety will eventually lead to a deterioration of the level of response. When anxiety develops as an abnormal state, not necessarily related to stress, it is regarded as a symptom or part of a broader-based psychiatric syndrome. It reaches a pathological degree only when it surpasses the inherent ability of the subject to bear it.

The physical manifestations of an anxiety state resemble those of fear, with excessive activity of the autonomic nervous system. There may be symptoms associated with any of the bodily systems e.g.:

Cardiac – tachycardia and palpitation

Respiratory – breathlessness and tightness of the chest

Gastro-intestinal – nausea, vomiting, diarrhoea and abdominal cramps

Genito-urinary – frequency, urgency, enuresis

Vasomotor – sweating, shivering and dizziness

Neuromuscular – weakness, tension

The anxious patient shows signs of apprehension and assumes a tense posture with furrowing of the brow and wringing of hands. The voice may be uneven or strained, and the pupils widely dilated. There may be sweating of the hands and face and weakness, nausea and tremor may be present.

In a moderate degree of emotional stress only a few of these signs and symptoms may be present. However, long-continued emotions of fear, shame, anger, resentment etc., may produce more symptoms and if they become exaggerated and established they may continue even after the original situation has disappeared and may eventually lead to structural changes in the organ or viscus through which the anxiety is expressed ('The sorrow which has no vent in tears may make other organs weep': Henry Maudsley). Disorders of bodily functions are the clinically dominant features and a patient will rarely complain or even recognize his anxiety, tension or depression.

Tension

Tension is a component of anxiety and may be confused with the effect of anxiety. It arises when an individual is torn between contradictory desires and strivings.

In tension the patient has a continuing feeling of tautness, both emotionally and in his muscles. He senses a restlessness, dissatisfaction and dread. He presents a strained, tense facial expression, has tremor of the hands and his movements are abrupt. He probably will complain of tightness or other unpleasant sensations in the head and other bodily pains – usually in the neck and shoulders, back and chest. The pain in the head may be described as 'dull', 'nagging', 'an ache', or 'tight' and occasionally 'stabbing'. There is usually difficulty in concentration, broken sleep and fatigue. Among other symptoms of tension are: abdominal pain (particularly in children), amenorrhoea, dysmenorrhoea, menorrhagia, constipation, diarrhoea, frequency of micturition, migraine, and various skin changes such as itching and flushing.

INFLUENCE OF EMOTIONAL FACTORS ON SOME SPECIFIC ILLNESSES

Rheumatoid arthritis

There are many theories concerning the cause of rheumatoid arthritis, none of which establishes sufficient proof to be fully acceptable.

Probably several factors, including infections, local trauma, debilitating states and emotional disturbances may precipitate or aggravate the disease. Often direct temporal relationships between the onset of the arthritic symptoms and emotional crises are observed, and exacerbations and remissions can often be linked with changes in the environmental stress under which the patient lives.

While some authorities hold the view that rheumatoid arthritis is an organic psychosomatic disease others suggest that the emotional factors apparently affecting the disease are only part of the picture, and should be looked upon as only one of several possibly provocative agents.

Sufferers from rheumatoid arthritis tend to fit into a particular personality pattern which is frequently associated with psychosomatic disorders. They show emotional inhibition, probably stemming from early childhood when they were shy and retiring, possibly due to restrictive overprotective parental influence in infancy. Many aspects of their emotional lives are repressed and they grow up into meticulously orderly, overconscientious people, well adjusted to emotional life, but showing restrictions of feelings and emotions.

Whatever the cause of the disease, or its exacerbations, it must be remembered that any chronically disabling disease is likely to produce serious emotional problems. Many patients develop a sense of hostility due to the threat of dependency, and the frustrations associated with the condition (disruption of social life, interference with earning power etc.) tend to produce neurotic symptoms. Others tend to cling to their position of dependency. Either of these reactions to the limiting factors of the disease is damaging to the confidence of relationships with others, even (or perhaps especially) those who are trying to help. The type of person whose mobility and muscular ability is essential to his adaptation will suffer deeply and have less inner strength to deal with the enforced regression which the limitations of the disease impose.

Asthma

Because of the close relationship between emotional tensions and respiratory function, as instanced by crying, laughing, screaming or speaking, it is probable that in most diseases of the respiratory system, psychological factors play an important role.

469

It has long been known that emotional factors play a large part in the asthmatic attack, although the spasm of the bronchioles, which is the immediate cause of the attack, is often precipitated by exposure to a specific allergen, such as pollen, animal fur, paint etc. Usually both these factors co-exist to produce an attack but either may be the precipitating factor.

The emotional disturbances leading to an asthmatic attack are many and varied, and include almost any sudden intensive emotional stimulus, such as anger, jealousy, rage, sexual excitement etc. It has been found that anything which threatens to separate the patient from the protective mother or her substitute is apt to precipitate an attack. For example, the birth of a sibling is often found to be the initiating factor of the asthmatic condition. This repressed dependence upon the mother is a constant feature around which different types of character defences may develop. Among asthma sufferers may be found many types of personalities – aggressive, ambitious, argumentative, or hypersensitive aesthetic types, all of which develop from the conflict surrounding the excessive unresolved dependence on the mother.

The theory has been advanced that the asthmatic attack represents symbolically both a protest against separation from the mother, and also the wish to re-establish this relationship through crying; this is considered equivalent to a repressed cry and in fact the sounds made in asthma resemble those of a whining cry or repressed sobbing. This view is substantiated by the fact that most asthma patients spontaneously report difficulty in crying and observe that asthmatic attacks have terminated when the patient could give vent to his feelings of crying.

In other patients, an asthmatic attack may occur as a conditioned reflex to a conditioned stimulus. For example, a patient who had previous attacks precipitated by pollen from a certain plant may develop further attacks when shown a picture of that plant.

Thus it can be seen that emotional factors play an important part in the production of the illness though the relative importance of the physiological and psychological elements is variable. Treatment is directed towards both these elements, though it has been found that the elimination of only one of them will usually effect a remission of symptoms.

470

SPECIAL ASPECTS OF PSYCHIATRIC PHYSIOTHERAPY

The physiotherapist working with psychiatric patients, whether in a small unit attached to a general hospital or in a large psychiatric hospital is not 'another being' in 'another world'. It is true that there are some small differences in the tasks before the physiotherapist but the basic situation is the same i.e. a patient is a person with an illness and the physiotherapist is a member of a team committed to restoring that person to full health.

With modern techniques and drugs in psychiatry the tendency is for more patients to be returned to the community and in a much shorter time; therefore the number of chronically sick is diminishing, although there will always be some patients who need constant and long-term care. With this in mind, the present policy is for patients with acute psychiatric illnesses to be treated in small units which form an integral part of the general hospitals, many of them attending as day patients, and returning home each evening. This, it is hoped, will help to banish the stigma which is still attached, to a greater or lesser degree, to being a psychiatric patient.

While the main function of the physiotherapist in psychiatry is still the management of the physical condition of the patients, she is also a member of the team whose function is to restore the patient to full mental and physical health. So she is concerned not only with the physical effects of treatment but also with the psychological, social and economic adjustment of the patient to illness and disability.

Nurses, physiotherapists, occupational therapists and other staff who are in constant personal contact with the patients are in an excellent position to observe any changes in their mood or behaviour, which may be caused by the pattern of the illness. Physical changes may be due to medication. Parkinsonism is a common side-effect of drugs. As an overall picture of the patient's behaviour is an essential part in the planning or changing of treatment schedules by the psychiatrists, any such change must be reported to them. Liaison among the staff is augmented by frequent inter-disciplinary meetings, in addition to the consultant's ward round.

All staff at these meetings know the personal as well as the medical background of each patient and so are able to note even small physical or mental changes. With this full knowledge of the patients' personal backgrounds, avoidance of over-involvement of any member of staff with any one patient is essential.

TREATMENTS

EXERCISES

Many psychiatric patients, either because of the nature of their illness or because of the drugs prescribed, need much firm persuasion to become involved in anything physically active. Apart from their natural reluctance to join in anything as 'childish' as organized games or class exercises, they often have a genuine feeling of lethargy or tiredness. Once persuaded, however (often by other patients who have previously had to overcome their own inertia), they usually enjoy the classes and the sense of well-being produced.

Classes of general exercises should be organized to suit the varying needs of the individual patients – grouped according to either age or general physical fitness. The aims of all such classes must be:

a. to prevent or overcome physical deterioration
b. to improve precision and co-ordination
c. to promote relaxation of tense muscles
d. to relieve feelings of aggression and hostility

Classes for older or less physically fit patients should consist of simple rhythmical exercises, perhaps performed to music. If music is used it should be carefully chosen, with a simple but positive rhythm and it should be borne in mind that a patient may occasionally be upset by a particular record, because of previous associations, but this cannot be foreseen, and the situation must be dealt with as it arises.

The scheme of exercises should include a selection for all parts of the body, special attention being paid to the muscles controlling head, neck and shoulders as it is in these muscles that tension associated with the majority of mental disorders is found. Free swinging exercises should be given at intervals throughout the session in an attempt to break the physical tension.

Sometimes patients on certain drugs find that head movements produce vertigo and even nausea, but this usually decreases as the medication is stabilized, and can be controlled by deep breathing exercises, which should form part of the programme.

Postural training in sitting and standing should also be included. Younger, fitter patients should have more vigorous exercises, more suited to their superior physical fitness, and ball games may be included; although it may be more beneficial both physically and psychologically for the more formal exercises to be performed at the beginning of the day, and ball games and apparatus work taken as an additional activity later in the day.

Apparatus work should be as varied and stimulating as possible, and include such things as weight-lifting, static rowing, punch ball as well as team games with small apparatus such as ropes, small balls or bean bags. Outdoor games are to be recommended wherever possible, as these give active youngsters the opportunity to 'let off steam' without disturbing other patients.

It is interesting to note how, at all levels, the performance of individual patients alters as the mental condition improves. Often the improvement noticed in the performance of exercises is one of the first indications that the patient is beginning to recover mentally.

RELAXATION

Relaxation therapy is an invaluable part of the treatment prescribed for many psychiatric patients, most of whom exhibit some signs of physical tension. Their diagnoses may vary considerably, from depressive illnesses to personality disorders or phobias, but tension is common to all.

The timing of the class is important as some patients, e.g. those with anxiety states, are most tense in the morning and improve as the day goes on, whereas others will derive more benefit from an afternoon session, as their tension increases as the day progresses.

Relaxation therapy may be requested by the psychologist for patients undergoing a course of aversion therapy, which is a treatment aimed at inducing a conditional aversion to, say, alcohol or drugs by associating the taking of them with repeated nausea and vomiting. In this case relaxation is given immediately prior to the treatment.

In general, patients who are very aware of their tensions, and have a strong desire to relax, are the ones who start to improve most quickly. They require a more concentrated effort to relax and usually learn the technique more readily. On the other hand some patients may increase their tension by trying too hard! If some time is devoted to explaining to the patient the particular relaxation technique to be used, before treatment commences, the stage is well set for the therapy to begin. The patient will accept the treatment more readily, and knowing what

473

is expected of him, will be in a less apprehensive, and therefore more receptive, frame of mind. Even so, it is unlikely that he will achieve relaxation at the first session. Often several sessions are required before the patient, having learnt the technique, is able to use it as a conscious weapon against the tensions arising in his muscles.

The physiotherapist will have her own relaxation technique, but the one most commonly used is the rhythmical contraction-relaxation movement of each group of muscles from toes to head. The patient must concentrate on each movement so that he learns to distinguish between the different feelings of tension and relaxation in each muscle group.

Whatever the technique used, the prerequisites are the same:

a. The patient must be lying comfortably! It is useless to try to teach a patient to relax if he is uncomfortable. The patient should choose his own lying position, though if the side-lying position is adopted, the top leg must be flexed and supported by a pillow, *not* by the other leg. Similarly, the lower arm should be behind the trunk, not having to support it, or be crushed by it. If the patient prefers to lie on his back, a pillow should be placed under the knees to avoid strain on the lumbar spine.

b. The mattress should be on a firm base, or even on the floor as long as there are no draughts.

c. The room should be darkened, as much as is consistent with the therapist's ability to observe the patient, and as quiet as possible.

d. The patient should be covered with a blanket, both for warmth and added security.

e. Commands should be given in a low, monotonous voice.

f. At the end of the instruction time, the patient should be encouraged to concentrate his thoughts on breathing in and out slowly. This in itself helps to promote relaxation, and channels the patient's thoughts away from any external factors which may produce tension.

g. The session should last for at least an hour, during which time the patient is observed for signs of increasing tension such as tightening of the face muscles. If this occurs the procedure should be repeated from the beginning. It may be necessary for a patient to leave before the full time has elapsed, as sometimes lying in a quiet, darkened room may increase the tension.

h. Treatment should be reviewed frequently, as some patients may derive more benefit from other forms of treatment, or relaxation sessions could become just an 'escape to sleep'.

474

i. Progression of relaxation from lying to sitting should be practised, so that if at any time the patient becomes aware of increasing muscular tension, he is able to relax at will, without the need for retiring to bed!

Facial massage may be a useful adjunct for extremely tense patients, sometimes with dramatic results. Some patients, however, are unable to tolerate any tactile stimulation, and derive no benefit from it.

ELECTRO-SLEEP THERAPY

There are many different types of electro-sleep apparatus at present in use in hospitals in this country. They have been designed for use in re-establishing a normal sleep pattern in a patient whose pattern has been disturbed by either physical or psychiatric illness. Most developments in this field have taken place in the U.S.S.R. and Germany over the past few years. It is not yet known how electrically-induced sleep works, but experiments have shown that the electrical impulses are carried into the central nervous system and have an inhibitory effect.

Electro-sleep therapy is used in the treatment of anxiety, tension and insomnia, and claims have been made for its beneficial use in many medical and surgical conditions, as well as in psychiatric conditions, and psychosomatic illnesses.

Sleep is induced by applying small modulated impulses to the skull, by means of three or four electrodes, usually incorporated in rubber goggles. The positive electrodes are placed on the closed eyelids, and the counter-electrodes placed on the mastoid processes. Some designs have only one counter-electrode, which is then placed at the nape of the neck.

The prerequisites of treatment are the same as those for relaxation therapy, but it is even more important here, for the procedure to be explained to the patient, and the expected effect. This is to minimize feelings of apprehension when the electrodes are applied. He will merely feel a slight tingling sensation under the electrodes, and (with some machines) hear a musical note throughout the treatment, designed to exclude any extraneous sounds. He will feel very relaxed during treatment, will become drowsy, and finally enjoy a relaxing sleep, though because of the initial apprehension this might not be so in the first treatment or two. It should be pointed out to the patient that the machine is independent of the mains current. When he is lying on the bed in the normal sleeping position, the rubber goggles are placed on the patient's head, and the connecting leads are plugged into the machine which is then switched on. The output control is turned up slowly until the patient reports that he can feel a tingling sensation under the electrodes, and then left. The first session should be of 20 minutes duration, this time being increased at each daily session until each session lasts one to two hours.

The number of sessions required varies with the individual, but optimum effect is usually reached in 10–15 sessions, though some patients need a longer course, and will continue to derive benefit even after 30–40 treatments.

As there are no side-effects to the treatment, it can be used to replace drugs for night sedation if the treatment is given at the normal bed-time, and a normal sleep pattern is re-established.

CONTINUOUS NARCOSIS

Treatment by continuous narcosis is sometimes used in states of acute anxiety which have followed recent severe stress, and modified narcosis may be used for drug-dependants who are being withdrawn from their drugs.

The treatment aims to produce light sleep for most of each 24 hour period, the sleep only being interrupted at 5-hourly intervals for feeding, toilet requirements, exercise and general nursing care. The duration of the treatment varies from a few days to a few weeks. Before the narcosis commences, breathing exercises are taught to the patient and practised at each waking interval thereafter. Care of the chest is of prime importance, as with the enforced inactivity secretions may collect in the lungs. Postural drainage with clapping and shaking is carried out daily. Simple abdominal and postural exercises are also given, and the treatment is concluded with a brisk walk. This improves circulation and reduces the risk of venous thrombosis. Nursing staff supervise the exercises and walking at each wakeful period when the physiotherapist is not on duty. A sudden drop in blood pressure sometimes occurs, which can cause severe vertigo, and this must be taken into account at all exercise sessions. Chest and circulatory disturbances are not uncommon in patients undergoing narcosis therapy.

OTHER TREATMENTS

Statistics show that there is a higher percentage of physical ailments among psychiatric patients than among the general population. All of these are treated in the prescribed manner, but it must be borne in mind that in these patients there may be more psychological overlay.

Hysterical paralysis must be mentioned, although physical treatment is usually contra-indicated for these patients, as is any treatment which draws further attention to the 'paralysed' limb or limbs. In some cases, however, treatment is prescribed in order to prevent muscular atrophy or contractures arising from disuse.

Any treatments planned by the psychiatric physiotherapist must take into account the possible side-effects of any drugs prescribed for the patient. Many of these drugs can produce side-effects such as heat or light sensitivity which are incompatible with normally acceptable physiotherapy procedures. For instance, treatment by ultraviolet light is contra-indicated for patients who are taking chlorpromazine and particular caution must be used in the application of any form of heat therapy to patients on antidepressants such as imipramine hydrochloride which also produces heat/light sensitivity.

CONCLUSION

The physiotherapist, being in such close and constant contact with the patient, is in an excellent position to recognize and elicit any signs of anxiety or tension and in many cases to allay the fears and apprehensions of the patient.

For example, in a general department, while it is no part of the physiotherapist's role to reveal the prognosis of a chronic or incurable disease, it is her duty to promote physical *and mental* rehabilitation, by demonstrating at an early stage of the illness that the patient can lead a life which is as full and independent as possible. It is also important that she is able to recognize that a 'simple' condition such as a Colles' fracture can produce, in some patients, as much anxiety and distress as an apparently more serious illness.

In a psychiatric hospital, the emphasis is shifted somewhat in that a diagnosis of an anxiety state or other psychiatric disorder has usually been made, and the physiotherapist's role is as a member of the psychiatric team whose aim is to restore the patient to a life of physical, mental and emotional stability. This means that, although a far smaller proportion of the day is concerned with physical treatments there is much closer involvement with the patients, their social background, and their overall treatment. This close involvement makes the work of the psychiatric physiotherapist a very stimulating and rewarding experience.

SOME TERMS USED IN PSYCHIATRY AND THEIR MEANINGS

Psychosis and Neurosis

These terms are used to differentiate between two groups of mental illnesses which correspond approximately to the commoner expressions 'madness' or insanity (psychosis) and the milder 'nervousness' (neurosis). The distinction between the two terms is by no means clear-cut, and it is often difficult to decide in which group a particular patient belongs.

However, the chief points of difference are as follows:

1. Psychosis is a severe disorder of the mind which seriously interferes with the patient's relationships with other people. Neurosis is a less severe disorder.

2. A psychosis may be brought about by organic factors, or by psychological factors, or by a combination of the two. A neurosis is brought on by psychological factors, e.g. a reaction to stressful circumstances in a personality predisposed as a result of adverse experiences in childhood.

3. A psychosis is usually characterized by the presence of one or more such specific symptoms as delusions, illusions or hallucinations. A neurosis is not usually characterized by these, but the clinical picture often includes one or more specific symptoms such as conversions, phobias and obsessions.

4. A psychosis involves severe disorganization of the various personality functions such as memory, perception, judgement etc. A neurosis involves decreased efficiency of one or more of these functions but less disorganization of them.

5. Psychotics are usually not aware of the fact that they are psychiatrically ill – they lack 'insight'. Neurotics are usually aware of their illness – they have 'insight'.

6. In psychosis there is a loss of contact with reality, whereas in neurosis there is normal contact.

Schizophrenia

This is a generic name for a group of mental disorders which have certain characteristics in common. It is probably the most common of all psychoses.

The condition is characterized by an emotional coldness and a loss of connection between thoughts, feelings and actions. It occurs in people with a particular type of temperament characterized by reticence, aloofness, and partial divorcement from reality. The schizoid personality experiences many adaptive difficulties from childhood onwards, and often becomes more and more aloof, and less interested in other people, or in events which interest other people. His shyness leads to exclusiveness and an inability to make human contacts. Not everyone with this type of personality breaks down into illness. Indeed, many manage to find a niche for themselves in which they can work and indulge in fantasy. The poorer the contact with reality the greater the liability to schizophrenic breakdown.

The onset of symptoms usually coincides with a period of emotional stress, such as that of puberty, though increasingly strange behaviour over a period of time has usually been noted by relatives. The patient appears preoccupied and withdraws interest from life. This inward attitude is often associated with the emergence of delusions of being watched or influenced in uncanny ways. His behaviour may become peculiar and unpredictable, and apathy and lack of interest in normal activities develop. This may be progressive throughout the course of the illness, and then contributes to the severe degree of deterioration found in so many chronic patients.

Diagnostic features include severe thought disorder, delusions supported by hallucinations, stupor alternating with frenzy, and in the later stages a marked emotional indifference.

Schizophrenic disorders are often classified into four varieties, the simple, hebephrenic, catatonic and paranoid types. There is often overlapping of symptoms from one type to another, and during the course of his life a patient may have a number of schizophrenic illnesses, the forms of which may vary and at different times may fit better into one category than another.

SIMPLE SCHIZOPHRENIA

In this disorder, which usually develops insidiously throughout adolescence and early adulthood, there are no highlights of gross behaviour disorder, hallucinations, or delusions. For some time the only manifestations may be lack of drive, an odd manner and an emotional impoverishment. The patient becomes increasingly solitary and detached and eventually may withdraw from society, refusing to go to work, and neglecting his appearance. His physical health may deteriorate as a result of lack of exercise and adequate nourishment and he may need admission to hospital. Many of these people, however, continue to exist in the community but often are alone, friendless and on a very low economic level.

HEBEPHRENIC SCHIZOPHRENIA

This disorder also tends to develop in young people, but is characterized by more obvious symptoms, and comes closer to the popular idea of 'madness'. Often after a period of insidious withdrawal, the patient enters a phase of wild excitement during which he shows many florid symptoms of mental disorder. Hallucinations are common and the patient may be preoccupied with voices which he hears, often accusing him of misdeeds, or ordering him to perform actions which he may consider to be quite alien to his nature. If he realizes that there is no one about, he tends to blame 'wireless' or 'electricity' for the voices. The voices may command him to perform antisocial actions, such as attacking others, and he may become so preoccupied with them that he is incapable of any normal activity.

Some patients find it difficult to express their ideas in words, and often thoughts do not follow each other in the normal manner and connections appear illogical and bizarre.

The episode of acute disturbance is usually short, and the patient is often left feeling bewildered and perplexed. With or without treatment the patient may recover sufficiently to resume normal life although relapses are likely to occur, each attack leaving him less well than the previous time, until finally he withdraws from reality and lives in a world of fantasy.

CATATONIC SCHIZOPHRENIA

This disorder comes on later than the previous two, but the first attack usually occurs in young adulthood. The prognosis is somewhat better, especially if the patient's previous personality was mature and well integrated. The extremes of catatonic behaviour are stupor, where the patient remains motionless in bed, apparently unaware of what is going on around him, and an attack of excitement and wild senseless activity. The transitions from one state to the other may be very sudden and occur almost without forewarning. These extremes of behaviour can, nowadays, usually be modified by treatment with appropriate drugs.

PARANOID SCHIZOPHRENIA

This disorder begins later in life, usually between 30 and 40 years. It is characterized by delusions of a fairly coherent nature, which may change rapidly. There is often a discrepancy between the disturbing delusions and hallucinations on the one hand, and the poor emotional response which they evoke on the other. The onset is usually gradual, and the personality is better preserved than in the other types of schizophrenia.

The prognosis in schizophrenic disorders is less favourable than in many other mental disorders, though with the aid of modern drugs, many patients recover from their acute schizophrenic attacks and remain apparently well for long periods, often leading a useful and happy existence in the community.

Dementia

Irreversible impairment of intellectual ability, memory and personality, due to permanent damage or disease of the brain, occurs in this disorder. It also accompanies degenerative changes which occur in some apparently hereditary conditions, like Huntington's chorea. The patient's performance in intelligence tests deteriorates, though his vocabulary usually remains good. He may retain the ability to solve concrete problems but is unable to think in the abstract. For example, he may be unable to add up figures, but able to count beads.

His understanding of other people's actions and feelings declines, and he may become irritable and stubborn, with rapid changes of mood. Often there is a decline in moral standards, and the patient eventually becomes helpless and totally dependent.

FURTHER READING

Ackner, B. *Handbook for Psychiatric Nurses.* Ballière Tindall.
Alexander, F. *Psychosomatic Medicine.* George Allen & Unwin, 1952.

Physiotherapy in some Psychiatric Conditions

Altschul, A *Psychiatric Nursing*. Ballière Tindall. 3rd ed. 1969.

Beccle, H. C. *Psychiatry: Theory and Practice for Students and Nurses*. Faber & Faber. 5th ed. 1962.

Fish, F. J. *An Outline of Psychiatry*. Wright, 2nd ed. 1968.

Hofling, C. K. *et al. Psychiatry for Medical Practice*. Lippincott, 1963.

Hollander, J. L. *et al. Arthritis*. Lea & Febinger, 1960.

Kolb, L. C. *Noyes Modern Clinical Psychiatry*. Saunders.

O'Neill, D. O. *A Psychosomatic Approach to Medicine*. Pitman Medical Publishing Co. Ltd., 1955.

Pearson, M. N. *Strecher's Fundamentals of Psychiatry*. Lippincott.

Stafford-Clark, D. *Psychiatry for Students*. George Allen & Unwin. 1964.

British Journal of Psychiatry, special publication No. 3. 'Studies of Anxiety'.

Appendix I

PHYSIOTHERAPY DEPARTMENT

Quality of Movement

The chart is intended to record the *quality* of the movements performed. All variations from normal patterns should be observed and noted.

This chart is *not* intended to record functional ability since functions can often be achieved with grossly abnormal patterns.

NAME   REFERRED BY

ADDRESS   DATE

OCCUPATION   HOSPITAL NO.

Date of Assessments

KEY

0 = Impossible
1 = Can be placed in position or moved passively
2 = Can assist when helped into position or through movement
3 = Cannot offer balance reactions
4 = Can produce the position or movement and react but abnormally
5 = Normal in all respects

A, B, C, D, E = Tick where appropriate

483

Test Applied	Score	A Tremor	B Weak- ness	C Stiff Joints	D Reflex Pattern	E Rigid- ity	Comments
Prone Lying Head turned, hands by side. Legs abducted and laterally rotated							
Obtaining elbow support. Prone lying							
Rolling Prone – Supine to right a) Head leading b) Upper limbs leading c) Lower limbs leading							
Rolling Supine to Prone to right a) Head leading b) Upper limbs leading c) Lower limbs leading							
Rolling Prone – supine to left a) Head leading b) Upper limbs leading c) Lower limbs leading							
Rolling Supine to Prone to left a) Head leading b) Upper limbs leading c) Lower limbs leading							
Side lying Balance reactions a) Conscious volitional b) Automatic							
Supine lying move to right side sitting Supine lying move to left side sitting	Not always suitable for elderly						

Appendix I

Test Applied	Score	A Tremor	B Weak- ness	C Stiff Joints	D Reflex Pattern	E Rigid- ity	Comments
Supine lying move to sitting over bed edge to right							
Supine lying move to sitting over bed edge to left							
High Sitting Balance a) Conscious volitional b) Automatic							
Right side sitting to prone kneeling Left side sitting to prone kneeling	Not always suitable for elderly						
Balance in prone kneeling a) Conscious volitional b) Automatic							
Sitting move to hand support and forwards stoop standing							
Left side sitting to kneeling upright Right side sitting to kneeling upright	Not always suitable for elderly						
Balance in kneeling a) Conscious volitional b) Automatic							
Kneeling – change to right half kneeling							

Appendix I

Test Applied	Score	A Tremor	B Weakness	C Stiff Joints	D Reflex Pattern	E Rigidity	Comments
Kneeling – change to left half kneeling							
Balance Right half kneel a) Conscious volitional b) Automatic							
Balance – Left half kneel a) Conscious volitional b) Automatic							
Right half kneeling move to hand support forwards stoop standing							
Left half kneeling move to hand support forwards stoop standing							
Upright Standing a) Stride b) Walk c) Oblique walk							
Balance reactions in standing a) Conscious volitional b) Automatic							
Walking a) Forwards b) Sideways c) Backwards							
Right step Standing							
Left standing							
Stairs a) Up b) Down							

Appendix I

NOTES AND ADDITIONAL COMMENTS

Appendix II

PHYSIOTHERAPY DEPARTMENT

Functional Ability

NAME   REFERRED BY

ADDRESS   DATE

OCCUPATION   HOSPITAL NUMBER

KEY

0 = Not possible
1 = Possible with assistance but difficult
2 = Possible with some assistance
3 = Possible without assistance but difficult (stand-by needed)
4 = Possible without assistance
5 = Normal

Bed examination	Date						
Turn over: prone to supine supine to prone							
Move to side of bed							
Move up bed							
Move down bed							
Sit over bed edge							
Balance in sitting							
Transfer: bed to chair chair to bed							

Appendix II

Wheelchair examination	Date							
Apply brake Release brake								
Propel chair on level: forwards backwards turn								
Negotiate doorway								
Slopes: up down								
Kerb: up down								
Transfer: Chair to chair Chair to toilet seat chair to floor floor to chair chair to bath or shower bath to chair								

Examination of gait	Date						
Balance in standing Stand up Sit down Get on to floor Get up from floor							
Walking – Crutches On level Slope up Slope down Rough ground							
Walking – Sticks On level Slope up Slope down Rough ground							
Walk – No sticks or crutches On level Slope up Slope down Rough ground							
Stairs 6 inches up 6 inches down 10 inches up 10 inches down							

NOTES

Index